Nursing and Global Healthcare

Nursing and Global Healthcare

Editor: Addison Holmes

MURPHY & MOORE
www.murphy-moorepublishing.com

www.murphy-moorepublishing.com

MURPHY & MOORE

Cataloging-in-Publication Data

Nursing and global healthcare / edited by Addison Holmes.
p. cm.
Includes bibliographical references and index.
ISBN 978-1-63987-774-4
1. Nursing. 2. Nursing--Practice. 3. Medical care. 4. Medicine--Practice. I. Holmes, Addison.
RT42 .E95 2023
610.73--dc23

Murphy & Moore Publishing
1 Rockefeller Plaza,
New York City,
NY 10020, USA

ISBN 978-1-63987-774-4

Contents

Preface....VII

Chapter 1 **Associations between Knowledge of the Causes and Perceived Impacts of Climate Change**....1
Lianping Yang, Wenmin Liao, Chaojie Liu, Na Zhang, Shuang Zhong and Cunrui Huang

Chapter 2 **On the Suitability and Potential of Nursing Care Discussion Forums as a Health Promotion Measure for Long-Distance Caregiving Relatives**....15
Tatjana Fischer and Markus Jobst

Chapter 3 **A Multicentre Study of Psychological Variables and the Prevalence of Burnout among Primary Health Care Nurses**....35
Elena Ortega-Campos, Guillermo A. Cañadas-De la Fuente, Luis Albendín-García, José L. Gómez Urquiza, Carolina Monsalve Reyes and E. Inmaculada de la Fuente-Solana

Chapter 4 **Nursing Students' Experiences of Clinical Practices in Emergency and Intensive Care Units**....45
María González-García, Alberto Lana, Paula Zurrón-Madera, Yolanda Valcárcel-Álvarez and Ana Fernández-Feito

Chapter 5 **Mishel's Model of Uncertainity Describing Categories and Subcategories in Fibromyalgia Patients**....59
Ana Fernandez-Araque, Julia Gomez-Castro, Andrea Giaquinta-Aranda, Zoraida Verde and Clara Torres-Ortega

Chapter 6 **Satisfaction with Social Support Received from Social Relationships in Cases of Chronic Pain: The Influence of Personal Network Characteristics in Terms of Structure, Composition and Functional Content**....72
Rosario Fernández-Peña, José Luis Molina and Oliver Valero

Chapter 7 **Association between Health Problems and Turnover Intention in Shift Work Nurses: Health Problem Clustering**....89
Jison Ki, Jaegeum Ryu, Jihyun Baek, Iksoo Huh and Smi Choi-Kwon

Chapter 8 **Workplace Violence and its Effects on Burnout and Secondary Traumatic Stress among Mental Healthcare Nurses**....101
Yudai Kobayashi, Misari Oe, Tetsuya Ishida, Michiko Matsuoka, Hiromi Chiba and Naohisa Uchimura

Chapter 9 **Individual Circadian Preference, Shift Work and Risk of Medication Errors** 112
Rosaria Cappadona, Emanuele Di Simone, Alfredo De Giorgi, Benedetta Boari, Marco Di Muzio, Pantaleo Greco, Roberto Manfredini, María Aurora Rodríguez-Borrego, Fabio Fabbian and Pablo Jesús López Soto

Chapter 10 **I am a Nursing Student but Hate Nursing: The East Asian Perspectives between Social Expectation and Social Context** 123
Luis Miguel Dos Santos

Chapter 11 **Living with the Memories—Parents' Experiences of their Newborn Child Undergoing Heart Surgery Abroad** 141
Ólöf Kristjánsdóttir, Annica Sjöström-Strand and Gudrún Kristjánsdóttir

Chapter 12 **Relief Alternatives during Resuscitation: Instructions to Teach Bystanders** 157
María José Pujalte-Jesús, César Leal-Costa, María Ruzafa-Martínez, Antonio Jesús Ramos-Morcillo and José Luis Díaz Agea

Chapter 13 **Analyzing the Job Demands-Control-Support Model in Work-Life Balance** 168
Virginia Navajas-Romero, Antonio Ariza-Montes and Felipe Hernández-Perlines

Chapter 14 **Prevalence of Comorbidities in Individuals Diagnosed and Undiagnosed with Alzheimer's Disease in León, Spain and a Proposal for Contingency Procedures to Follow in the Case of Emergencies Involving People with Alzheimer's Disease** 185
Macrina Tortajada-Soler, Leticia Sánchez-Valdeón, Marta Blanco-Nistal, José Alberto Benítez-Andrades, Cristina Liébana-Presa and Enrique Bayón-Darkistade

Chapter 15 **Experiences of Homeless Families in Parenthood** 200
Filipa Maria Reinhardt Andrade, Amélia Simões Figueiredo, Manuel Luís Capelas, Zaida Charepe and Sérgio Deodato

Chapter 16 **Nurse Manager Core Competencies: A Proposal in the Spanish Health System** 214
Alberto González García, Arrate Pinto-Carral, Jesús Sanz Villorejo and Pilar Marqués-Sánchez

Chapter 17 **Experiences of Nursing Students during the Abrupt Change from Face-to-Face to E-Learning Education during the First Month of Confinement Due to COVID-19** 229
Antonio Jesús Ramos-Morcillo, César Leal-Costa, José Enrique Moral-García and María Ruzafa-Martínez

Permissions

List of Contributors

Index

Preface

Nursing is a profession that involves the practice of caring for the ill and infirm. It plays a critical role in health-care delivery. It also encourages the well-being of patients and influences positive patient outcomes. It is an important part of the global healthcare systems, since it provides support and care, enables rehabilitation, promotes health, and educates the patients and public on the prevention of illnesses and injuries. It is also involved in forming a patient-centered design that promotes hospital environment safety, health and well-being. The constant attention, presence and observation skills which are a part of nursing enable doctors to make accurate diagnosis and recommend effective treatments. Early warning symptoms of impending emergencies such as respiratory failure or cardiac arrest are also observed within the field of nursing in order to save the lives of people. This book explores all the important aspects of nursing and its relevance in global healthcare in the present day scenario. It presents researches and studies performed by experts across the globe. This book will serve as a reference to a broad spectrum of readers.

This book unites the global concepts and researches in an organized manner for a comprehensive understanding of the subject. It is a ripe text for all researchers, students, scientists or anyone else who is interested in acquiring a better knowledge of this dynamic field.

I extend my sincere thanks to the contributors for such eloquent research chapters. Finally, I thank my family for being a source of support and help.

Editor

Associations between Knowledge of the Causes and Perceived Impacts of Climate Change

Lianping Yang [1,†], Wenmin Liao [1,†], Chaojie Liu [2], Na Zhang [1], Shuang Zhong [3,*] and Cunrui Huang [1,*]

1 School of Public Heath, Sun Yat-sen University, Guangzhou 510080, China; yanglp7@mail.sysu.edu.cn (L.Y.); liaowm3@mail2.sysu.edu.cn (W.L.); zhangn23@mail2.sysu.edu.cn (N.Z.)

2 School of Psychology and Public Health, La Trobe University, Melbourne 3086, Australia; c.liu@latrobe.edu.au

3 Center for Chinese Public Administration Research, School of Government, Sun Yat-sen University, Guangzhou 510275, China

* Correspondence: amigo-008@163.com (S.Z.); huangcr@mail.sysu.edu.cn (C.H.)

† These authors contributed equally to this work.

Abstract: This study aimed to measure the knowledge and perceptions of medical, public health, and nursing students about climate change and its impacts, and to identify associations between the knowledge and perceptions. Data were from a nationwide cross-sectional survey of 1387 students sampled in five different regional universities in China (April–May 2017). The knowledge and perceptions of the participants were collected by self-administered questionnaires. We found that most respondents believed that climate change is generally "bad" (83%) and bad for human health (88%), while 67% believed that climate change is controllable. The vast majority of respondents acknowledged illness conditions resulting from poor air quality (95%), heat stress (93%), and extreme weather events (91%) as potential impacts of climate change. Nevertheless, only 39% recognized malnutrition as a consequence of food deprivation resulting from climate change. Around 58% of respondents could correctly identify the causes of climate change. The knowledge of the causes of climate change was not associated with the ability to recognize the health consequences of climate change. However, the knowledge of causes of climate change was a significant predictor of increased awareness of the negative impacts of climate change between the medical and nursing students, although this was not the case among their public health counterparts. Poor knowledge about the causes of climate change is evident among students in China. They are able to recognize the direct links between weather events and health, but less likely to understand the consequences involving complicated pathways. Research and training into the underlying mechanisms of health impacts of climate change needs to be strengthened.

Keywords: climate change; health impact; knowledge; perception; university students

1. Introduction

Climate change is imposing one of the biggest global health threats in 21st century [1–3]. A lack of adequate response to climate change can undermine the last half century of gains in global health [1]. The health impacts of climate change can be a direct effect of weather events, such as heat stress, floods, drought and storms, and/or an indirect effect as a consequence of displacement and mental disorders, air pollution, spread of disease vectors, food insecurity, and malnutrition [1,4,5].

Health professionals are supposed to play a critical role in mitigating the health risks of climate change [6,7]. Physicians, nurses, public health specialists, and health officials should be equipped with high expertise and take essential responsibilities in protecting populations from the harm of climate change [8]. Millions of patients all over the world seek consultations and treatments from physicians every day. Physicians also enjoy a high level of recognition and trust in the society. They are well positioned to exert influence on the society for the common good, advocating for environment-friendly lifestyles and pro-health public policies [9]. Nurses are bound by both clinical practices and professional ethics to address concerns of their patients and prevent adverse health outcomes [10]. Public health specialists have endeavored to have a broad view on population health. They can support the implementation of programs and policies in ways that enhance physical and social environments at the local, national, and international levels [8]. Therefore, the preparedness of health professionals forms a critical part of the global response to climate change.

University education is a good starting point for preparing health professionals. Mitigation and adaptation strategies in response to climate change can be taught in universities under the umbrella of sustainability. Higher education has been widely considered to be critical for the sustainable development of the world [11–13]. Sustainability-related issues, like environmental pollution, climate change, overconsumption, and exploitation of resources are often addressed through various curricula. Zsoka et al. [14] explored the impacts of environmental education on the environmental knowledge, attitudes, and "greening" daily activities of high school and university students, and found out that the focus of environmental education is essential in shaping the attitudes of the students toward sustainable consumptions. But it remains a great challenge in developing proper strategies for priming medical students into a "medical mode" that can alter their opinions on the scientific merit of nonmedical issues [15]. Ng et al. highlighted the importance of emphasizing the ethical aspects of corporate social responsibility in undergraduate education programs for the future professional accounts [16]. However, there is a shortage of research documenting effective ways of teaching about sustainability in universities. University students are still forming their values and beliefs. A one-fits-for-all approach in acquiring sustainability competences is not feasible [17]. Environmental education for students in health-related disciplines, for example, has to consider the specific contexts of their professions. Without proper education, they may hold naïve awareness of the potential impact of individual contributions and feel disempowered for actively engaging in sustainability efforts [11]. Chaplin and Wyton pointed out the importance of understanding and addressing the value-action gap in motivating university students to engage with sustainability [12]. Kagawa suggested that future studies should be directed towards identifying various means of facilitating pro-sustainability behaviors [18].

Knowledge is a key driver of global actions on climate change [19]. Empirical evidence shows that the public concern about climate change is shaped by their acquired knowledge [19–21]. Climate-relevant knowledge appeared important for the public's willingness to change behaviors and to accept climate change policies [21]. However, not all dimensions of knowledge are equally influential. Knowledge about the causes of climate change is perhaps the most powerful driver of concerns about and actions on climate change, although it has been subject to serious debates over the past few decades in the public and political arenas [22,23]. A cross-country survey conducted by Shi and colleagues revealed that a higher level of concerns from the general public on climate change is associated with their understanding on the causes of climate change [19]. Bord et al. found that causal knowledge of global warming is associated with beliefs and behavioral intentions about climate change [24]. Similar results were also found in a study that was conducted by Tobler et al. [25]. Based on these findings, Shi and colleagues argued that climate change campaigns should have a strong focus on promoting knowledge about the causes of climate change [21].

There is paucity in the literature documenting the importance of causal knowledge on raising awareness and competency of health workers in response to the health impacts of climate change. Although medical, nursing, and public health students are likely to engage in or be exposed to climate change debates, little is known about how these students incorporate climate change knowledge into their professional learning. There has been an increasing call for teaching about climate change in medical education [26]. Some medical schools, such as those in the USA, have indeed started to offer coursework on "climate change and health". However, it is by no means arranged as a standard requirement [27]. There is a lack of consensus about what should be taught about climate change in medical, nursing, and public health curricula.

This study aimed to fill the literature gap by conducting a survey in a representative sample of medical, nursing, and public health students in China. The preparedness of health workforce in actions on climate change is particularly important for China, because China is highly vulnerable to global climate change due to its large population size and rapid transition in economic and social development. Findings of this study may help educational providers to better incorporate climate change components into their teaching deliveries.

2. Materials and Methods

A nationwide cross-sectional questionnaire survey was conducted on medical, nursing, and public health students in a representative sample in China during April and May in 2017.

2.1. Study Participants

Senior university students majoring in clinical medicine, nursing, and public health were eligible to participate in this study. The participants were restricted to those who had one more year to finish their undergraduate studies: year four in clinical medicine and public health; and, year three in nursing. These students had already completed all required coursework and were ready for the final year practice placements. Their completed coursework usually contained two parts: half in relation to basic biomedicine subjects and half in relation to clinical/professional subjects [28].

A multistage stratified cluster sampling method was adopted to recruit participants. China has been officially divided into five geographic regions. One university in each region was identified: Harbin Medical University in the north, Sichuan University in the west, Sun Yat-sen University in the south, Fujian Medical University in the east, and Huazhong University of Science and Technology in the central region. We estimated that a minimal sample size of 250 from each participating university would be able to meet the requirements of sub-group statistical tests and regression analyses: 110 in clinical medicine; 80 in public health; and, 60 in nursing in line with the proportion of enrolled students for each degree program. Students in these participating universities studied in groups from beginning to completion, each comprising 30–40 members. These groups formed the basic unit for sampling. We randomly selected two or three groups of students for each major in each participating university and invited all of the group members to participate in the survey.

2.2. Data Collection

A questionnaire was developed based on the theories of KAP (knowledge, attitudes, and practice) and rational choice action. These theories hypothesize that individuals may choose a particular course of action that is in line with their beliefs and preferences, and knowledge plays a crucial role in shaping these beliefs and preferences [12,29,30]. Human beings are characterized by pursuing the causal structure of the world that supports cognitive achievements [31]. Causal knowledge plays a central role in the human thoughts [32]. It allows people to provide an explanation on the occurrence of an event and to predict the future events and even the consequences of counterfactuals. This forms the foundation of reasoning and rational actions.

The questionnaire comprised three sections, with items deriving from the existing literature [10,19,33–36] (Table S1). Section One tapped into the general perceptions of the respondents on the nature and impacts of climate change. Example questions included "whether climate change is controllable" and "whether climate change is bad for human health". Respondents were asked to rate their opinions on a six point Likert scale without a neutral midpoint. Such an approach was recommended by Maibach et al. to better capture the inclination of the participants [37]. Section Two asked the respondents to identify the health impacts of climate change from a list of 12 health-related problems. These 12 aspects of problems have been widely accepted as potential important health impacts of climate change [10,34]. Section Three investigated the knowledge of respondents about the causes of climate change. A list of four statements [19] were presented and the respondents were asked to judge whether they are true or false. Example statements included "Climate change is mainly caused by human activities" and "The global CO_2 concentration in the atmosphere has increased during the past 250 years".

The questionnaires were distributed by our trained investigators to the classrooms of the selected groups of students. They were asked to complete the questionnaires independently and returned the questionnaires to a collection box when they left the classrooms. A total of 1436 questionnaires were disseminated and 1387 (response rate, 97%) were returned and valid for data analyses.

2.3. Data Analyses

Perceptions on the nature and impacts of climate change were recoded into binary data ("yes vs. no" or "correct vs. incorrect") for the purpose of data analyses. The percentage of positive or correct responses in relation to each item was compared between different streams of students using χ^2 tests.

The ability of respondents to identify the health impacts of climate change was assessed using the percentage of correct answers related to the 12 listed problems, which was further categorized into high ($\geq$50%) and low (<50%) levels. We also calculated a summed score (0–12), reflecting the total number of problems that were correctly identified by the respondents. This served as an indication of the overall ability of an individual to identify climate change related health problems.

Similarly, knowledge of the causes of climate change was assessed using the percentage of correct answers related to the four tested statements, which was further categorized into high ($\geq$50%) and low (<50%) levels. A summed score (0–4) was calculated to reflect the overall understanding of an individual on the causes of climate change.

Multivariate logistic regression models were established to examine the associations between knowledge of the causes of climate change (high vs. low) and perceived impacts of climate change ("yes or no" on seven questions), controlling for variations in social demographic characteristics (gender, age, location, household income, and health status). Because multiple indicators (perceived impacts of climate change as dependent variables) were used in the logistic regression tests, we used the Bonferroni procedure to adjust the p values in regard to the statistical significance of the adjusted odds ratios (AORs) of causes knowledge [38]. We also performed sensitivity tests by introducing the summed score (0–4) of causes of knowledge into the regression models.

3. Results

3.1. Characteristics of Participants

Of the 1387 respondents, 69% were 21–22 years old and 67% were female. The majority (>80%) rated their health status as good or very good. The nursing students were more likely to be female ($p < 0.01$) and reported lower household income ($p < 0.01$) (Table 1).

Table 1. Demographics of participants by different majors.

Characteristics	All (n = 1387)		Medical (n = 644)		Public Health (n = 430)		Nursing (n = 313)	
	n	(%)	n	(%)	n	(%)	n	(%)
Region								
East	258	18.6	117	18.2	80	18.6	61	19.5
North	308	22.2	156	24.2	79	18.4	73	23.3
Central	248	17.9	107	16.6	84	19.5	57	18.2
West	262	18.9	120	18.6	83	19.3	59	18.9
South	311	22.4	144	22.4	104	24.2	63	20.1
Gender								
Female	926	66.8	328	50.9	319	74.2	279	89.1
Male	461	33.2	316	49.1	111	25.8	34	10.9
Age								
≤20	126	9.5	38	6.1	20	5.0	68	23.1
21–22	913	68.9	419	66.7	302	74.8	192	65.3
>22	287	21.6	171	27.2	82	20.3	34	11.6
Monthly household income per capita (¥)								
<1000	154	11.2	62	9.8	51	12.0	41	13.1
1000–1999	284	20.7	112	17.6	95	22.4	77	24.6
2000–4999	514	37.5	239	37.6	155	36.6	120	38.3
5000–9999	293	21.4	146	23.0	89	21.0	58	18.5
≥10,000	127	9.3	76	12.0	34	8.0	17	5.4
Self-rated health								
Very good	303	21.9	156	24.2	80	18.6	67	21.4
Good	858	61.9	378	58.7	275	64.0	205	65.5
Medium or poor	226	16.3	110	17.1	75	17.4	41	13.1

3.2. Perceived Impacts of Climate Change

About 67% of respondents believed that climate change is controllable, as compared with 13% who believed it is uncontrollable. The majority of respondents (>80%) agreed that climate change has negative impacts on the public in general and for human health specifically. Over 85% of respondents anticipated serious health impacts of climate change in the next 20 years at the local, national, and international levels. These perceptions were consistent across different streams of students, except that the public health students were more likely ($p < 0.01$) to believe climate change is controllable (Table 2).

Overall, the respondents were able to identify on average 9.5 problems (SD 2.3) out of a total of 12 related to climate change. The vast majority of respondents acknowledged illness conditions and service disruptions resulting from poor air quality (95%), heat stress (93%), and extreme weather events (91%) as potential health impacts of climate change. Nonetheless, only 39% recognized malnutrition and 64% recognized mental health illness as a consequence of climate change. About 20–30% of respondents believed that the list of problems were exhaustive. The medical students were more likely to be able to recognize water-borne infectious disease, food-borne infectious disease, mental health illness, and malnutrition as a consequence of climate change as compared to their nursing and public health counterparts (Table 2).

Table 2. Perceived impacts of climate change from medical, public health and nursing students.

Perceived Impacts of Climate Change	Medical (n = 644)		Public Health (n = 430)		Nursing (n = 313)		All (n = 1387)		p
	n	(%)	n	(%)	n	(%)	n	(%)	
Climate change is controllable	418	64.9	321	74.7	196	62.6	935	67.4	<0.01
Overall, climate change is bad	546	84.8	359	83.5	253	80.8	1158	83.5	0.30
Climate change is bad for human health	575	89.3	381	88.6	266	85.0	1222	88.1	0.15
Climate change will be serious in my local community	576	89.4	368	85.6	282	90.1	1226	88.4	0.09
Climate change will be serious in China	619	96.1	413	96.1	298	95.2	1330	95.9	0.79
Climate change will be serious in the world	609	94.6	410	95.4	299	95.5	1318	95.0	0.76
Health consequences of climate change									
Air quality-related illness	604	93.8	413	96.1	299	95.5	1316	94.9	0.22
Heat-related illness	596	92.6	407	94.9	283	90.4	1286	92.8	0.07
Disruption of health services by extreme weather events	585	90.8	396	92.1	282	90.1	1263	91.1	0.62
Cold-related illness	570	88.5	385	89.5	276	88.2	1231	88.8	0.82
Flooding-related displacement	550	85.5	375	87.4	259	82.8	1184	85.5	0.20
Illness related with shortage of water supply	556	86.5	352	82.2	269	86.2	1177	85.1	0.13
Vector-borne infectious disease	541	84.0	359	83.9	249	79.8	1149	83.0	0.23
Water-borne infectious disease	544	84.6	328	76.6	249	79.6	1121	81.0	<0.01
Other health impacts of climatic change	479	76.4	348	82.1	234	76.0	1061	78.1	0.06
Food-borne disease	472	73.4	250	58.1	226	72.2	948	68.4	<0.01
Mental health conditions	443	68.8	255	59.3	185	59.1	883	63.7	<0.01
Malnutrition	282	43.9	141	32.8	117	37.4	540	39.0	<0.01
Total score (Mean ± SD)	9.70 ± 2.39		9.36 ± 2.20		9.36 ± 2.27		9.52 ± 2.31		0.03

3.3. *Knowledge about the Causes of Climate Change*

Overall, the respondents achieved a mean score of 2.31 and 58% correctly identified all of the answers about the causes of climate change. About 53% medical students, 50% public health students, and 41% nursing students achieved a high level of knowledge about the causes of climate change: the differences appeared to be statistically significant ($\chi^2 = 11.06$, $p < 0.01$).

Most respondents accepted the general truth of increasing earth temperature (64%), increasing CO_2 in the atmosphere (75%), and the contribution of human activities to climate change (77%). However, only 16% of respondents were able to identify details about the change in CO_2 concentrations over the past few centuries (Table 3).

Table 3. Correct answers on the causes of climate change from medical, public health, and nursing students.

Causes of Climate Change	All		Medical		Public Health		Nursing		p
	n	%	n	%	n	%	n	%	
Climate change is mainly caused by human activities	1071	77.3	508	78.9	333	77.4	230	73.7	0.17
The global CO_2 concentration in the atmosphere has increased during the past 250 years	1034	74.7	484	75.2	321	75.0	229	73.2	0.80
The last century's global increase in temperature was the largest during the past 1000 years	880	63.6	420	65.2	285	66.4	175	56.5	0.01
Today's global CO_2 concentration in the atmosphere has already occurred in the past 650,000 years	217	15.7	94	14.6	75	17.5	48	15.4	0.45
Total score (Mean ± SD)	2.31 ± 1.01		2.34 ± 1.02		2.36 ± 1.01		2.18 ± 0.98		0.02

3.4. Associations between Knowledge on the Causes and Perceived Impacts of Climate Change

The logistic regression models showed that there was no significant association between the knowledge on the causes of climate change and the ability of the respondents to recognize climate change related health problems (Table 4).

However, a higher level of knowledge about the causes of climate change was a significant predictor of increased awareness of the negative impacts of climate change, in particular among the medical students (with an AOR ranging from 1.83 for "climate change is controllable" to 9.18 for "health impacts of climate change will be serious in China"). However, among the public health students, knowledge on the causes of climate change did not appear as a significant predictor of increased awareness on the negative impacts of climate change. Among the nursing students, the knowledge level was only a significant predictor of the overall perception on the negative impacts of climate change. The sensitivity tests produced consistent results, although the AORs changed (Tables S31–S34).

Table 4. Associations between understandings of the causes of climate change and perceived impacts of climate change: results from logistic regression analyses [1].

Perceived Impacts of Climate Change	Adjusted Odds Ratio (95% Confidence Interval) of Respondents with a High (vs. Low) Level of Understanding on the Causes of Climate Change			
	All	Medical	Public Health	Nursing
Climate change is controllable (yes vs. no)	1.68 ** (1.32–2.14)	1.83 ** (1.29–2.60)	1.38 (0.85–2.25)	1.81 (1.07–3.06)
Overall, climate change is a bad thing (yes vs. no)	2.16 ** (1.57–2.96)	1.98 ** (1.24–3.17)	2.33 (1.28–4.24)	2.94 ** (1.44–5.99)
Climate change is bad for human health (yes vs. no)	1.83 ** (1.28–2.60)	2.18 ** (1.27–3.75)	1.47 (0.75–2.85)	2.11 (1.00–4.50)
Health impacts of climate change will be serious in my local community (yes vs. no)	2.07 ** (1.44–2.99)	3.45 ** (1.93–6.17)	1.16 (0.62–2.15)	2.08 (0.85–5.07)
Health impacts of climate change will be serious in China (yes vs. no)	5.40 ** (2.60–11.24)	9.18 ** (2.65–31.76)	2.86 (0.83–9.87)	5.55 (1.12–27.49)
Health impacts of climate change will be serious in the world (yes vs. no)	4.00 ** (2.17–7.39)	6.30 ** (2.47–16.02)	1.97 (0.68–5.67)	4.29 (0.87–21.17)
Ability to recognize health consequences of climate change (high vs. low)	1.30 (1.04–1.64)	1.45 (1.03–2.04)	1.27 (0.83–1.95)	1.22 (0.74–2.01)

[1] Controlled for influences of region, gender, age, discipline (only in the model involving all respondents), income, and health status. ** Bonferroni adjusted $p < 0.01$.

4. Discussion

There was an overwhelming belief in the respondents that climate change is generally "bad" and bad for human health. However, only 60% of the respondents could correctly identify the causes of climate change. On average, the respondents identified nine health problems that were related to climate change out of a total of 12 in the list. Knowledge on the causes of climate change is not associated with the ability to recognize the health consequences of climate change. Nevertheless, it is a significant predictor of increased awareness of the medical and nursing students on the overall negative impacts of climate change.

Higher education can and should play an important role in raising awareness and shaping the attitudes and practices of the new generations toward actions on sustainability. The values and behaviors of university students with the sustainability agenda are important within the climate change context. There are some university initiatives that are known as greening the curriculum [39]. Chaplin and Wyton found that university students tend to accept the importance of sustainable living, yet their understanding is usually at a very low level and there is a shortage of actions [12]. It is critical to close the gap between knowledge, values, and actions [11].

4.1. *Perceptions about Climate Change and Its Health Impacts*

Overall, perceptions on the impacts of climate change are consistent across the three streams of students. They all anticipated increasing consequences of climate change in the near future at the local, national, and international levels. However, the immediate health challenges that are associated with extreme weather events (e.g., heat stress and service disruptions) are more likely to attract their attentions when compared with those indirect, more complex, and long lasting health consequences (e.g., changing ecosystem).

It appears that it is less likely that these students would adopt a global view on the impacts of climate change. Mental health conditions and malnutrition, which are often a result from population displacement (e.g., climate refugees), came to the bottom on the list of recognized health challenges that are associated with climate change. This phenomenon is not unique in China. People's concerns are naturally connected with their past experiences and the environment in which they grow up. Empirical evidence shows that the world is experiencing increasing catastrophic weather events over the past few decades. However, these events appear in various forms in different locations [1]. Air quality related illness is the most recognizable health problem in this study, perhaps because air pollution has been an extraordinary environmental problem in China [40]. By contrast, in Ethiopia, health science students reported flooding, drought, and increasing temperature as the most prominent impacts of climate change [41]. In the USA, local health officers considered extreme hot weather and wildfire as the most serious threat of climate change [34].

The medical and nursing students in this study demonstrated a lower level of confidence on the prospect of controlling climate change than their public health counterparts. This may be a reflection of the limitations of their professional training: medical and nursing students are usually better equipped with skills for individual actions than those for collective actions [18]. The weak confidence on collective actions may eventually jeopardize the ability of medical and nursing professionals to play an imperative role in the debate of and actions on climate change [42]. On the other hand, we found that the public health students were less likely to be able to identify water-borne infectious disease, food-borne infectious disease, mental health conditions, and malnutrition as a consequence of climate change as compared with their medical and nursing counterparts. This is not surprising given the recent trend of public health education, shifting from a focus on disease prevention to a focus on health promotion. Public health professionals are becoming more interested in social, environmental and behavioral determinants of health, which are usually associated with multiple disease conditions. Internationally, there are increasing numbers of public health professionals without a qualification of biomedical training [10,34].

4.2. *Low Level of Knowledge on the Causes of Climate Change*

Overall, the students demonstrated a low level of knowledge about the causes of climate change, with 58% giving correct answers to all of the four knowledge questions as compared with an average of 60% in the general public revealed in a cross-country study [19]. The nursing students had a lower level of knowledge than their medical and public health counterparts. It is not clear whether this is caused by the differences in educational programs or the differentiations in professional functions and cultures.

There has been a strong consensus in the scientific community that global warming has increased significantly in the last century due to human activities [43]. Nonetheless, we found a significant level of disagreement in the student respondents with the scientific conclusion: more than 35% disagreement on global warming and more than 25% disagreement on CO_2 changes in the past 250 years. Internationally, there are around 17% of the public respondents (age over 20) that do not think the CO_2 concentration changed and 36% that do not perceive the temperature increase [19]. Therefore, university students did not show higher correct consensus when compared to the general public.

4.3. Higher Level of Knowledge on the Causes of Climate Change Is Associated with Higher Awareness of the Negative Impacts of Climate Change

Some researchers argued that a good understanding about the causes of climate change is essential for motivating health professionals to embrace eco-friendly practices and advocate for green and healthy lifestyles: they have to believe in human causes to climate change [43,44]. In Pakistan, the public perception on climate change is shaped by their knowledge relating to heat waves within a climate change context [45]. Medical students should be educated to endorse the importance of containing CO_2 emissions so that they can develop confidence and be empowered to play an active role in global actions on climate change [1,27]. Indeed, a higher level of knowledge on the causes of climate change is a significant predictor of increased awareness on the negative impacts of climate change. This is particularly true for medical students, as revealed in this study. Knowledge and perceptions are usually considered as prerequisites for the general public to adapt to climate change [46].

However, knowledge on the causes of climate change by itself is not enough to enhance the skills of medical, public health, and nursing students in recognizing and mitigating health harms resulting from climate change. We found that knowledge on the causes of climate change is not associated with the ability of the students to recognize climate change related health problems. Kahan and colleagues [47] also found that knowledge has limited effects on people's perceptions on climate change, let alone behavioral changes. Grimm [31] concluded that causal knowledge can lead to skill gains, but only under certain conditions. Hagmayer and Witteman proposed a Causal-explanation-based Decision Making (CDM) framework, which describes when and how causal knowledge and reasoning should be used in decision making for better outcomes [32]. They pointed out that the CDM framework aligns well with the clinical reasoning of health professionals. It is important to note that the causal knowledge about climate change measured in this study does not entail understandings about the underlining mechanisms of the potential health impacts of climate change. Our limited understanding on these mechanisms may jeopardize the effect of the causal knowledge on the skill gains of the students in recognizing climate change related health problem.

It appears that knowledge on the causes of climate change may have varied effects on different health professionals. In this study, we found that the knowledge on the causes of climate change has no significant associations with perceived impacts of climate change in public health students. However, it is a significant predictor of perceived negative impacts of climate change in medical students, as is consistent with findings of a study on the general public across six countries [19]. Since different health professionals play a different role in climate change actions, some researchers have called for developing different approaches, such as teaching, learning, and assessment approaches in integrating climate change topics into the teaching curricula for medical, nursing, and public health students [27,48,49].

4.4. Implications on Teaching and Research into Health Impacts of Climate Change

Health professionals can play various roles at different levels in global actions on climate change [50]. At the individual level, they identify the patients and those who are in high risks of developing health problems as a consequence of climate change. They take consideration of the environmental factors in treating and preventing relevant disease conditions. At the practice level, they need to be conscious of the environmental impacts of their business operations and engaged in reduction of CO_2 footprints. At the population level, they are role models of the community and they advocate social and environmental actions for improving population health [50,51].

Obviously, different skill sets are required for competent performance of the above roles [48]. It is evident from this study that the students lack a global and systems view on health impacts of climate change despite high awareness of the negative impacts of climate change. They have difficulties in recognizing health problems that are indirectly linked to climate change through more complex pathways, including those that are associated with population displacement and changing ecosystems. In the literature, there have been discussions about how to reinforce knowledge on the interaction between climate change and human health in medical education [48]. However, such education programs have to adopt a global view. It is not ethical for health professionals to constrain services to the concerns of their local patients only, and ignore the broader problems that are experienced by those from the "other parts of the world" as a result of climate change [51]. Meanwhile, teaching into climate change has to be meaningful and bear close connections with the reality the health professionals are facing [26]. China is not a migrant country. The concept of climate refugee may sound alien to many health professionals in China. However, the recent transition of China's economy has witnessed dramatic growth in population movements (e.g., rural-to-urban and region-to-region migrations) and changes in ecosystems (e.g., the three gorges dam). In recent years, China has also accelerated its international health assistance activities to other countries. As a result, health professionals in China have been increasingly exposed to many health challenges that are similar to some of the problems resulting from climate change. It would be a reasonable choice to combine the considerations of development and climate change in teaching deliveries [26].

No doubt, climate change should be integrated into the curricula for medical, public health, and nursing students [52]. Nevertheless, this is by no means a simple and straightforward task. There are a number of challenges: (1) Medical curricula have already been overcrowded [27]; (2) We need to apply different pedagogies in teaching for different health professionals [44]; (3) Our understanding on the mechanisms of health impacts of climate change is still limited; and, (4) There is a serious shortage of academic staff in medical, public health, and nursing schools who are competent in teaching and research into the area of climate change. At this stage, most "climate change" education programs have restricted contents to the trend and causes of climate change. Although this is important for raising awareness and building motivations for actions, it is far less than enough to empower health professionals to engage in actions on climate change. Research into the underlying mechanisms of health impacts of climate change needs to be strengthened. There is also a need to change the culture of professional practices: health professionals need to see themselves as an integral part of the global action on climate change. Environmental education is important [53,54], but it needs to be integrated into the professional education programs as a higher order of learning beyond the confines of professional knowledge and skills [16]. Teaching about climate change typically takes a wider sustainability focus [18,48]. The Higher Education Academy (HEA) in the UK developed some examples about skills and knowledge that are necessary for an "action-oriented, sustainability literate" graduate [18].

To our knowledge, this is the first national study to explore the knowledge and perceptions on climate change of medical, public health and nursing students in China. Similar studies are also limited in the international literature. There are some limitations in this study. The study instrument was developed based on the few available literature. The reliability and validity of the instrument are subject to further scrutiny. The study adopted a cross-sectional design. No causal relationships can be drawn from the results. In addition, perceptions can be shaped by many factors, including culture, values and religious belief, just to name a few. Unfortunately, many of these data were either unavailable or hard to measure due to a lack of reliable measurement instruments. Furthermore, this study was undertaken in China. Precautions should be taken in attempts to generalize the findings to other countries. However, China's medical education system has borrowed experiences from many other countries. It has become increasingly aligned with international standards. Lobell et al. point out that Asia and Africa are likely to suffer similar problems due to the same likelihood of large food-insecure human populations [55]. Future studies are warranted to explore the effective ways of incorporating climate change contents into medical curricula. There is also a need to develop a more comprehensive instrument to assess competencies of health professionals in dealing with climate change and its health impacts.

5. Conclusions

Medical, public health, and nursing students in China are highly aware of the negative impacts of climate change; but, it is evident that they have poor knowledge about the causes of climate change. The students are able to recognize the direct links between weather events and health; but, they are less likely to be able to understand the consequences of climate change involving complicated pathways. A higher level of knowledge on the causes of climate change is a predictor of increased awareness on the negative impacts of climate change; but, the ability to recognize health consequences of climate change is not associated with knowledge on the causes of climate change. Although a good understanding on the causes of climate change by itself is important, it is not enough to get health professionals prepared to cope with climate change consequences. Training and research into the underlying mechanisms of health impacts of climate change needs to be strengthened.

Author Contributions: Conceptualization, L.Y., S.Z. and C.H.; Data curation, W.L. and N.Z.; Formal analysis, L.Y. and C.L.; Funding acquisition, S.Z. and C.H.; Methodology, L.Y., W.L., C.L. and C.H.; Writing–original draft, L.Y.; Writing–review & editing, C.L. and N.Z. All authors approved the final version to be published.

Acknowledgments: This work was supported by grants from the National Key R&D Program of China (2018YFA0606204); National Natural Science Foundation of China (No. 71603292); Guangdong Natural Science Foundation (No. 2016A030310162); Guangdong Special Fund for Science and Technology Development (No. 2017A070707002) and Guangdong Province Medical Science and Technology Research Foundation (A2016245).

References

1. Watts, N.; Adger, W.N.; Agnolucci, P.; Blackstock, J.; Byass, P.; Cai, W.; Chaytor, S.; Colbourn, T.; Collins, M.; Cooper, A.; et al. Health and climate change: Policy responses to protect public health. *Lancet* **2015**, *386*, 1861–1914. [CrossRef]
2. Robbins, A. Health consequences of climate change interventions. *Lancet* **2015**, *386*, 1819. [CrossRef]
3. McIver, L.; Kim, R.; Woodward, A.; Hales, S.; Spickett, J.; Katscherian, D.; Hashizume, M.; Honda, Y.; Kim, H.; Iddings, S.; et al. Health Impacts of Climate Change in Pacific Island Countries: A Regional Assessment of Vulnerabilities and Adaptation Priorities. *Environ. Health Perspect.* **2015**, *124*, 1707–1714. [CrossRef] [PubMed]
4. Astrom, C.; Orru, H.; Rocklov, J.; Strandberg, G.; Ebi, K.L.; Forsberg, B. Heat-related respiratory hospital admissions in Europe in a changing climate: A health impact assessment. *BMJ Open* **2013**, *3*, e001842. [CrossRef] [PubMed]
5. Tawatsupa, B.; Yiengprugsawan, V.; Kjellstrom, T.; Seubsman, S.A.; Sleigh, A.; Thai Cohort Study Team. Heat stress, health and well-being: Findings from a large national cohort of Thai adults. *BMJ Open* **2012**, *2*, e001396. [CrossRef] [PubMed]
6. Gill, M.; Stott, R. Health professionals must act to tackle climate change. *Lancet* **2009**, *374*, 1953–1955. [CrossRef]
7. Roberts, I.; Stott, R. Doctors and climate change. *Lancet* **2010**, *376*, 1801–1802. [CrossRef]
8. Winkler, M.S.; Roosli, M.; Ragettli, M.S.; Cisse, G.; Muller, P.; Utzinger, J.; Perez, L. Mitigating and adapting to climate change: A call to public health professionals. *Int. J. Public Health* **2015**, *60*, 631–632. [CrossRef] [PubMed]
9. Moser, A.M.; Stigler, F.L.; Haditsch, B. Physicians' responsibility for planetary health. *Lancet Planet. Health* **2017**, *1*, e56. [CrossRef]
10. Polivka, B.J.; Chaudry, R.V.; Mac Crawford, J. Public health nurses' knowledge and attitudes regarding climate change. *Environ. Health Perspect.* **2012**, *120*, 321–325. [CrossRef] [PubMed]
11. Whitley, C.T.; Takahashi, B.; Zwickle, A.; Besley, J.C.; Lertpratchya, A.P. Sustainability behaviors among college students: An application of the VBN theory. *Environ. Educ. Res.* **2018**, *24*, 245–262. [CrossRef]

12. Chaplin, G.; Wyton, P. Student engagement with sustainability: Understanding the value-action gap. *Int. J. Sustain. High. Educ.* **2014**, *15*, 404–417. [CrossRef]
13. Eagle, L.; Low, D.; Case, P.; Vandommele, L. Attitudes of undergraduate business students toward sustainability issues. *Int. J. Sustain. High. Educ.* **2015**, *16*, 650–668. [CrossRef]
14. Zsoka, A.; Szerenyi, Z.M.; Szechy, A.; Kocsis, T. Greening due to environmental education? Environmental knowledge, attitudes, consumer behavior and everyday pro-environmental activities of Hungarian high school and university students. *J. Clean. Prod.* **2013**, *48*, 126–138. [CrossRef]
15. Prasad, V.; Thistlethwaite, W.; Dale, W. Effect of clinical vignettes on senior medical students' opinions of climate change. *South. Med. J.* **2011**, *104*, 401–404. [CrossRef] [PubMed]
16. Ng, A.W.; Leung, T.C.H.; Lo, J.M.K. Developing Sustainability Competence for Future Professional Accountants: The Integrative Role of an Undergraduate Program. *World Sustain. Ser.* **2017**. [CrossRef]
17. Lambrechts, W.; Ghijsen, P.W.T.; Jacques, A.; Walravens, H.; Van Liedekerke, L.; Van Petegem, P. Sustainability segmentation of business students: Toward self-regulated development of critical and interpretational competences in a post-truth era. *J. Clean. Prod.* **2018**, *202*, 561–570. [CrossRef]
18. Kagawa, F. Dissonance in students' perceptions of sustainable development and sustainability: Implications for curriculum change. *Int. J. Sustain. High. Educ.* **2007**, *8*, 317–338. [CrossRef]
19. Shi, J.; Visschers, V.H.M.; Siegrist, M.; Arvai, J. Knowledge as a driver of public perceptions about climate change reassessed. *Nat. Clim. Chang.* **2016**, *6*, 759–762. [CrossRef]
20. Corner, A. Psychology: Science literacy and climate views. *Nat. Clim. Chang.* **2012**, *2*, 710–711. [CrossRef]
21. Shi, J.; Visschers, V.H.; Siegrist, M. Public Perception of Climate Change: The Importance of Knowledge and Cultural Worldviews. *Risk Anal.* **2015**, *35*, 2183–2201. [CrossRef] [PubMed]
22. Krosnick, J.A.; Holbrook, A.L.; Lowe, L.; Visser, P.S. The origins and consequences of democratic citizens' policy agendas: A study of popular concern about global warming. *Clim. Chang.* **2006**, *77*, 7–43. [CrossRef]
23. Lorenzoni, I.; Pidgeon, N.F. Public views on climate change: European and USA perspectives. *Clim. Chang.* **2006**, *77*, 73–95. [CrossRef]
24. Bord, R.J.; O'Connor, R.E.; Fisher, A. In what sense does the public need to understand global climate change? *Public Underst. Sci.* **2000**, *9*, 205–218. [CrossRef]
25. Tobler, C.; Visschers, V.H.M.; Siegrist, M. Consumers' knowledge about climate change. *Clim. Chang.* **2012**, *114*, 189–209. [CrossRef]
26. Maxwell, J.; Blashki, G. Teaching about Climate Change in Medical Education: An Opportunity. *J. Public Health Res.* **2016**, *5*, 673. [CrossRef] [PubMed]
27. Friedrich, M.J. Medical Community Gathers Steam to Tackle Climate's Health Effects. *JAMA* **2017**, *317*, 1511–1513. [CrossRef] [PubMed]
28. Jing, M.A.; Yue, Y.-G. Medical Education System in European and American Countries Enlightenments on the Current Medical Education Reform in Our Country. *Med. Innov. China* **2014**, *11*, 75–78.
29. James, H.; Handu, S.S.; Al Khaja, K.A.J.; Otoom, S.; Sequeira, R.P. Evaluation of the knowledge, attitude and practice of self-medication among first-year medical students. *Med. Princ. Pract.* **2006**, *15*, 270–275. [CrossRef] [PubMed]
30. Johnston, J.M.; Leung, G.M.; Fielding, R.; Tin, K.Y.K.; Ho, L.M. The development and validation of a knowledge, attitude and behaviour questionnaire to assess undergraduate evidence-based practice teaching and learning. *Med. Educ.* **2003**, *37*, 992–1000. [CrossRef] [PubMed]
31. Grimm, S.R. Understanding as Knowledge of Causes. *Synth Libr.* **2014**, *366*, 329–345. [CrossRef]
32. Hagmayer, Y.; Witteman, C. Chapter Four- Causal Knowledge and Reasoning in Decision Making. In *Psychology of Learning and Motivation*; Ross, B.H., Ed.; Academic Press: Cambridge, MA, USA, 2017; Volume 67, pp. 95–134.
33. Lee, T.M.; Markowitz, E.M.; Howe, P.D.; Ko, C.Y.; Leiserowitz, A.A. Predictors of public climate change awareness and risk perception around the world. *Nat. Clim. Chang.* **2015**, *5*, 1014–1020. [CrossRef]
34. Bedsworth, L. Preparing for climate change: A perspective from local public health officers in California. *Environ. Health Perspect.* **2009**, *117*, 617–623. [CrossRef] [PubMed]
35. Wei, J.; Hansen, A.; Zhang, Y.; Li, H.; Liu, Q.; Sun, Y.; Bi, P. Perception, attitude and behavior in relation to climate change: A survey among CDC health professionals in Shanxi province, China. *Environ. Res.* **2014**, *134*, 301–308. [CrossRef] [PubMed]

36. Roser-Renouf, C.; Maibach, E.W.; Li, J. Adapting to the Changing Climate: An Assessment of Local Health Department Preparations for Climate Change-Related Health Threats, 2008–2012. *PLoS ONE* **2016**, *11*, e0151558. [CrossRef] [PubMed]
37. Maibach, E.W.; Kreslake, J.M.; Roser-Renouf, C.; Rosenthal, S.; Feinberg, G.; Leiserowitz, A.A. Do Americans Understand That Global Warming Is Harmful to Human Health? Evidence from a National Survey. *Ann. Glob. Health* **2015**, *81*, 396–409. [CrossRef] [PubMed]
38. McDonald, J.H. *Handbook of Biological Statistics*, 3rd ed.; Sparky House Publishing: Baltimore, MD, USA, 2014.
39. Hopkinson, P.; Hughes, P.; Layer, G. Sustainable graduates: Linking formal, informal and campus curricula to embed education for sustainable development in the student learning experience. *Environ. Educ. Res.* **2008**, *14*, 435–454. [CrossRef]
40. Lancet, O. Climate change and non-communicable diseases. *Lancet Oncol.* **2016**, *17*, 1. [CrossRef]
41. Nigatu, A.S.; Asamoah, B.O.; Kloos, H. Knowledge and perceptions about the health impact of climate change among health sciences students in Ethiopia: A cross-sectional study. *BMC Public Health* **2014**, *14*, 587. [CrossRef] [PubMed]
42. Duvivier, R.J.; Watts, N.R.; Rukavina, S.; Kaduru, C.J. Doctors talk climate change–students take action. *Lancet* **2011**, *377*, 995. [CrossRef]
43. Ding, D.; Maibach, E.W.; Zhao, X.Q.; Roser-Renouf, C.; Leiserowitz, A. Support for climate policy and societal action are linked to perceptions about scientific agreement. *Nat. Clim. Chang.* **2011**, *1*, 462–466. [CrossRef]
44. Green, E.I.; Blashki, G.; Berry, H.L.; Harley, D.; Horton, G.; Hall, G. Preparing Australian medical students for climate change. *Aust. Fam. Physician* **2009**, *38*, 726–729. [PubMed]
45. Rauf, S.; Bakhsh, K.; Abbas, A.; Hassan, S.; Ali, A.; Kachele, H. How hard they hit? Perception, adaptation and public health implications of heat waves in urban and peri-urban Pakistan. *Environ. Sci. Pollut. Res. Int.* **2017**, *24*, 10630–10639. [CrossRef] [PubMed]
46. Akompab, D.A.; Bi, P.; Williams, S.; Grant, J.; Walker, I.A.; Augoustinos, M. Heat Waves and Climate Change: Applying the Health Belief Model to Identify Predictors of Risk Perception and Adaptive Behaviours in Adelaide, Australia. *Int. J. Environ. Res. Public Health* **2013**, *10*, 2164–2184. [CrossRef] [PubMed]
47. Kahan, D.M.; Peters, E.; Wittlin, M.; Slovic, P.; Ouellette, L.L.; Braman, D.; Mandel, G. The polarizing impact of science literacy and numeracy on perceived climate change risks. *Nat. Clim. Chang.* **2012**, *2*, 732–735. [CrossRef]
48. Bell, E.J. Climate change: What competencies and which medical education and training approaches? *BMC Med. Educ.* **2010**, *10*, 31. [CrossRef] [PubMed]
49. Leffers, J.; Levy, R.M.; Nicholas, P.K.; Sweeney, C.F. Mandate for the Nursing Profession to Address Climate Change through Nursing Education. *J. Nurs. Scholarsh.* **2017**, *49*, 679–687. [CrossRef] [PubMed]
50. Kreslake, J.M.; Sarfaty, M.; Roser-Renouf, C.; Leiserowitz, A.A.; Maibach, E.W. The Critical Roles of Health Professionals in Climate Change Prevention and Preparedness. *Am. J. Public Health* **2017**, *108*, S68–S69. [CrossRef] [PubMed]
51. Shin, G.Y.; Manuel, R.J. Healthcare professionals must "think globally, act locally" on climate change. *BMJ* **2016**, *355*, i5686. [CrossRef] [PubMed]
52. Shaman, J.; Knowlton, K. The Need for Climate and Health Education. *Am. J. Public Health* **2017**, *108*, S66–S67. [CrossRef] [PubMed]
53. Varela-Losada, M.; Vega-Marcote, P.; Perez-Rodriguez, U.; Alvarez-Lires, M. Going to action? A literature review on educational proposals in formal Environmental Education. *Environ. Educ. Res.* **2016**, *22*, 390–421. [CrossRef]
54. Mosher, H.R.; Desrochers, M. The effects of information regarding sustainability issues and behavioral self-management instruction on college students' energy conservation. *Int. J. Sustain. High. Educ.* **2014**, *15*, 359–370. [CrossRef]
55. Lobell, D.B.; Burke, M.B.; Tebaldi, C.; Mastrandrea, M.D.; Falcon, W.P.; Naylor, R.L. Prioritizing climate change adaptation needs for food security in 2030. *Science* **2008**, *319*, 607–610. [CrossRef] [PubMed]

2

On the Suitability and Potential of Nursing Care Discussion Forums as a Health Promotion Measure for Long-Distance Caregiving Relatives

Tatjana Fischer [1,*] and **Markus Jobst** [2]

[1] Institute of Spatial Planning, Environmental Planning and Land Rearrangement, University of Natural Resources and Life Sciences Vienna, Peter-Jordan-Straße 82, 1190 Vienna, Austria

[2] Department for Geodesy and Geoinformation, Research Group Cartography, Vienna University of Technology, Erzherzog-Johann-Platz 1/120-6, 1040 Vienna, Austria; markus@jobstmedia.at

* Correspondence: tatjana.fischer@boku.ac.at

Abstract: *Background*: The number of persons who have to overcome extensive geographical distances for caring for their older parent(s), hereinafter referred to as long-distance caregiving relatives (LDCs), is rising. However, in the non-English-speaking Global North, little is known about the LDCs' health literacy and the design of tailor-made health promotion measures for this target-group. Using the example of nursing care discussion forums (NCDF), this paper reflects the requirements and (future) potential of professionally-lead support groups for LDCs on the case-study example of Upper Austria. *Methods*: In order to approach this unexplored topic considering spatial-related aspects, a qualitative-explorative study design was chosen, focusing on the providers' perspective. A written survey among all NCDF-group leaders was carried out. *Results*: LDCs do not make use of NCDFs at present. It is considered that this is above all for time constraints, lack of information and location-based problems of fit. This applies for urban as well as rural contexts. *Conclusions*: LDCs need more attention in public health. Suitable NCDFs have to be located in the LCDs' residential municipalities and have to fulfill different requirements from those of local caregiving relatives, particularly with regard to purpose and scope.

Keywords: long-distance caregiving relatives; health promotion; nursing care discussion forums; requirements; problems of fit; location planning; spatial context; expert survey; Upper Austria

1. Introduction

Due to demographic aging—caused by an increase in life expectancy and declining birth rates [1,2]—the discussion on financing care services for the elderly and the fact that nursing careers differently takes long [3], especially in the Global North, family caregiving relatives have become a target group of public health [4,5]. This is because caregiving relatives are an essential pillar of domestic care for older family members [5,6] and help to fulfill the central wish of older people—namely, staying at home as long as possible [7]. Providing (informal) domestic care is linked with physical strains as well as psychological strains and affects both the caregiver's well-being and—in the long run—health [8–14]. The impacts on health and well-being vary individually, because caregiving related overloads and burdens are linked to personality such as the degree of emotional involvement and ability to distance oneself from expectations of others, coping strategies and health literacy, the life-cycle position related to employment and child-care, as well as the amount of accompanying support related to domestic care for the elder family member(s).

In order to support caregiving relatives, over time, a number of support and relief measures have been developed. These health promotion measures comprise a variety of information and counseling services for dealing with the care situation and finding external (professional) support [4,5,11,15]. Among them and in comparison to other relief measures such as holiday offers for informal caregivers and offers for replacement care, are Austria nursing care discussion forums (NCDFs), which have a long tradition and serves as short breaks from caregiving [5] and primarily address local caregiving relatives who are either living together with the cared-for person under a single roof or next to the cared-for person [5].

Thus far, the efficiency of professionally-led support groups or NCDFs and their added value for psychological well-being and health of caregivers of cared-for elder persons of different clinical pictures is discussed controversially [16–22], while the issue of demand and location planning as well as the design of health promotion and public health measures—in comparison to local caregiving relatives [14,23–28]—are disregarded. It is precisely the latter aspect that needs attention regarding a considerable proportion of informal caregivers whose amount will increase in the future [25,29], namely long-distance caregivers. This also applies for their coping strategies, health literacy and use of health promotion measures [24,25].

Aim of the Paper and Research Questions

In order to reach the United Nations Sustainable Development Goals' overarching aim to leave no one behind and in order to preserve good health and well-being to all regardless of gender, age and place of residence according to the Shanghai Declaration 2016 [30], this paper deals in the context of target-group appropriate social infrastructure planning with the requirements and potential of nursing care discussion forums as a health promotion measures for LDCs. The spatial reference framework is Upper Austria, a province of Austria. Austria is a high-income member state of the European Union, but faces an increasing polarization between rapidly growing urban areas on the one hand and aging rural or alpine peripheries on the other hand [31,32]. LDCs are a neglected target group in public health and sound empirical evidence on health literacy and making use of existing health promotion measures including NCDFs is missing [33,34].

This paper addresses LDCs who belong to the second generation of caregiving relatives, namely daughters and sons as well as daughters-in-law and sons-in-law. The reason for this scoping lies in the fact of an increasing imbalance related to the distribution and age-structure of the population, the trends towards the beanpole family [35] and the spatially differentiated potential of family care due to (Upper) Austria's growing spatial heterogeneity between (infra-)structurally strong and weak areas [34,36]. These factors are strongly linked and have already led to a decrease of supportive caregiving members within the families themselves on the one hand and a growing number of LDCs in Austria [34] on the other hand. In turn, it can be assumed that this already may have led and still will lead to the LDCs' increased focus on care for their parent(s).

Taking into account the LDCs'-specific burdens and constraints, three research questions are posed, in order to assess the present offer and if necessary, to derive prerequisites to raise the NCDFs' suitability:

1. What do we know about the LDCs' attendance of NCDFs in different spatial settings?
2. What kinds of (spatial-related) factors determine the LDCs' use of NCDFs?
3. Do present NCDFs meet the requirements of LDCs and what can be done to increase the attractiveness of this health promotion measure for this target group?

2. Literature Review: Nursing Care Discussion Forums and Long-Distance Caregiving

2.1. Nursing Care Discussion Forums as a Support Measure for Informal Caregivers

For this paper nursing care discussion forums (NCDFs) are defined as a type of support group for informal caregivers of (older) people in need of care in order to maintain or enhance the caregivers' mindfulness—a focal component of psychological health [37]—well-being and stress coping capacity [18].

NCDFs take place in secure surroundings, are led by nursing or health care professionals and offer space for mutual exchange among caregivers, provide emotional support, information and counseling [16] and require experienced and highly-skilled group leaders in order to be able to sufficiently deal with particular caregiving situations [18]. Moreover, NCDFs helps to build communities among caregivers [16].

It was found that non-mixed NCDFs related to the clinical picture of the cared-for (older) person of the participants [ibid] and a small group size [18] are relevant factors for success of this intervening support measure. For this reason, over the years a range of NCDFs came into existence, above all focusing on informal caregivers of persons who suffer from Alzheimer and dementia [18,19].

2.2. Long-Distance Caregiving Family Members—A Particular Target Group in Health Promotion

Caregiving relatives are a heterogeneous group related to availability for caregiving reasons and the spatial constellation related to the places of residence of the caregivers on the one hand and the cared-for-family member(s).

Spatially spoken, caregiving relatives can be split into two groups: local caregivers and distance caregivers. The latter mostly belong to the second generation of carers (daughters, sons) [14,35] and among them, there is a subgroup called long-distance caregivers (LDCs), who have a time expose of at least one hour in order to overcome a geographical distance of at least 50 miles (80 kilometers) between their place of residence and those of their cared-for parent(s) [38,39].

Due to an ongoing spatial concentration of higher education facilities and labor markets in urban agglomerations and mostly rural-urban directed internal and international migration flows [27,40], as well as due to retirement migration [26], overcoming (extensive) distances for caregiving reasons has become a widespread phenomenon internationally and overcoming extensive geographical distances is an obstacle for those relatives who are willing to engage (more) in domestic care for their parent(s) [1,24,29,41]. International research on LDCs—mainly from the US—shows that the necessity to overcome extensive geographical distances impacts the intensity as well as the kind of support or care for the older parent(s), but not the strength of emotional bonds [ibid]. Long-distance caregiving results in different kinds of involvement related to the care situation itself [26]. LDCs take on different tasks such as coordination and organization of professional domestic care, financial donations, provide support for those caring family members who bear the main burden of care [23,39–42].

LDCs suffer from completely different challenges compared to local caregivers [26,29]. These include: time exposure and financial expenses of (regularly) commuting between at least two places of residence, being torn between perceived obligation, the desire to give something back and the actual opportunity to engage in domestic care, as well as living with uncertainties related to information on the actual status of well-being and health of the older parent(s), being condemned to observe the older parent(s) physical and mental deterioration from afar and experience conflicts with other family members who provide most of the care locally [24–26,29,39,43].

Life and stress situations of LDCs individually differ and depend on the degree of care need, the clinical picture, particularly cancer and dementia, which are becoming more and more relevant [23,42,44], the availability of formal and informal support on-site [45] and the LDCs' attitude or readiness to commute, as well as the geographical distance itself [25,46]. In addition, it was found that women tend to be more willing to overcome longer geographical distances for caregiving reasons than men [1]. It can be assumed that the care situation is particularly stressful for middle-aged female LDCs.

Nevertheless, there is a wide range of support or health promotion measures for LDCs [28] covering comprising on-site or face-to-face support measures (e.g., peer support) and web-based measures.

Since it has been shown that the availability of direct contact to the cared-for person at any time has a calming effect to LDCs and promotes their well-being [46], a variety of web-based support measures has been developed over the years, focusing primarily on bridging geographical distance associated with communication between LDCs and the cared-for person (e.g., by means of video telephony [40] and virtual exchange between LDC, the cared-for person and formal caregivers [23]). All these web-based solutions are advertised on relevant internet platforms.

Additionally, there are a number of online-guides addressing amongst others two core issues: (1) providing effective care from distance [47] and (2) the presentation of coping strategies for dealing with this challenging situation [48,49]. They contain various advice for dealing with care at a distance and to provide an overview of other contact addresses and web links.

3. Materials and Methods

The present paper deals with a new topic in public health in Austria, and because of its complexity, a mixed-methods-approach was applied [50]. The selected information sources were as follows:

- An existing dataset that originates from an explorative-qualitative written survey of group leaders of the Upper Austrian NCFDs conducted in 2017.
- Secondary and statistical data comprising (1) a summary list of all NCDFs in Upper Austrian NCDFs, including information on location municipalities, provided by the provincial administration of Upper Austria, (2) statistical data on care allowance recipients in Upper Austria, provided by the provincial administration of Upper Austria and (3) the official dataset on the spatial types of the Austrian municipalities, namely the Urban-Rural-Typology of the Austrian municipalities, provided by Statistics Austria [51].

This section describes the information sources including reasons for selection, procedure of data collection, data analysis and triangulation.

3.1. Information Sources, Handling of Data and Data Analysis

3.1.1. Information Source 1: Results of a Written Survey of Group Leaders of the Upper Austrian NCDFs Conducted in 2017

In summer 2017, the first author of this paper received an invitation to contribute to the anthology "Fair opportunities for healthy aging" on the occasion of the 20th anniversary of the Fund for a Healthy Austria. The initial consideration was to draft a conceptual contribution on LDCs in Austria in order to introduce this target group to the relevant stakeholder in public health. At the same time, an employee of the provincial administration of Upper Austria—also invited to contribute—was interested in writing an article about NCDFs and their relevance for caregivers in Upper Austria. Within the scope of a telephone conversation, both ideas were linked. Due to the fact that in Austria LCDs have not yet been explored before, it was decided to conduct a cross-sectional qualitative-explorative written survey with the group leaders of the Upper Austrian NCDFs in order to understand the providers' perspective referring to the interrelations of demand, supply and location issues that determine the use of NCDFs of two different groups of caregiving relatives: local caregivers and LDCs. It turned out that a target group-specific analysis went beyond the editor's scope of the publication. With regard to LDCs, the joint publication [33] concluded by pointing out the necessity to fathoming the relevance of NCDFs as a health promotion measure for LDCs.

In the following, the procedure of data collection and data analysis of the dataset are described; intending to collect as much information as possible on LDCs, it was aimed to attract as many NCDF-group leaders as possible for the written survey. The employee of the Upper Austrian provincial administration—second author of the above mentioned publication [ibid]—who is professionally responsible for the supervision of the Upper Austrian NCDFs and over the years has stayed in good contact with the NCDF-group leaders, invited all of them (there were 77 Upper Austrian NCDFs as of 2017) by mail to participate in a written survey.

Due to the lack of literature on the service-specific suitability of NCDFs in the context of long-distance caregiving and the lack of information on LDCs in the Austrian context in general as well as on the concrete schedule of NCDFs and on how the NCDF-group leaders document each session, a theoretically-led formulation of categories for closed-questions seemed to be inappropriate. In order to provide the opportunity to respond narratively and spontaneously, it was decided for mostly open-ended questions [51] addressing target group-specific (local caregiving relatives as well as LDCs) issues as follows:

- The actual catchment area of the NCDFs.
- The target group-specific (LDCs') actual demand.
- Ideas on ideal health promotion for LDCs.
- The suitability of NCDFs for LDCs.

A questionnaire consisting of 25 questions (see Table 1) was prepared by the first author of this paper and the employee of the Upper Austrian provincial administration. The latter also took on the task of validation of the questionnaire related to content and wording due to her educational background in nursing and responsibility for the quality assurance of the Upper Austrian NCDFs.

Table 1. Structure and content of the questionnaire for the written expert survey.

Structure of Questionnaire	Subjects
thematic block no. 1: demographic profile of NCDF-group leaders	• sex • age (two closed questions)
thematic block no. 2: organization and catchment area of NCDFs	• name of eponymous and partner municipalities • location • day of the week, time, duration, frequency of place-taking • catchment areas related to attendees • changes in demand • advertising • cooperation with other municipalities (nursing care discussion cluster) (11 open-ended questions)
thematic block no. 3: demographic profile of participants places of residence of participating caregiving relative and cared-for person	• sex • age • number of participants • family relationship between attendee and cared-for person • places of residence of NCDF-participant and cared-for person (3 closed and 2 open-ended questions)
thematic block no. 4: NCDF-group leaders' assessment of the NCDFs' health-promoting effects	• expectations of participants • strains, burdens and concrete concerns of participants • explicit contribution on the participants' health and well-being (4 closed questions)
thematic block no. 5: knowledge on burdens related to long-distance caregiving and considerations related to target-group-specific support and relief measures (including NCDFs)	• challenges and concerns related to extensive commuting distances • considerations on the reachability of long-distance caregiving relatives by NCDFs • considerations on the characteristics of ideal support and relief measures for long-distance caregivers • considerations on the relevance and location planning of NCDFs (3 open-ended questions)

In fall 2017, in a second e-mail, the questionnaire—attached in the form of a Word document—was sent to the NCDF group leaders. They were asked to insert the questions directly into the Word document and to send it back within a period of three weeks. In a cover letter written by the employee of the Upper Austrian provincial administration, it was pointed out that non-participation was fully respected. Since the written survey was conducted with official permission of the appropriate department of the Upper Austrian provincial administration and did not address investigative medical research, no ethic approval from an ethics committee was required. Nonetheless, compliance with all international research standards—above all, warranting voluntary participation without fear of negative consequences in case of refusal; and confidential handling of data—was met.

By the end of November 2017, 47 out of 77 NCDF-group leaders (61%) took part in the survey and submitted the completed questionnaires by e-mail, mail or fax.

3.1.2. Information Source 2: Summary List of Upper Austrian NCDFs

This summary list in form of a Word document was provided by the Upper Austrian provincial administration. It contained current information on the number and the catchment areas of the NCDFs (as of 2017). Two different types of NCDFs can be distinguished: (1) NCDFs with a catchment area that is limited to the location municipality, hereafter referred to as eponymous municipalities, and (2) NCDFs with regional catchment, namely the eponymous municipality and the participating partner municipalities, hereafter referred to as nursing care discussion clusters.

3.1.3. Information Source 3: Urban-Rural-Typology of Statistics Austria

All municipalities where NCDFs were located were categorized, using the Urban-Rural Typology of Statistics Austria [52], which offered 10 different spatial categories based on several indicators, such as the number of inhabitants, commuter relationships between municipalities, reachability of urban centers and the level of infrastructure facilities. In order to be able to carry out a spatial-related analysis of the NCDFs, all Austrian municipalities were grouped into the following four spatial categories: urban centers, regional centers, suburban municipalities and rural municipalities.

3.2. Mapping the NCDFs' Coverage and Catchment Areas

In order to map the coverage of the Upper Austria with NCDFs the information from the summary list were transferred to a table and merged with geographic information. The process of data wrangling precedes the integration of the NCDF and geoinformation. Whereas the NCDF table requested a manual harmonization of the indicator identifiers according to their way of writing and temporal validity, the requested geoinformation had to be extracted and validated for the proposed time of survey. Although all data are accessible in Austria, the given quality did not prevent from manual data wrangling.

In order to be able to estimate the representativeness of the response rate regarding to the NCDFs' theoretical catchment referring to caregiving relatives of domestically cared-for older people, administrative data from Upper Austria on the recipients of care allowance were used. These data refer to the number of care allowance recipients at the municipal level, but are not classified according to age or sex of the recipients for reasons of data protection.

In order to determine the proportion of domestically cared-for older people among all care allowance recipients, the following assumptions were made: firstly, it was assumed that the share of older people made up 98%; secondly, 80% of these older people received care or support from their relatives.

3.3. Assessment of the Current NCDF-Offer for LDCs and Implications

In a first step, the questionnaires were numbered chronologically according to their receipt. The registered answers—the quality of information referring to questions decidedly addressing LDCs (see Figure 1) ranged from a few notes to short sentences and paragraphs—were transferred verbatim to an Excel file (version 26 for Windows). The closed questions were coded in a binary form (0 = no/not appropriate, 1 = yes/appropriate; missing answers = 99).

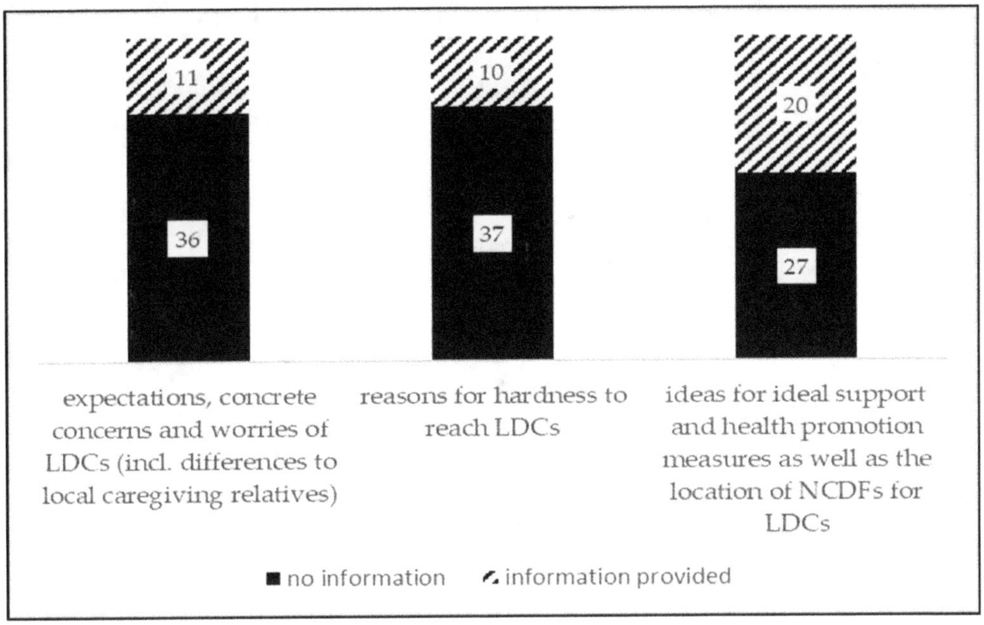

Figure 1. Available information on LDCs.

In a second step, categories were developed according to the comparative method of Glaser and Strauss [53]. For this purpose, the information related to the open-ended questions were binary coded (0 = no/not appropriate, 1 = yes/appropriate; missing answers = 99), then transformed to an SPSS database (version 24 for Windows, IBM, Armonk, NY, USA).

In a third step, in order to assess the data, they were analyzed theme-centered according to Boyatzis [54].

The LCD-related responses (see Figure 1) formed the starting point for reflecting the demand, supply and location issues and further LCD-suitable NCDF-development. In order to be able to assess the suitability of the current NCDF-offer, the gathered information referring to LDCs was compared to those for local caregiving relatives.

On this basis, the LCD-suitability of the current NCDF-offer was considered including implications for necessary or possible improvement by comparing the NCDF-requirements for LDCs and local caregiving relatives.

As Figure 1 shows, LCD-related questions have been answered by comparatively few NCDF-group leaders: 21 out of 47 responding NCDF-group leaders at least have answered one out of three questions related to LDCs, four group leaders have answered all three questions. In order to reliably assess the Upper Austrian situation, it was decided to conduct a descriptive statistical analysis and to discuss the results—if possible and suitable—with (international) literature.

4. Results

In 2017, NCDFs were located in 195 out of the then 442 Upper Austrian municipalities. It was found that:

- With the exception of NCDFs located in regional centers, all other spatial types of NCDF-municipalities were covered by the expert survey, namely 50 % of the urban NCDFs, 75% of the suburban NCDFs and 60% of the rural NCDFs (see Table 2).
- Out of all Upper Austrian municipalities, 57% were eponymous municipalities or partner municipalities, that built a Nursing Care Discussion Cluster (see Figure 2).
- The coverage related to the theoretical catchment area of the NCDFs referring to domestically cared-for older persons: 70% of the theoretical catchment could be recorded (see Figure 2).

- From the written expert survey, information on 61% out of all 77 Upper Austrian NCDFs could be obtained (see Table 2).

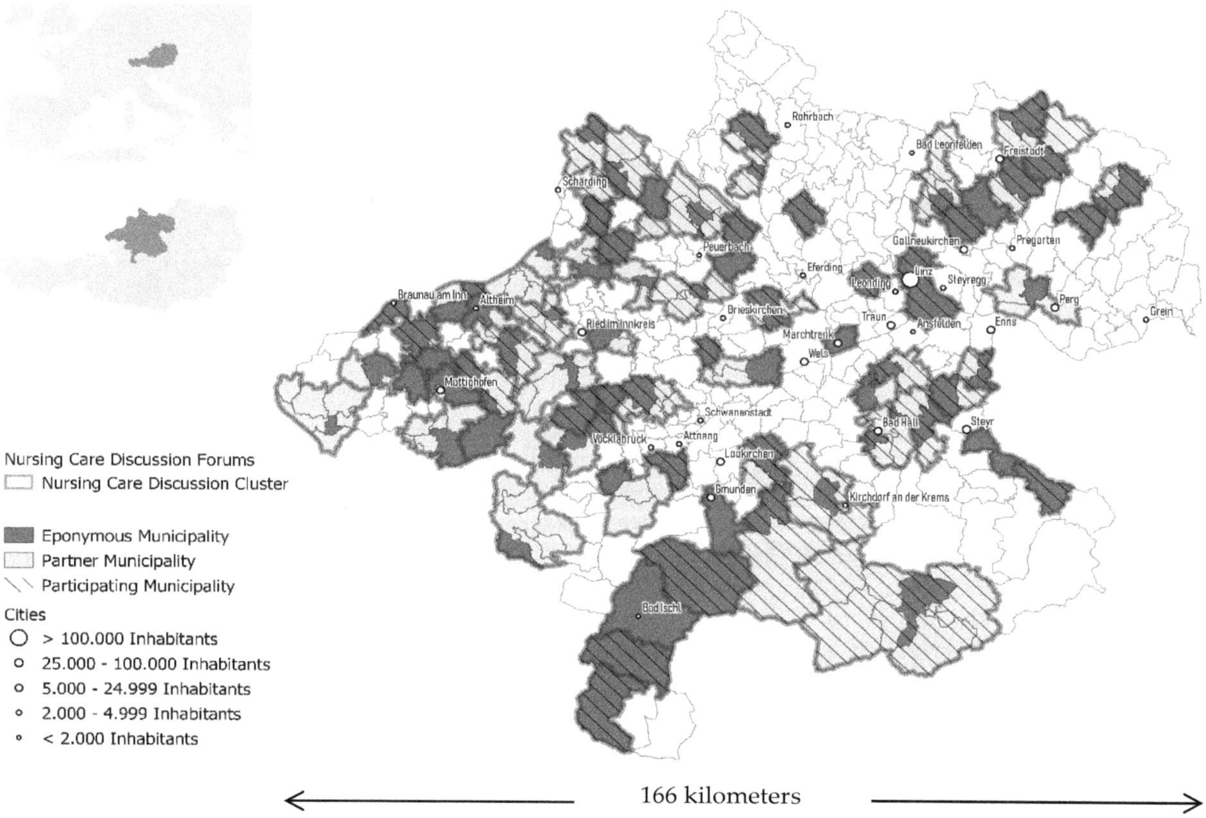

Figure 2. Spatial organization structure of the Upper Austrian NCDFs (as of 2017). The dark colored and bordered areas (referred to as eponymous municipalities) show NCDF-municipalities without further cooperation municipalities. The light gray colored municipalities (referred to as partner municipalities) together with the respective eponymous municipalities (=dark colored areas) constitute a nursing care discussion cluster (=regional NCDF-cooperation). The borders mark the delimitation of the nursing care discussion clusters which consist of neighboring municipalities. The hatched areas in turn, designate those NCDF-municipalities or nursing care discussion clusters which are covered by the written survey.

Table 2. Structure and content of the questionnaire for the written expert survey.

Spatial Typology of Upper Austria's NCDF-Municipalities	In Total	Covered in the Written Survey [%]
urban centers	10	5 [50%]
regional centers	2	0 [0%]
suburban municipalities	20	15 [75%]
rural municipalities	45	27 [60%]
in total	77	47 [61%]

4.1. Result 1: Catchment and Reachabilityof NCDFs

NCDFs are health promotion measures located near to the places of residence of the participants and mostly are of local reach. Although being intensively advertised, only a small number of caregivers make use of this offer. The participants mostly live in the same municipality as the cared-for older person(s) or parent(s). Joining NCDFs apparently justifies a short break from caregiving obligations. There are no LDCs among the NCDF-participants.

4.1.1. A Portrait of NCDFs

NCDFs are run by highly skilled health and nursing staff, especially women, and are places of personal, professional and confidential exchange of caregivers' central concerns and worries. NCDFs are held in selected locations such as restaurants, suitable rooms in the municipal office as well as in nursing homes. Normally, NCDFs take place once or twice a month, usually during the week and in the evening [33] (see Table 3). The NCDF-group leaders receive a small expense allowance for this service.

Table 3. Breakdown of basic information on NCDFs.

Basic Information on Group Leaders and Organization of NCDFs	**In Urban Centers**	**In Suburban Municipalities**	**In Rural Municipalities**
age of group leaders	aged 43–58	aged 33–62	aged 42–68
sex of group leaders	entirely women	entirely women	mainly women (24 out of 27)
sharing their function as group leaders	mainly yes (4 out of 5)	no	mainly not (22 out of 27)
frequency of place-taking	mostly once a month (4 out of 5) in one case: twice a month	mostly once a month (12 out of 15) in one case: twice a month in two further cases: bimonthly	mostly once a month (26 out of 27) in one case: twice a month
day of the week	during the week (Mon, Tue or Thu)	during the week (Mon, Tue, Wed or Thu)	during the week (Mon, Tue, Wed or Thu)
start time	between 6 and 7 p.m.	mostly between 7 and 8 p.m. (13 out of 15) in one case: 2 p.m. in one further case: between 5 and 7 p.m.	between 7 and 8 p.m.
duration	2 h	0.5–2 h	2–2.5 h

4.1.2. NCDFs' Catchment Areas

The catchment areas of the NCDFs correspond to the places of residence of the caregivers. In none of these cases, the actual catchment area extends beyond the nursing care discussion cluster or cooperating neighbor municipalities. 29 out of 47 NCDFs are designed as nursing care discussion clusters comprising at least two neighboring municipalities in which the NCDFs are alternately held. In 26 out of 29 cases, one NCDF-group leader is responsible for all involved municipalities. The theoretical catchment area of the 47 NCDFs or nursing care discussion clusters comprises 82 municipalities, including about 18,700 domestically cared-for older people supported by family members. In contrast, the actual catchment area comprises 37 municipalities with about 15,000 domestically care-for older people who are cared for at home by family members.

The actual catchment area of the NCDFs covers 45% of the involved municipalities and 80% of the domestically cared-for older people who receive (care) support from relatives. Referring to the latter aspect, there are differences related to the spatial type of the eponymous NCDF-municipalities (see Table 4): this is just under 100% for NCFDs located in urban municipalities, 4% for the suburban and 56% for the rural NCDFs. This means that the deviations between the theoretical and the actual catchment area of rural NCDFs are greatest or rather that the catchment area of an NCDF is tended to be limited to the eponymous municipality.

Table 4. Theoretical and actual catchment areas of NCDFs (eponymous and nursing care discussion clusters) related to the number of domestically cared-for older persons living in NCDF location municipalities.

NCDFs' Catchment Area	Spatial Type of NCDF Eponymous Municipality	Number of NCDFs	Theoretical Catchment Area of NCDFs Related to Domestic Cared-for Older Persons *)	Actual Catchment Area of NCDFs Related to Domestic Cared-for Older Persons *)	Relation between Theoretical and Actual Catchment Area [in %]
limited to eponymous municipality	urban centers	4	9300	9300	100%
	suburban municipalities	5	500	500	100%
	rural municipalities	9	1300	1300	100%
comprising partner municipalities	urban centers	1	200	<100	10%
	suburban municipalities	10	2600	1800	69%
	rural municipalities	18	4700	2100	44%
related to all NDFs	urban centers	5	9500	9200	98%
	suburban municipalities	15	3100	2300	74%
	rural municipalities	27	6100	3400	56%
in total		47	18,700	15,000	80%

* Values rounded to 100s.

4.1.3. Profile of NCDF-Participants

Looking at the profile of the NCDF-participants, it can be seen that they belong to the first and second generation of caregiving relatives and are aged 45 to 70 years. The participants are mainly women supporting or caring for their parent(s) or parent(s)-in-law. The NCDF-participants live primarily in the same municipality as the cared-for older relative, except for one urban NCDF, which cannot be explained on the basis of the information available. LDCs cannot be found among the participants [33]. Moreover, NCDFs are relevant for a small number of caregivers and show a tendency to decline regarding their use [ibid] (see Table 5). With regard to these facts and to the sociodemographic profile of the NCDF-participants, the NCDFs in urban, suburban as well as in rural municipalities hardly differ from each other.

Table 5. Profile of NCDF-participants belonging to the second generation of caregiving relatives.

Profile of Participants	NCDFs in Urban Centers	NCDFs in Suburban Municipalities	NCDFs in Rural Municipalities
participants per NCDF	4–5 (5 out of 5)	4–8 (15 out of 15)	3–15 (25 out of 27)
development of NCDF-attendance	trending downwards (3 out of 5)	trending downwards (8 out of 15)	trending downwards (12 out of 27)
age of participants	aged 50–60 (5 out of 5)	aged 50–70 (15 out of 15)	aged 45–70 (27 out of 27)
sex of participants	mainly women (4 out of 5)	mainly women (13 out of 15)	mainly women (24 out of 27)
relationship of places of residence of participants and their cared-for older relative/s	mostly living in the same municipality (3 out of 5)	mostly living in the same municipality (11 out of 15)	mostly living in the same municipality (22 out of 27)
kinship of participants and older cared-for person/s	daughter > daughter-in-law (5 out of 5)	daughter > daughter-in-law (15 out of 15)	daughter > daughter-in-law (27 out of 27)
older cared for person/s	mother > father > parent-in-law (5 out of 5)	mother > parent-in-law > father (15 out of 15)	mother > mother-in-law > father/father-in-law (27 out of 27)

To sum up, NCDFs particularly are a health promotion measure for local caregiving relatives.

4.1.4. Advertising Channels and Reachability of LDCs

Irrespective, of whether or not NCDFs are located in urban, suburban or rural municipalities, according to the NCDF-group leaders' statements, NCDFs are advertised using various channels (see Figure 2 and Table 6). Overall, 20 different advertisement channels could be distilled from empirical data. These channels, in turn, can be clustered into four groups, taking into account the geographical scope and the way in which caregivers are contacted:

- Advertisement channels of local scope.
- Advertisement channels of regional scope.
- Directly addressing of caregiving relatives.
- Unspecified advertisement channels in terms of both, their (spatial) scope and contact building with caregiving relatives.

Table 6. Advertising NCDFs.

	NCDFs in Urban Centers	**NCDFs in Suburban Municipalities**	**NCDFs in Rural Municipalities**	**Number of Advertisement Channels in Total**
being advertised (information provided: 44 out of 47 NCDF-group leaders)	yes: 5 out of 5	yes: 14 no, no longer: 1	yes: 25 no, no longer: 2	
most relevant advertisement channels of local scope (number of channels)	organized by municipality (municipal newspapers, homepage) > leaflets (community physician, pharmacy) > information provided by hospital (5 cases)	municipal newspapers > community physician/pharmacy > announcements of the church (10 cases)	community physician/pharmacy > nursing homes/day-care centers for elderly people > leaflets of the municipality > announcements of the church (10 cases)	11 in total
most relevant promotion channels of regional scope (number of channels)	regional newspapers (1 case)	regional newspapers > health fairs/health days (3 cases)	regional newspapers > announcements of the initiative "healthy communities" (4 cases)	4 in total
directly contacting caregiving relatives (number of channels)	personal acquaintance/telephone contact, written invitation, word-of-mouth advertising (3 cases)	personal acquaintance/telephone contact, written invitation, word-of-mouth advertising (1 case)	personal acquaintance/telephone contact, written invitation, word-of-mouth advertising > SMS, Facebook, Whatsapp (2 cases)	4 in total
most relevant promotion channels not specified scope (number of channels)	none	posters, events (1 case)	posters, events (1 case)	1 in total
ranking of promotion channels related to relevance	information with local scope > direct contacts to caregiving relatives > information channels of regional scope	information with local scope > information channels of regional scope > direct contacts to caregiving relatives	information with local scope > direct contacts to caregiving relatives > information channels of regional scope	

It turns out that the advertisement of the NCDFs primarily focuses on the local level. In total, NCDFs were advertised through 11 different advertisement channels, including:

- Promotion activities on the part of the NCDF-municipalities themselves.
- Insertion of flyers in medical practices or pharmacies.
- Promotion activities by nursing homes and day care centers.

Advertisement channels of a regional scope mainly comprised regional newspapers. All NCDF-group leaders describe directly addressing to caregiving relatives as very important way to promote NCDFs, either by telephone contact or via Facebook or SMS.

Differences related to the variety and the spatial scope of the advertisement channels arose taking into account the spatial typology of the eponymous municipality. As far as the variety of information channels used is concerned, rural NCDF-municipalities stand out. Urban NCDF-municipalities were most imaginative with regard to directly addressing to caregiving relatives. Nevertheless, all NCDF-municipalities failed to reach LDCs. At this point, it should be noted that there is no information on how comprehensively contact building takes place and whether LDCs as a subgroup of caregiving relatives explicitly are contacted. This is in-line with a statement of a NCDF-group leader of a rural municipality that said the reason for failure is that LDCs do not know about the existence of NCDFs.

Nine further NCDF-group leaders referred to the non-attendance of LDCs and time constraints schedule clashes as the main reasons of LCDs not to be able to attend NCDFs (from urban, suburban and rural NCDFs-municipalities), and the fact that the caregiving relative cannot leave the cared-for person alone (mentioned by a rural NCDF-group leader).

37 of the 47 respondents explained why they could not answer this question. The main reasons were that on the one hand, NCDF-group leaders have too little information on this target group, and on the other hand, representatives of the group of LDCs do not participate in NCDFs.

4.2. Result 2: Knowledge on LDCs Strains and Assessment of LDCs' Demand for NCDFs

The written expert survey brought into light that little is known about the strains of LDCs by NCDF-group leaders. Nevertheless, time constraints are assumed as the main obstacle for the demand for and participating in NCDFs.

Eleven out of 47 NCDF-group leaders addressed questions related to LDCs' strains and burdens and presumed expectations related to NCDFs, and in this context, mainly referred to the challenge of overcoming extensive geographical distances between the places of residence of the LDC and the cared-for older parent(s). The answers of the respondents can be summarized to the following statements or conclusions:

- The necessity to overcome distances leads to time constraints and a state of emotional disorder (mentioned three times in total, including one urban and two rural NCDF-group leaders).
- Geographical distance creates uncertainty about the actual physical and psychological condition of the cared-for older parent(s) (mentioned two times in total, comprising one group leader each from a suburban and a rural NCDF-municipality).
- LDCs have more efforts with regard to the organization of care within the family [55] (two mentions in total, including one urban and one suburban NCDF-group leader).
- LDCs are plagued by ambivalent feelings [56]: on the one hand, geographical distance leads to an increase of emotional distance; on the other hand, geographical distance causes more worries (mentioned by a group leader of a rural NCDF-municipality).
- Travel expenses are a burden, especially in winter (mentioned by a group leader of a rural NCDF-municipality).
- One group leader of a rural NCDF-municipality is of the opinion that geographical distance furthermore makes it easier to talk about one's (LDC-related) problems.
- Again, the reasons for the little information on this issue are that LCDs are out of the NCDF-group leaders' sight.

4.3. Result 3: On the Potential of NCDFs as a Health Promotion Measure for LDCs

From the perspective of the NCDF-group leaders, NCDFs are thought to have a certain potential as a health promoting measure for LCDs. It significantly depends on the location of NCDFs if they will become a suitable and attractive offer for LDCs.

The following results are based on the information of 20 out of 47 NCDF-group leaders.

4.3.1. Suggestions on Suitable Health Promotion or Support Measures for LDCs

The NCDF-group leaders' suggestions relate to three different types of support measures:

1. Support measures that are linked with active involvement of LDCs. This includes the creation of a balanced care support mix, consisting of informal neighborhood assistance and professional care, mainly through mobile social and care services (mentioned three times in total, one from a group leader of an urban and two from group leaders of rural NCDFs); the willingness of LDCs to make use of existing offers (mentioned four times in total, all from group leaders of rural NCDFs); trying to organize care while the NCDF is taking place (mentioned by a group leader of a rural NCDF); the reduction of working time and claiming for more support from the social environment of the cared-for person (mentioned by a group leader from a rural NCDF).
2. Concessions from outside by taking into account the specific situation and strains of LDCs, e.g., in the context of medical appointments in order to save time (mentioned by two group leaders of each one suburban and rural NCDF).
3. The development of a particular telephone counseling offer (suggestions from two NCDF-group leaders, one suburban and one rural).

4.3.2. Considerations on the Ideal Location for LDCs' Nursing Discussion Forums

Under the condition that LDCs recognize NCDFs as an appropriate support measure—four out of 20 group leaders from all spatial types of NCDF-municipalities think so—we assume the importance of the right location to be a key factor for use.

While two group leaders of rural NCDFs, or rather nursing care discussion clusters, plead for locating NCDFs in the municipality where LDCs live, two further NCDF-group leaders (one from a suburban and one from a rural NCDF) suggest to establish NCDFs there, where "most of the efforts are". Unfortunately, this statement is not explained in more detail.

5. Discussion

5.1. Appropriateness of Study Design, Representativenes and Reliability of Empirical Findings

Since LDCs are a neglected target-group in the public health sector in Austria [33,34], an explorative-qualitative case-study based approach, exploring the suitability of the current offer of NCDFs for LDCs in one of the nine provinces of Austria was chosen addressing the "providers'" perspective. For time exposure reasons, the geographical dispersion [57], of the NCDFs and due to the fact that there was no opportunity for third-party funding for this research, it was decided to conduct a written survey of all NCDF-group leaders in this province.

The results are based on a written survey of the NCDF-group leaders only show one side of the coin and call for research on the opinions of the LCDs relating to their support needs and ideas on the design of suitable NCDFs.

Nonetheless, related to the empirical findings a high representativeness is ensured due to a response rate of 61% out of all 77 Upper Austrian NCDFs. We can only speculate about the reasons for non-participation.

Given the fact that usually only one group leader is responsible for the NCDFs, in a way, the group leaders who have responded also reflect the situation in NDFs that, geographically speaking, have a regional dimension. It cannot be implied whether the results are true for the other eight Austrian provinces.

In addition, the limited information on LDCs indicates that the respondents know little about this target group and their health literacy and making use of health promotion offers. This, in turn, implies frankness in answering the questions and indicates reliability. Furthermore, the NCDF-group leaders cite the reasons for their knowledge deficit.

Since the NCDF-group leaders were not asked to unfold their assessment rules related to the life and strain situations of LDCs, it remains entirely open whether professional expertise and private experiences were mixed up.

However, it can be assumed that this is closely related to the fact that there still is a large knowledge gap on this target group in Austria [34].

5.2. Interrelations between the Profile and Advertisment of the Current NCDF-Offer and the Lack of Reachability of LDCs

At this point, first of all it should be noted that in general caregiving persons are less likely to use health-promoting measures compared to non-carers [9]. Referring to LDCs, one always has to keep in mind that time constrains are the focal obstacle that (could) hinder LDCs from making use of face-to-face and on-site health promotion offers. Besides that, the empirical results of the Upper Austrian case-study—in line with international findings [5,26]—show that a lack of information about availability of NCDFs [56] and the inappropriateness of the existing offer may explain the lack of reachability of LDCs.

Interestingly, the respondents did not interrelate reachability of LDCs with advertising efforts. This is quite comprehensible, as NCDFs are intensively advertised in urban and suburban, as well as in rural municipalities in a variety of ways, above all focusing the local level and directly addressing caregiving relatives—as was the case in 24 out of 47 cases—by telephone, Facebook or mail.

However, it must be recognized that the NCDF-group leaders neither have information on the procedure of the so-called "direct communication with LCDs", nor are they able to assess the success of direct communication with the members of this specific target group.

5.3. On the Potential of NCDFs as a Health Promotion Measure and Requirements for a LDC-Suitable NCDF-Offer

Aside from the general problem of the measurability of the immediateness of effects of health-promotion measures [58], basing on the survey results, first of all it can be assumed that an ideal support, relief or health promoting measure never will exist due to the impossibility considering the great diversity of the LDCs' living and caregiving situations [10]. At best, NCDFs will become a health promoting measure among others, above all web-based offers [36].

For the heterogeneous collective of LDCs, it is difficult to estimate the need for professionally-led support groups such as the NCDFs, because the caregiving situations, including the amount of formal, or rather professional (health and care), and of informal (future) family support on-site, as well as the degree of personally experienced strains associated to strategies differ from case to case. Considering this, sound empirical data on the use of health promotion measures by LDCs are still missing [25], but are urgently needed.

In addition, we still know little about the LDCs' health literacy and self-awareness as a target group for health promotion, and in general. There is a knowledge gap on the meaning of professionally led on-site support groups for LDCs. Moreover, against the backdrop of time constraints, we do not know about whether LDCs give precedence to an informal chat with a friend with a cup of coffee over a professionally led conversation. It can be assumed that this decision also essentially depends on the content of the conversation (professional advice versus speaking something from one's soul). Both in Austria and elsewhere, an in-depth discussion considering a wide-spread geographical scope on the issues of what is currently being discussed in NCDFs and—as far as LDCs are among the participants—what is burning in the soul of LDCs is needed.

Assuming that LDCs are or rather would be interested in face-to-face professionally led group-discussions on-site—regardless of whether the cared-for parent(s) is or are living at home or in a nursing home—based on the findings for the local caregiving relatives, only a small number of actual demanders can be expected. At this point, it is recalled that (1) the small number of participants of mainly female caregiving relatives (spouses) belonging to the first generation of caregiving relatives as well as the interrelation between the decline of use of health promotion measures and increasing age [4], (2) the small number of participants belonging to the second generation of caregiving relatives (daughters, daughters-in-law) as well as the observed declining trend of utilization and (3) the downwards trending NCDF-attendance [33].

Findings from the written survey referring to the differences between the strains and requirements of local caregiving relatives and LDCs and from literature can serve as a starting point for conceptualizing LDC-suitable NCDFs (see Table 7).

Although both target groups suffer from time constraints, physical distress dominates in local caregivers, whereas today's LDCs are more likely to be psychologically overstrained [26,29,55]. It is to be expected that the psychological burdens of those LDCs, whose parent(s) in need of care are living in rural areas, will increase in the near future, because due to the continuing trend towards the beanpole family, the support potential within the family will decrease [35]. This, in turn, will raise particularly the loneliness among the very old [59]. Furthermore, in rural areas, the provision of daily goods and services, including mobile social and health care is thinning out and the accessibility of age-specific infrastructure facilities becomes more and more challenging [60–62]. These developments affect especially those LDCs who are on the one hand are single children, and whose spouses or partners experience the same caregiving situation on the other hand.

Since LDCs perceive geographical distances differently—on the one hand, they are experienced liberating and relieving, on the other hand, they can enhance the psychological pressure on LDCs—the perceived emotional pressure on LDCs also depends on their cared-for-older parents' understanding for the demanding caregiving-situation and caregiving limitations [26]. Against this backdrop, the question arises of whether NCDFs for LDCs (in the future will) take over the function of "a safe haven" (according to justification and serving as time-outs from caregiving), focusing on exchanging personal caregiving experiences with others. Here, further healthcare research needs to focus more on health promotion measures from the perspective of the different target groups [10]. Due to the fact that non-carers are more likely to use health promotion measures than caregivers [9], and the assumption that work-life-balance becomes more important in society as well as it is predicted that health promotion will gain a higher social value in the future [63], referring to the potential of NCDFs as a health promotion measure, it is important to consider the following three questions:

1. Where should NCDFs be located in order to save time?
2. To what extent and at which locations could a handful of LDCs be brought together?
3. What are the requirements for tailor-made NCDFs in terms of organization and scope?

Based on the NCDF-group leaders' assessments, the following conceptual relations can be derived (see Table 7), which need to be evaluated in the course of future quantitative-oriented studies exploring both the provider's (NCDF-group leaders) and the "consumer's" (LDCs') perspective (see Table 7):

1. The profile of the NCDF-participants is as follows: women and men in midlife, of different marital status.
2. LDCs living in cities or towns with older parent(s) in need of care living in rural municipalities are not likely to make us of NCDFs located in their parents' rural residential municipality. This may be due to the "fact" that LDCs only come for caregiving reasons and exclusively dedicate each minute to their parent(s). NCDFs are to be designed as a location-based offer in the residence municipalities or (urban) working places of LDCs.

3. Urban NCDFs might have a larger catchment area of LDCs and a larger number of (potentially interested) LDCs in comparison to NCDFs in rural municipalities.
4. At the moment, we can only speculate about the scope of tailor-made NCDFs for LDCs. Basing on evidence on the burdens and strains of LDCs, dealing with guilt and responsibility may be focal issues.
5. LDCs approach to NCDFS with different concerns in comparison to local caregivers. That is why it should be considered to offer target-group-specific and LDC-specialized NCDF-offers regardless of the spatial setting.

Table 7. Considerations on the requirements for LDCs' and local caregiving relatives' suitable NCDFs.

Information Derived from Expert Survey and Literature	NCDFs for Long-Distance Caregiving Relatives	NCDFs for Local Caregiving Relatives
current demand of NCDFs	still unknown	to a limited extent
relevance and further (quantitative) development of the target group	increasing	increasing
further development of psychological burdens	rising	rising
demand for professionally led-discussion groups	still unknown	to a limited extent
relevance of web-based alternative services	probably relevant	increasing
future demand for NCDFs	still unknown	unknown or in decline
appropriate name of offer	"Supervised Discussion Forums for LDCs"	"Regular's Tables for Caregiving Relatives"
assumed motivation for participation	mutual exchange with similarly affected caregiving relatives supervised speaking-from-the-soul getting in touch with health and care professionals staying informed about support measures and developments in domestic care	time-outs / short breaks from domestic care gaining personal distance exchange with similarly affected caregiving relatives information and counseling
demographic profile of (future) NCDF-participants	women (and men) caregiving relatives of the second generation (particularly daughters/sons)	women (and men) caregiving relatives of the first and second generation
relation LDCs/local caregivers	solely LDCs	solely local caregiving relatives
assumed number of participants per NCDF	a couple of people	as at present
regularity of participation [57]	useful, but still unknown	useful, but still unknown
appropriate advertising channels	word-of-mouth advertising information (leaflets) in medical practices directly being contacted by care and nursing professionals information channels with super-regional scope (e.g., newspapers, internet platforms)	as at present
catchment area	local (residential municipalities of LDCs)	local (residential municipalities of local caregiving relatives) or small-scaled (neighbor municipalities)
appropriate location municipality for NCDFs	residential municipality of the LDC: mostly in the urban or suburban	residential municipality of the local caregiving relative: urban, suburban, as well as rural
location/meeting place	at the workplace attractive meeting places (e.g., cafes)	attractive meeting points (cafes)
organization structure depending on location	on demand, during the week during lunch breaks, in the afternoon and (early) evening	on demand, during the week, in the (early) evening
assumed scope of NCDFs (scope/discussed issues)	constructing identity as caregivers [55] developing mindfulness coping with guilt and feelings of obligation and responsibility	dealing with "unlimited" availability
relevance and function of care and nursing expert (=NCDF-group leader)	Informant, counselor mediator trainer	link between oneself and the cared-for older parent(s)

6. Conclusions

First of all, in view of the fact that we are still fishing in murky waters in many respects—among others due to the lack of statistical recording and the absence of other case-study based sound

LDC-related empirical databases—and in order to limit the margin of interpretation, we must not be tempted to mix up factual data and private caregiving experiences when considering the suitability of NCDFs as a health promotion measure for the particular and heterogeneous target-group of LDCs. Referring to the results discussed above, the risk of overestimating of pithy single statements is substantial. Furthermore, at this time, there are no sufficient empirical findings in order to reflect the Austrian-wide situation, nor to judge the situation in other socioeconomically and socio-culturally comparable countries.

Moreover, LDCs are still an underexplored target group in the context of the perception and reception of health promotion measures such as NCDFs. Relating to the location planning of NCDFs, we have to admit that we still know little on the (future) profile of LDCs. A present, we only know where they are living or probably will live in the near future—their places of residence will further concentrate in urban municipalities (cities, small towns). However, what we do not know is whether and to what extent the next generation of LCDs will continue to feel obliged to care for their older parent(s) and whether their parent(s) will expect them to do so. For this reason, we do not know to what extent the NCDFs' non-reachability of LDCs is or rather will remain a problem of fit or a problem of missing perception in terms of availability and receipt in terms of frequency [17].

That is why, in the future, the analysis of problems of fit—particularly related to NCDFs—must take into account: (a) the relevance of self-perception of LDCs as caregiving relatives, their feelings of belonging to a target-group, as well as their needs for emotional and informative support, (b) the state of knowledge and perceived attractiveness of different health promotion or support measures and (c) the (potential) competitive impact or complementary function of web-based, virtual support services and information platforms.

In a way this pilot study may serve as a starting-point for forming hypotheses on the suitability and future of NCDFs in the context of long-distance caregiving. What is needed here is another methodological approach, namely a quantitative investigation of LDCs, including their migration patterns, followed by an interdisciplinary interpretation of findings linked to demand and location planning of health promotion measures such as NCDFs.

On the assumption that professionally-led (group) support measures are or will always be very important to a small number of LDCs, too [11,38,48], NCDFs may experience a renaissance or generally gain importance as a health promotion measure. In order for this to work, public health needs to take the following steps:

1. Care and nursing professionals must be trained for the target-group of LDCs [34,55,57].
2. The target group of LDCs must be made visible to public. Thereby, NCDF-group leaders can act as multipliers.
3. LDCs must be given time to develop self-awareness as a target group of health promotion measures. For that reason, NCDFs can serve as on-site platforms for the development of mindfulness, health literacy and community building. In turn, all three are important prerequisites for making use of health promotion measures [64].
4. Pilot projects ("NCDFs for LDCs") should be initiated in different spatial settings and accordingly advertised in order to make LDCs aware of this kind of support or health promotion offer [58]. As a first step, it would be interesting to explore what (currently) is being debated in the NCDFs of other provinces of Austria, in order to identify the support needs of LDCs and to be able to sharpen ideas on the demand, organization and scope of (future) suitable offers. It should to be kept in mind that NCDFs cannot eliminate distress and burdens that directly are related to overcoming extensive geographical distances, but nevertheless may improve quality of life [60].
5. After running for a reasonable period, NCDFs need to be evaluated and linked to basic research on intervention programs for informal caregivers [55]. Only then it will become apparent whether NCDFs may be a suitable health promotion measure for LDCs and may exist alongside web-based offers.

Author Contributions: Conceptualization, T.F.; Data curation, T.F. and M.J.; Formal analysis, T.F. and M.J.; Investigation, T.F.; Methodology, T.F. and M.J.; Project administration, T.F.; Software, T.F. and M.J.; Supervision, T.F.; Validation, T.F..; Visualization, T.F. and M.J.; Writing—original draft, T.F.; Writing—review and editing, T.F. and M.J.

Acknowledgments: The authors would like to thank the Upper Austrian provincial administration, namely Kasberger, MSc for supporting the written expert survey and providing the summary list on NCDFs in Upper Austria and Schöfecker, for providing statistical data. The open access publishing was supported by BOKU Vienna Open Access Publishing Fund.

References

1. Joseph, A.E.; Hallman, B.C. Over the hill and far away: Distance as a barrier to the provision of assistance to elderly relatives. *Soc. Sci. Med.* **1998**, *46*, 631–639. [CrossRef]
2. Collins, W.L.; Holt, T.A.; Moore, S.E.; Bledsoe, L.K. Long-distance caregiving: A case study of an African-American family. *Am. J. Alzheimers Dis. Other Dement.* **2003**, *18*, 309–316. [CrossRef] [PubMed]
3. Gaugler, J.E.; Kane, R.L.; Kane, R.A.; Clay, T.; Newcomer, R.C. The Effects of Duration of Caregiving on Institutionalization. *Gerontologist* **2005**, *45*, 78–89. [CrossRef]
4. Kummer, K.; Budnick, A.; Blüher, S.; Dräger, D. Gesundheitsförderung für ältere pflegende Angehörige: Ressourcen und Risiken—Bedarfslagen und Angebotsstrukturen. *Präv. Gesundheitsförd.* **2010**, *5*, 89–94. [CrossRef]
5. Courtin, E.; Jemiai, N.; Mossialos, E. Mapping support policies for informal carers across the European Union. *Health Policy* **2014**, *118*, 84–94. [CrossRef]
6. Van den Berg, B.; Fiebig, D.G.; Hall, J. Well-being losses due to care-giving. *Health Econ.* **2014**, *35*, 123–131. [CrossRef]
7. Lehnert, T.; Heuchert, M.; Hussain, K.; König, H.H. Stated preferences for long-term care: A literature review. *Ageing Soc.* **2019**, *39*, 1873–1913. [CrossRef]
8. Sisk, R.J. Caregiver burden and health promotion. *Int. J. Nurs. Stud.* **2000**, *37*, 37–43. [CrossRef]
9. Acton, G.J. Health-Promoting Self-Care in Family Caregivers. *West. J. Nurs. Res.* **2002**, *24*, 73–86. [CrossRef]
10. Wiles, J. Daily geographies of caregivers: Mobility, routine, scale. *Soc. Sci. Med.* **2003**, *57*, 1307–1325. [CrossRef]
11. Zarit, S.; Femia, E. Behavioral and Psychosocial Interventions for Family Caregivers. *Am. J. Nurs.* **2008**, *108*, 47–53. [CrossRef]
12. Innes, A.; Morgan, D.; Kostineuk, J. Dementia care in rural and remote settings: A systematic review of informal/family caregiving. *Maturitas* **2011**, *68*, 34–46. [CrossRef] [PubMed]
13. Zigante, V.; European Commission, Directorate-General for Employment, Social Affairs and Inclusion; London School of Economics and Political Science. Informal Care in Europe: Exploring Formalisation, Availability and Quality. 2018. Available online: http://publications.europa.eu/publication/manifestation_identifier/PUB_KE0418543ENN (accessed on 30 July 2019).
14. Larkin, M.; Henwood, M.; Milne, A. Carer-related research and knowledge: Findings from a scoping review. *Health Soc. Care Commun.* **2018**, *27*, 55–67. [CrossRef] [PubMed]
15. Toseland, R.W.; Rossiter, C.M.; Labrecque, M.S. The Effectiveness of Peer-Led and Professionally Led Groups to Support Family Caregivers. *Gerontologist* **1989**, *29*, 465–471. [CrossRef]
16. Hornillos, C.; Crespo, M. Support groups for caregivers of Alzheimer patients: A historical review. *Dementia* **2011**, *11*, 155–159. [CrossRef]
17. Del-Pino-Casado, R.; Frías-Osuna, A.; Palomino-Moral, P.A.; Ruzafa-Martínez, M.; Ramos-Morcillo, A.J. Social support and subjective burden in caregivers of adults and older adults: A meta-analysis. *PLoS ONE* **2018**, *13*, e0189874. [CrossRef]
18. Chien, L.Y.; Chu, H.; Guo, J.L.; Liao, Y.M.; Chang, L.L.; Chen, C.H.; Chou, K.R. Caregiver support groups in patients with dementia: A meta-analysis. *Int. J. Geriatr. Psychiatry* **2011**, *26*, 1089–1098. [CrossRef]
19. Gräßel, E.; Trilling, A.; Donath, C.; Luttenberger, K. Support groups for dementia caregivers–predictors for utilisation and expected quality from a family caregiver's point of view: A questionnaire survey part I. *BMC Health Serv. Res.* **2010**, *10*, 219. [CrossRef] [PubMed]

20. Tak, Y.; Song, J.; Woo, H.; An, J. Realist Review: Understanding Effectiveness of Intervention Programs for Dementia Caregivers. *Asian Nurs. Res.* **2019**, *13*, 11–19. [CrossRef]
21. Dam, A.E.; de Vugt, M.E.; Klinkenberg, I.P.; Verhey, F.R.; van Boxtel, M.P. A systematic review of social support interventions for caregivers of people with dementia: Are they doing what they promise? *Maturitas* **2016**, *85*, 117–130. [CrossRef] [PubMed]
22. Aksoydan, E.; Aytar, A.; Blazeviciene, A.; van Bruchem-Visser, R.L.; Vaskelyte, A.; Mattace-Raso, F.; Acar, S.; Altintas, A.; Akgun-Citak, E.; Attepe-Ozden, S.; et al. Is training for informal caregivers and their older persons helpful? A systematic review. *Arch. Gerontol. Geriatr.* **2019**, *83*, 66–74. [CrossRef]
23. Douglas, S.L.; Mazanec, P.; Lipson, A.; Leuchtag, M. Distance caregiving a family member with cancer: A review of the literature on distance caregiving and recommendations for future research. *World J. Clin. Oncol.* **2016**, *7*, 214. [CrossRef]
24. Cagle, J.G.; Munn, J.C. Long-Distance Caregiving: A Systematic Review of the Literature. *J. Gerontol. Soc. Work* **2012**, *55*, 682–707. [CrossRef]
25. Bledsoe, L.K.; Moore, S.E.; Collins, W.L. Long Distance Caregiving: An Evaluative Review of the Literature. *Ageing Int.* **2010**, *35*, 293–310. [CrossRef]
26. Koerin, B.B.; Harrigan, M.M.P. PS I Love You: Long-Distance Caregiving. *J. Gerontol. Soc. Work* **2003**, *40*, 63–81. [CrossRef]
27. Bischofberger, I.; Otto, U.; Franke, A.; Schnepp, W. Pflegebedürftige Angehörige über Landesgrenzen hinweg unterstützen: Erkenntnisse aus zwei Fallstudien. *Pflege Ges.* **2017**, *22*, 84–93.
28. Franke, A.; Kramer, B.; Pirkko, M.J.; van Holten, K.; Zentgraf, A.; Otto, U.; Bischofberger, I. Aktuelle Befunde zu "distance caregiving". Was wissen wir (noch) nicht? *Z. Gerontol. Geriatr.* **2019**, *52*, 521–528. [CrossRef] [PubMed]
29. Harrigan, M.P.; Koerin, B.B. Long-distance caregiving: Personal realities and practice implications. *Reflections* **2007**, *13*, 5–16.
30. World Health Organization (WHO). Shanghai declaration on promoting health in the 2030 Agenda for Sustainable Development. *Health Promot. Int.* **2017**, *32*, 7–8. [CrossRef]
31. EUROSTAT. Demographic Balance, 2018. Available online: https://ec.europa.eu/eurostat/statistics-explained/index.php?title=File:Demographic_balance,_2018_(thousands).png (accessed on 21 July 2019).
32. Österreichische Raumordnungskonferenz. *Austrian Spatial Development Concept (ÖREK) 2011*; ÖROK: Vienna, Austria, 2011; p. 101.
33. Fischer, T.; Kasberger, D. Der Stammtisch für betreuende und pflegende Angehörige und sein Beitrag zur Gesundheitsförderung: Dargestellt am Beispiel Oberösterreich. In *Faire Chancen Gesund zu Altern. Beiträge zur Förderung Gesundheitlicher Chancengerechtigkeit Älterer Menschen in Österreich*; Gesundheit Österreich GmbH, Geschäftsbereich Fonds Gesundes Österreich: Vienna, Austria, 2018; pp. 209–2016. (In German)
34. Fischer, T. Multilokalität—Eine zentrale Herausforderung für sorgende Angehörige. *Österreichische Pflegez.* **2019**, *5*, 34–37. (In German)
35. Bengtson, V.L.; Rosenthal, C.J.; Burton, L.M. Families and aging: Diversity and heterogeneity. In *Handbook of Aging and the Social Sciences*, 3rd ed.; Binstock, R., George, L., Eds.; Academic Press: New York, NY, USA, 1990; pp. 263–287.
36. Hat, K.; Stöglehner, G. How Resilient is Growth? Resilience Assessment of Austrian Municipalities on the Basis of Census Data from 1971 to 2011. *Sustainability* **2019**, *11*, 1818. [CrossRef]
37. Keng, S.L.; Smoski, M.J.; Robins, C.J. Effects of mindfulness on psychological health: A review of empirical studies. *Clin. Psychol. Rev.* **2011**, *31*, 1041–1056. [CrossRef] [PubMed]
38. Schoonover, C.B.; Brody, E.M.; Hoffman, C.; Kleban, M.H. Parent Care and Geographically Distant Children. *Res. Aging* **1988**, *10*, 472–492. [CrossRef]
39. Roff, L.L.; Martin, S.S.; Jennings, L.K.; Parker, M.W.; Harmon, D.K. Long Distance Parental Caregivers' Experiences with Siblings: A Qualitative Study. *Qual. Soc. Work* **2007**, *6*, 315–334. [CrossRef]
40. Benefield, L.E.; Beck, C. Reducing the distance in distance-caregiving by technology innovation. *Clin. Interv. Aging* **2007**, *2*, 267–272.
41. Parker, M.W.; Call, V.R.A.; Dunkle, R.; Vaitkus, M. "Out of Sight" But Not "Out of Mind": Parent Contact and Worry Among Senior Ranking Male Officers in the Military Who Live Long Distances from Parents. *Mil. Psychol.* **2002**, *14*, 257–277. [CrossRef]

42. Edwards, M. Distance Caregivers of People with Alzheimer's Disease and Related Dementia: A Phenomenological Study. *Br. J. Occup. Ther.* **2014**, *77*, 174–180. [CrossRef]
43. Sahlstein, E.M. Relating at a distance: Negotiating being together and being apart in long-distance relationships. *J. Soc. Pers. Relatsh.* **2004**, *21*, 689–710. [CrossRef]
44. World Health Organization (WHO). Supporting Informal Caregivers of People with Dementia. 2015. Available online: http://www.who.int/mental_health/neurology/dementia/dementia_thematicbrief_informal_care.pdf (accessed on 18 September 2019).
45. Wilks, S.E.; Croom, B. Perceived stress and resilience in Alzheimer's disease caregivers: Testing moderation and mediation models of social support. *Aging Ment. Health* **2008**, *12*, 357–365. [CrossRef]
46. Bevan, J.L.; Sparks, L. Communication in the context of long-distance family caregiving: An integrated review and practical applications. *Patient Educ. Couns.* **2011**, *85*, 26–30. [CrossRef]
47. Brossoie, N. Long-Distance Care-Giving: Five Steps to Providing Effective Care. 2019. Available online: https://www.pubs.ext.vt.edu/350/350-231/350-231.html (accessed on 18 September 2019).
48. Family Caregiver Alliance. Handbook for Long-Distance Caregivers. An Essential Guide for Families and Friends Caring for Ill or Elderly Loved Ones. 2003. Available online: https://www.caregiver.org/content/pdfs/op_2003_long_distance_handbook.pdf (accessed on 8 July 2019).
49. National Institute on Aging. Long-Distance Caregiving: Twenty Questions and Answers. 2016. Available online: https://order.nia.nih.gov/publication/long-distance-caregiving-twenty-questions-and-answers- (accessed on 8 July 2019).
50. Kuckartz, U. *Mixed Methods: Methodologie, Forschungsdesigns und Analyseverfahren*; Springer Fachmedien: Wiesbaden, Germany, 2014; p. 162. (In German)
51. Statistics Austria. Urban-Rural Typology by Statistics Austria. Available online: https://www.statistik.at/web_en/classifications/regional_breakdown/urban_rural/index.html (accessed on 6 July 2019).
52. Fowler, F.J., Jr.; Fowler, F.J. *Improving Survey Questions: Design and Evaluation*; Sage Publications Ltd.: London, UK, 1995; p. 191.
53. Glaser, B.G.; Strauss, A.L. *Grounded Theory. Strategien Qualitativer Forschung*, 1st ed.; Huber: Bern, Switzerland, 1998; p. 270. (In German)
54. Boyatzis, R.E. *Transforming Qualitative Information: Thematic Analysis and Code Development*, 1st ed.; Sage Publications: Thousand Oaks, CA, USA, 1998; p. 184.
55. Wagner, M.; Franke, A.; Otto, U. Pflege über räumliche Distanz hinweg. Ergebnisse einer Datenanalyse des Survey of Health, Ageing and Retirement in Europe. *Z. Gerontol. Geriatr.* **2019**, *52*, 529–536. [CrossRef]
56. Zentgraf, A.; Jann, P.M.; Myrczik, J.; van Holten, K. Pflegen auf Distanz? Eine qualitative Interviewstudie mit "distance caregivers". *Z. Gerontol. Geriatr.* **2019**, *52*, 539–545. [CrossRef]
57. Palgrave, M.M.; Watson, M.; Coombes, L. Surveys. In *Research Methods of Health and Social Care*, 1st ed.; Neale, J., Ed.; Palgrave Macmillan: London, UK, 2009; p. 308.
58. Nutbeam, D. Evaluating Health Promotion—Progress, Problems and solutions. *Health Promot. Int.* **1998**, *13*, 27–44. [CrossRef]
59. Dykstra, P.A. Older adult loneliness: Myths and realities. *Eur. J. Ageing* **2009**, *6*, 91–100. [CrossRef] [PubMed]
60. Kenney, G.M. Is access to home health care a problem in rural areas? *Am. J. Public Health* **1993**, *83*, 412–414. [CrossRef] [PubMed]
61. Ricketts, T.C. Health care in rural communities. *West. J. Med.* **2000**, *173*, 294–295. [CrossRef] [PubMed]
62. Bacsu, J.; Jeffery, B.; Abonyi, S.; Johnson, S.; Novik, N.; Martz, D.; Oosman, S. Healthy Aging in Place: Perceptions of Rural Older Adults. *Educ. Gerontol.* **2014**, *40*, 327–337. [CrossRef]
63. Shroufi, A.; Chowdhury, R.; Aston, L.M.; Pashayan, N.; Franco, O.H. Measuring health: A practical challenge with a philosophical solution? *Maturitas* **2011**, *68*, 210–216. [CrossRef]
64. Nutbeam, D. Health Promotion Glossary. *Health Promot. Int.* **1998**, *13*, 349–364. [CrossRef]

3

A Multicentre Study of Psychological Variables and the Prevalence of Burnout among Primary Health Care Nurses

Elena Ortega-Campos [1], Guillermo A. Cañadas-De la Fuente [2], Luis Albendín-García [2,*], José L. Gómez-Urquiza [2], Carolina Monsalve-Reyes [3] and E. Inmaculada de la Fuente-Solana [4]

1 Faculty of Psychology, University of Almería. Carretera de Sacramento s/n, 04120 Almería, Spain
2 Faculty of Health Sciences, University of Granada, Avenida de la Ilustración, 18016 Granada, Spain
3 Departamento de Ciencias Sociales, Universidad Católica de La Santísima Concepción, Avenida Alonso de Ribera, 2850 Concepción, Chile
4 Brain, Mind and Behaviour Research Center (CIMCYC), University of Granada, Campus Universitario de Cartuja, 18071 Granada, Spain
* Correspondence: lualbgar1979@ugr.es

Abstract: Nurses in primary health care (PHC) have multiple responsibilities but must often work with limited resources. The study's aim was to estimate burnout levels among PHC nurses. A Quantitative, observational, cross-sectional, multicentre study of 338 nurses working in PHC in the Andalusian Public Health Service (Spain) is presented. A total of 40.24% of the nurses studied had high levels of burnout. The dimensions of emotional exhaustion and depersonalisation were significantly associated with anxiety, depression, neuroticism, on-call duty and seniority-profession and inversely related to agreeableness. In addition, depersonalisation was significantly associated with gender, and emotional exhaustion correlated inversely with age. Personal achievement was inversely associated with anxiety and depression and positively correlated with agreeableness, extraversion and responsibility. There is a high prevalence of burnout among nurses in PHC. Those most likely to suffer burnout syndrome are relatively young, suffer from anxiety and depression and present high scores for neuroticism and low ones for agreeableness, responsibility and extraversion.

Keywords: anxiety; burnout; depression; nursing; occupational health; personality factors; public health service

---

1. Introduction

Primary health care (PHC) can be defined as basic, essential health care that is accessible to all members of a community. The cost of the service must be affordable to the participants, the community and the country. These considerations were highlighted at an international conference in this respect held in Alma-Ata in September 1978, where the urgent need was expressed for all governments and personnel involved in the development and promotion of health care to work for its universal availability [1]. According to a recent study, countries which emphasise the provision of PHC are better able to achieve their sustainable development goals and to promote the fairness and social justice on which the provision of universal health care is based [2].

Maslach and Jackson [3] provided the most widely accepted definition of burnout, describing it as a three-dimensional syndrome in which a worker experiences emotional exhaustion (EE), or feelings of physical overexertion and emotional fatigue as a result of the continuous interactions required between the worker and users of the service; depersonalisation (D) or the existence of cynical attitudes and responses towards the persons to whom services are provided; and a sensation of low personal achievement (PA) or the loss of confidence and the appearance of a negative self-concept due to encounters with unrewarding situation [4]. Among the various instruments proposed for assessing burnout, one of the most commonly used is the Maslach Burnout Inventory (MBI) [3]. Those affected by burnout usually work in contact with the public, as is the case of the health professions, and within this group, nurses are especially prone to burnout [5]. This syndrome not only impacts on workers but can also reduce the quality of care provided [6,7]. In recent years, the question of burnout syndrome has been addressed in literature reviews [8–11] and empirical studies [4,5], and work continues in this field, highlighting its importance in society [12].

In this context, an important consideration is that hospital nurses work in a specific clinical environment. Thus, the tasks performed regularly by nurses working in A & E, oncology or paediatrics departments, for example, differ greatly from those carried out in PHC [9,13–15].

The impact of burnout syndrome is normally analysed by reference to the different variables related to its presence. These may be sociodemographic (age, sex, marital status, number of children, etc.), employment-related (the hospital service in question, seniority in the workplace, seniority in the profession, etc.) or psychological (anxiety, stress, depression, personality traits, etc.). Identification of the variables/factors that influence the development of burnout syndrome would contribute to determining risk profiles for the nursing profession [16].

Little empirical research has been conducted into burnout syndrome in PHC nurses, in comparison with other hospital settings [17,18]. Further investigation in this respect, therefore, would help determine the prevalence of burnout in PHC nurses and facilitate its prevention [19].

This study has the following aims: (1) to estimate the level of burnout among nurses working in PHC in the Andalusian Public Health Service; (2) to determine the phases of burnout that most affect these nurses; (3) to analyse the relationship between sociodemographic, employment-related and personality variables and the burnout syndrome suffered by this group of persons.

2. Materials and Methods

2.1. Participants

The study sample was composed of 338 PHC nurses working in the Andalusian Public Health Service (Spain). These nurses were specialists or generalists who worked in community health centers, serving the entire community. The participants' average age was 45.92 years (SD = 7.51), and 58% were female. All had university studies in nursing and were employed in this capacity. The response rate was 84.5%.

2.2. Variables, Instruments and Data Collection

A research questionnaire was used to record the data compiled. The sociodemographic variables studied were gender (male-female), age (years), marital status (single, married, separated/divorced, widowed) and number of children (none, one, two, three or more). The employment-related variables considered were work pattern (fixed or rotating shifts), on-call obligation (yes-no); seniority in the workplace (months) and seniority in the profession (months).

Burnout syndrome was measured using the MBI [3] in a version adapted to a Spanish-speaking population [20]. The instrument consisted of 22 items, scored on a seven-point Likert-scale, from zero (never) to six (every day), with respect to three dimensions: EE (nine items), D (five items) and PA (eight items). Cut-off points for the presence of burnout were defined by reference to established values for the Spanish population, namely, EE > 24, D > 9 and PA < 33. The estimated coefficients of reliability for these MBI scales were EE ($\alpha = 0.91$), D ($\alpha = 0.72$) and PA ($\alpha = 0.86$).

The revised NEO personality inventory (NEO-FFI) instrument [21], adapted for use with a Spanish-speaking population [22], was also used. This instrument is composed of five personality factors: neuroticism, agreeableness, responsibility, extraversion and openness. Twelve items were considered for each of these dimensions (total, 60 items), and scored on a five-point Likert scale. The following reliability coefficients were obtained for the NEO-FFI dimensions: neuroticism ($\alpha = 0.83$), agreeableness ($\alpha = 0.80$), responsibility ($\alpha = 0.84$), extraversion ($\alpha = 0.82$) and openness ($\alpha = 0.67$).

The Educational-Clinical Questionnaire on Anxiety and Depression (CECAD), proposed by Lozano, García-Cueto and Lozano [23], was used to measure symptoms of anxiety and depression, in accordance with the DSM-IV criteria. This questionnaire consists of 45 items scored on a five-point Likert scale, with 19 items for anxiety and 26 for depression. The following reliability coefficients were obtained for the CECAD dimensions: anxiety ($\alpha = 0.94$) and depression ($\alpha = 0.96$).

To obtain the necessary data, the investigators first contacted the Spanish Nursing Union (SATSE), whose staff then worked in conjunction with the research team to inform PHC nurses in the Andalusian Public Health System about the study and to request their participation, which was totally voluntary, individual and anonymous. It was estimated that each nurse would require 45 min to complete the study questionnaire. The data were compiled from January to June 2017. The study was approved by the Ethics Committee of the University of Granada (393/CEIH2017) and was conducted in full compliance with the ethical considerations of the Declaration of Helsinki (2008). All study data were treated in accordance with the relevant Spanish legislation on data protection (LOPD, 1999) [24].

2.3. Study Design

This study is quantitative, observational, cross-sectional and multicentre.

2.4. Data Analysis

Descriptive statistics (mean, standard deviation, minimum and maximum) were calculated for the quantitative variables, and frequencies and percentages for the qualitative ones. Hypothesis tests for independent groups were conducted to determine differences in MBI dimensions and in the qualitative variables. Pearson correlation coefficients were estimated for the quantitative variables. All analyses were performed using SPSS 23.0 statistical software (IBM, Armonk, NY, USA).

3. Results

3.1. Data, Levels of Burnout and Prevalence

Table 1 shows the percentages and frequencies obtained for the qualitative variables included in the study. Regarding the participants, 58% were women, 78.6% were married and 84.6% had at least one child. With respect to employment patterns, 76.6% worked a fixed shift (morning, afternoon or evening) and 86.8% performed on-call duties.

Table 1. Descriptive data for the qualitative study variables.

Variable	% (*n*)	Variable	%(*n*)
Gender (*n* = 338)		Marital status (*n* = 336)	
Male	42 (142)	Single	14 (47)
Female	58 (196)	Married	78.6 (264)
Shift (*n* = 334)		Separated/Divorced	6.3 (21)
Fixed	76.6 (256)	Widower	0.9 (3)
Variable	23.4 (78)	Children (*n* = 332)	
On-call (*n* = 337)		None	15.4 (51)
Yes	68.8 (232)	One	19 (63)
No	31.2 (105)	Two	45.5 (151)
		Three or more	20.1 (67)

Table 2 presents the descriptive statistics (mean, standard deviation, minimum and maximum) obtained for the quantitative variables. Among the data for employment-related variables, the nurses had been employed for an average of 127.67 months (SD = 99.84) in the position and had an average of 273.66 months (SD = 91.38) of professional seniority as nurses. The following average scores were obtained for the NEO-FFI subscales: neuroticism 27.96 (SD = 8.33); extraversion 42.19 (SD = 7.90); openness 38.84 (SD = 6.68); agreeableness 44.80 (SD = 7.54); responsibility 46.73 (SD = 7.37). In the ECCAD dimensions, the mean scores obtained were 36.43 (SD = 11.66) for anxiety and 50.05 (SD = 17.03) for depression. Finally, the mean MBI scores were 17.70 (SD = 11.92) for EE, 7.59 (SD = 6.25) for D and 36.59 (SD = 8.90) for PA.

Table 2. Descriptive data for the quantitative study variables.

Variable	Mean (SD)	Min-Max
Age (n = 337)	45.92 (7.510)	25–64
Seniority: Workplace (n = 326)	127.67 (99.84)	1–444
Seniority: Profession (n = 338)	273.66 (91.38)	12–504
NEO-FFI		
Neuroticism (n = 332)	27.96 (8.33)	12–53
Extraversion (n = 336)	42.19 (7.90)	20–60
Openness (n = 333)	38.84 (6.68)	20–57
Agreeableness (n = 330)	44.80 (7.54)	19–60
Conscientiousness (n = 334)	46.73 (7.37)	20–60
CECAD		
Anxiety (n = 334)	36.43 (11.66)	19–69
Depression (n = 329)	50.05 (17.03)	26–102
MBI		
Emotional exhaustion (n = 335)	17.70 (11.92)	0–54
Depersonalisation (n = 335)	7.59 (6.25)	0–29
Personal Accomplishment (n = 335)	36.59 (8.90)	2–48

CECAD = Educational-Clinical Questionnaire on Anxiety and Depression; MBI = Maslach Burnout Inventory; NEO-FFI = Revised NEO Five Factor Inventory; SD = Standard deviation; Seniority = presented in months.

In relation to the EE dimension of burnout, 48.1% of the nurses presented a low level, 25.4% a moderate level and 26.6% a high level. For D, the corresponding figures were 35.1%, 27.6% and 37.2%, while for PA they were 43%, 28.7% and 28.4%.

Following the model proposed by Golembiewski, Munzenrider and Carter [25], the nurses were classified according to the stage of evolution of burnout syndrome. Phases 6, 7 and 8 of this model reflect a high level of burnout. According to this parameter, 40.24% (n = 134) of the nurses in our sample presented a high level of burnout (Table 3).

Table 3. Prevalence of burnout according to the stages of the Golembiewski model.

Phase	1	2	3	4	5	6	7	8
EE	L	L	L	L	H	H	H	H
D	L	H	L	H	L	H	L	H
PA	L	L	H	H	L	L	H	H
n	41	26	89	24	19	86	20	28
(%)	(12.31)	(7.81)	(26.73)	(7.21)	(5.7)	(25.83)	(6)	(8.41)

H = High; L = Low; EE = Emotional exhaustion; D = Depersonalisation; PA = Personal accomplishment.

3.2. *Exploratory Models and Factors Associated with Each of the Dimensions of Burnout*

The linear correlation coefficients between the MBI scales, the NEO-FFI scales and the anxiety and depression scores were also calculated. The EE scale presented the following statistically significant correlations with the NEO-FFI scores: neuroticism (r = 0.62), extraversion (r = −0.43), agreeableness (r = −0.45) and responsibility (r = −0.42). Significant correlations were also obtained with the CECAD scores for anxiety and depression (r = 0.67 and r = 0.69, respectively). On the D scale, statistically significant relationships were found with the following NEO-FFI and CECAD scores: neuroticism (r = 0.48), extraversion (r = −0.38), openness (r = −0.21), agreeableness (r = −0.49), responsibility

($r = -0.44$), anxiety ($r = 0.47$) and depression ($r = 0.48$). Finally, statistically significant correlations were found between the PA scale and the following NEO-FFI and CECAD scores: neuroticism ($r = -0.42$), extraversion ($r = 0.49$), openness ($r = 0.25$), agreeableness ($r = 0.49$), responsibility ($r = 0.55$), anxiety ($r = -0.40$) and depression ($r = -0.45$) (Table 4).

Table 4. Correlation coefficients between psychological variables and Burnout.

PV	EE	D	PA
NEO-FFI			
Neuroticism	0.62 **	0.48 **	−0.42 **
Extraversion	−0.43 **	−0.38 **	0.49 **
Openness	−0.08	−0.21 **	0.25 **
Agreeableness	−0.45 **	−0.49 **	0.49 **
Conscientiousness	−0.42 **	−0.44 **	0.55 **
CECAD			
Anxiety	0.67 **	0.47 **	−0.40 **
Depression	0.69 **	0.48 **	−0.45 **

PV = Psychological variables; EE = Emotional exhaustion; D = Depersonalisation; PA = Personal accomplishment; CECAD = Educational-Clinical Questionnaire on Anxiety and Depression; NEO-FFI = Revised NEO Five Factor Inventory; ** = $p < 0.001$.

The difference of the means test was conducted for the variables gender, shift work, on-call duties, marital status and children, against the MBI dimensions. Statistically significant differences were found in the D scale between men and women ($t_{(331)} = 2.52$, $p = 0.012$, $d = 0.28$), with men presenting higher levels. With respect to on-call duties, statistically significant differences were found in the EE scale ($t_{(232,646)} = 1.98$, $p = 0.048$, $d = 0.23$) and D ($t_{(330)} = 2.85$, $p = 0.005$, $d = 0.31$), with higher scores recorded for EE and D by the nurses who performed on-call duties.

Multiple linear regression models were estimated for each of the MBI dimensions. For the EE dimension, the variables age (B = −0.31, $p = 0.024$), seniority in the profession (B = 0.02, $p = 0.046$), neuroticism (B = 0.32, $p \leq 0.001$), agreeableness (B = −0.17, $p = 0.013$), anxiety (B = 0.30, $p = 0.001$) and depression (B = 0.14, $p = 0.035$) were statistically significant predictors. For goodness of fit, the model presented a value $R^2 = 0.553$, meaning that 55.3% of the variability of EE was explained by the model.

With respect to the D dimension, the variables age (B = −0.09, $p = 0.027$), seniority in the position (B = 0.01, $p = 0.027$), neuroticism (B = 0.12, $p = 0.013$), agreeableness (B = −0.26, $p \leq 0.001$) and anxiety (B = 0.11, $p = 0.001$) were predictors in the model. The model explained 35.4% of the variance of the variable D.

Finally, in the PA dimension, the variables agreeableness (B = 0.19, $p = 0.004$), responsibility (B = 0.38, $p \leq 0.001$), extraversion (B = 0.22, $p \leq 0.001$) and depression (B = −0.06, $p = 0.030$) were predictors. 40.2% of the variability in PA was explained by the model (Table 5).

Table 5. Multiple linear regression.

Regression	B	Standard Error	Beta	t	p	CI 95%
EE						
Intercept	6.16	5.82		1.05	0.291	(−5.29, 17.62)
Age	−0.31	0.13	−0.19	−2.26	0.024	(−0.58, −0.04)
Seniority: Profession	0.02	0.01	0.17	2.00	0.046	(0.00, 0.04)
Neuroticism	0.32	0.07	0.23	4.25	<0.001	(0.17, 0.47)
Agreeableness	−0.17	0.07	−0.11	−2.48	0.013	(−0.31, −0.03)
Anxiety	0.30	0.09	0.30	3.22	0.001	(0.12, 0.49)
Depression	0.14	0.06	0.20	2.11	0.035	(0.01, 0.27)
$R^2 = 0.553$						
D						

Table 5. *Cont.*

Regression	B	Standard Error	Beta	t	p	CI 95%
Intercept	15.40	3.34		4.60	<0.001	(8.83, 21.98)
Age	−0.09	0.04	−0.11	−2.22	0.027	(−0.17, −0.01)
Seniority: Workplace	0.01	0.00	0.11	2.22	0.027	(0.00, 0.01)
Neuroticism	0.12	0.04	0.16	2.48	0.013	(0.02, 0.21)
Agreeableness	−0.26	0.04	−0.31	−5.71	<0.001	(−0.35, −0.17)
Anxiety	0.11	0.03	0.20	3.31	0.001	(0.04, 0.17)
$R^2 = 0.354$						
PA						
Intercept	3.76	4.49		0.83	0.402	(−5.07, 12.60)
Agreeableness	0.19	0.06	0.16	2.91	0.004	(0.06, 0.32)
Conscientiousness	0.38	0.07	0.31	5.46	<0.001	(0.24, 0.52)
Extraversion	0.22	0.06	0.19	3.58	<0.001	(0.10, 0.34)
Depression	−0.06	0.02	−0.11	−2.17	0.030	(−0.11, −0.01)
$R^2 = 0.402$						

B = Estimated parameter; CI = Confidence interval; EE = Emotional exhaustion; D = Depersonalisation; PA = Personal accomplishment.

4. Discussion

PHC is considered less stressful than other hospital services, with patients who are more stable and present fewer complications [19]. In our study sample, although the percentage of male nurses was higher than in other studies, the group was sufficiently representative of the PHC nursing population. In terms of employment patterns, these nurses had considerable responsibilities, with most working a fixed shift (either mornings or afternoon/evenings) and, in addition, subject to on-call obligations ranging from 17 to 24 h per day. As a result, the work overload was significant, an adverse condition that contributed to the high levels of burnout prevalence observed among this population [26].

EE is the most representative dimension of burnout. This outcome becomes more acute with greater age and seniority in the position, due to the stress and monotony encountered and/or job dissatisfaction [19,27]. In addition, in our study sample, a significant proportion of the nurses were married. This factor, representing additional family commitments, also increases EE [27,28]. Our analyses highlight the existence of an important relationship between EE, anxiety, depression and personality traits. The skills required of the nurses and their heavy workload (especially as concerns on-call duties) are directly related to the dimension of responsibility [29,30]. The resulting stress and anxiety, moreover, contribute to feelings of neuroticism [26,31], such that some nurses consider abandoning the profession and, in the most extreme cases, may become suicidal [19]. In this respect, openness and extraversion are protective factors, mediating in stress and work-related problems [31,32].

Depression is another common manifestation of burnout among nurses. When levels of PA are high (for instance, due to the empathy and accompaniment implicit in caring for chronic patients), D is not usually very severe [30] but as with EE, it increases with age and the resulting lack of motivation [27] and this, in turn, decreases extraversion [31]. When nurses are subjected to heavy workloads, with an inefficient distribution of tasks and insufficient resources, they may view the environment as hostile [17,33] and experience anxiety, feelings of vulnerability, stress, lack of responsibility and depression, all of which increase the sensation of burnout [11,19,26,29,31,32,34]. Furthermore, agreeableness and openness—protective factors that would otherwise contribute to averting burnout–are both adversely affected [31,32].

In PHC, although nursing personnel may have considerable job satisfaction, it is not uncommon to find low levels of PA, since the degree of responsibility is high [29]. Nursing is a highly vocational profession [35] and so agreeableness plays an important role in this dimension, and this helps moderate the stress experienced [32]. On the other hand, some aspects of nursing work are viewed very negatively, especially the obligation to perform on-call duties. Not all nurses are psychologically or physically prepared for this obligation, which can generate stress, anxiety and lack of adaptation [26,31], frustration and work overload [30] and, sometimes, depression [19]. Adverse employment conditions can also cause extraversion and openness to be diminished, reducing nurses' ability to cope with problems that may arise [31].

In view of the results obtained, risk profiles for PHC nurses can be established. Persons who present high scores for EE and D and low ones for PA tend to be younger and to suffer from anxiety and depression. Moreover, their limited experience and exposure to organisational problems and even a hostile work environment can provoke negative attitudes [11,19,36,37].

With respect to personality factors, the results show that PHC nurses who obtain high scores for neuroticism and low ones for agreeableness, responsibility and extraversion are also at risk of presenting burnout syndrome. When a nurse has a high level of neuroticism, this is usually associated with an increased severity and frequency of personal problems [38]. Such an individual will often form part of the hierarchical structure of the organisation but not involve themselves in the job and will frequently be dissatisfied with it [5]. Low levels of agreeableness, responsibility and extraversion often mean less involvement and a decreased quality of care [5], poorer social skills [38] or unsatisfactory work conditions [11,26,29,30], all of which can result in reduced self-efficacy, increased hostility and a bad nurse–patient relationship [4]. These outcomes are consistent with the findings of previous studies, according to which the greater the number of negative personality traits in a nurse, the greater their risk of suffering from burnout [38].

One of the objectives of the study was to determine the burnout phase in which the nurses are. According to the data, the group of nurses surveyed present high levels of burnout. Based on Golembiewski's model [25] 40% are in the highest stages of burnout. These results are in line with recent studies [4,13,19]. The Golembiewski classification [25] is not widely used in studies on burnout, it would be advisable to include it because it provides important information especially regarding the classification and diagnosis of burnout syndrome.

The prevention of burnout helps create a positive working environment, promotes the autonomy of nurses and facilitates achievement of their objectives [37]. Psychological and organisational interventions in this respect [31], especially for younger and less experienced staff [36,38] would significantly contribute to reducing burnout among PHC nurses. Such interventions might include mindfulness programmes, the provision of social support and/or the development of protocols against violence in the workplace [17,33,34,39,40]. These initiatives could enhance personal protective factors, such as extraversion, agreeableness and openness [19,32,38] and organisational ones such as teamwork and job satisfaction, in an environment that can be very demanding and where resources are often insufficient [11,29].

Future research should analyse the influence of these burnout risk factors through longitudinal studies to establish causality relationships. Other variables, such as biochemical factors that may help the clinical diagnosis of burnout, should also be taken into account. Finally, it would be interesting to analyse the effect of some interventions on the reduction of burnout in primary care nurses.

5. Conclusions

The prevalence of burnout is high among PHC nurses, especially those who are younger, suffer from anxiety and depression and present high levels of neuroticism and low ones of agreeableness, responsibility and extraversion. This profile of PHC nurses that may be more prone to burnout syndrome should be taken into account by healthcare managers to establish preventive measures. The implementation of measures to improve the working conditions of PHC nurses would reduce levels of burnout and, therefore, enhance the quality of care provided.

Author Contributions: All authors listed meet the authorship criteria and are in agreement with the submission of the manuscript. All of them have made substantial contributions to the conception and/or design of the study. All authors were involved in drafting the text or in revising it critically for important intellectual content; all authors have given their approval to the version to be published, and all authors agree to be accountable for all aspects of the study, ensuring that questions related to the accuracy or integrity of any part of the work may be appropriately investigated and resolved. Conceptualization: G.A.C.-D.l.F. and E.I.d.l.F.-S.; methodology: E.O.-C., J.L.G.-U. and E.I.d.l.F.-S.; software: L.A.-G. and J.L.G.-U.; validation: G.A.C.-D.l.F., L.A.-G. and J.L.G.-U.; formal analysis: E.O.-C. and E.I.d.l.F.-S.; investigation: G.A.C.-D.l.F., L.A.-G., J.L.G.-U., C.M.-R. and E.I.d.l.F.-S.; resources: G.A.C.-D.l.F. and E.I.d.l.F.-S.; data curation: E.O.-C., L.A.-G. and C.M.-R.; writing—original draft preparation: E.O.-C., G.A.C.-D.l.F., L.A.-G. and C.M.-R.; writing—review and editing: G.A.C.-D.l.F., C.M.-R. and E.I.d.l.F.-S.; visualization: G.A.C.-D.l.F., C.M.-R. and E.I.d.l.F.-S.; supervision: E.I.d.l.F.-S.; project administration: G.A.C.-D.l.F. and E.I.d.l.F.-S.; funding acquisition: E.I.d.l.F.-S.

Acknowledgments: The authors wish to acknowledge the Spanish Nursing Union (SATSE) for their help in questionnaire administration and data collection and all those who participated in this study.

References

1. Vilaseca, J.M.; Sans, M. Alma Ata 40th anniversary: Milestones of primary health care. *Med. Clin.* **2018**, *151*, 441–443. [CrossRef] [PubMed]
2. Hone, T.; Macinko, J.; Millett, C. Revisiting Alma-Ata: What is the role of primary health care in achieving the Sustainable Development Goals? *Lancet* **2018**, *392*, 1461–1472. [CrossRef]
3. Maslach, C.; Jackson, S.E. The measurement of experienced burnout. *J. Organ. Behav.* **1981**, *2*, 99–113. [CrossRef]
4. Ramírez-Baena, L.; Ortega-Campos, E.; Gómez-Urquiza, J.L.; Cañadas-De la Fuente, G.R.; De la Fuente-Solana, E.I.; Cañadas-De la Fuente, G.A. A multicentre study of burnout prevalence and related psychological variables in medical area hospital nurses. *J. Clin. Med.* **2019**, *8*, 92. [CrossRef] [PubMed]
5. Cañadas-De la Fuente, G.A.; Vargas, C.; San Luis, C.; García, I.; Cañadas, G.R.; De la Fuente, E.I. Risk factors and prevalence of burnout syndrome in the nursing profession. *Int. J. Nurs. Stud.* **2015**, *52*, 240–249. [CrossRef]
6. Davey, D.M.; Cummings, G.; Newburn-Cook, C.V.; Lo, E.A. Predictors of nurse absenteeism in hospital: A systematic review. *J. Nurs. Manag.* **2009**, *17*, 312–330. [CrossRef]
7. Spence, L.H.K.; Leiter, M.P. The impact of nursing work environments on patient safety outcomes: The mediating role of burnout/engagement. *J. Nurs. Adm.* **2006**, *36*, 259–267. [CrossRef]
8. Albendín, L.; Gómez, J.L.; Cañadas-de la Fuente, G.A.; Cañadas, G.R.; San Luis, C.; Aguayo, R. Prevalencia bayesiana y niveles de burnout en enfermería de urgencias. Una revisión sistemática [Bayesian prevalence and burnout levels in emergency nurses. A systematic review]. *Rev. Lat. Am. Psicol.* **2016**, *48*, 81–146.
9. Cañadas-De la Fuente, G.A.; Gómez-Urquiza, J.L.; Ortega-Campos, E.; Cañadas, G.R.; Albendín-García, L.; De la Fuente-Solana, E.I. Prevalence of burnout syndrome in oncology nursing: A meta-analytic study. *Psychooncology* **2018**, *27*, 1426–1433. [CrossRef]
10. Gómez-Urquiza, J.L.; Aneas-López, A.B.; Fuente-Solana, E.I.; Albendín-García, L.; Díaz-Rodríguez, L.; Cañadas-De la Fuente, G.A. Prevalence, risk factors, and levels of burnout among oncology nurses: A systematic review. *Oncol. Nurs. Forum.* **2016**, *43*, E104–E120. [CrossRef]
11. Gómez-Urquiza, J.L.; De la Fuente-Solana, E.I.; Albendín-García, L.; Vargas-Pecino, C.; Ortega-Campos, E.; Cañadas-De la Fuente, G.A. Prevalence of burnout syndrome in emergency nurses: A meta-analysis. *Crit. Care. Nurs.* **2017**, *37*, E1–E9. [CrossRef] [PubMed]
12. Schaufeli, W.B.; Leiter, M.P.; Maslach, C. Burnout: 35 years of research and practice. *Career Dev. Int.* **2009**, *14*, 204–220. [CrossRef]
13. De la Fuente-Solana, E.I.; Gómez-Urquiza, J.L.; Cañadas, G.R.; Albendín-García, L.; Ortega-Campos, E.; Cañadas-De la Fuente, G.A. Burnout and its relationship with personality factors in oncology nurses. *Eur. J. Oncol. Nurs.* **2017**, *30*, 91–96. [CrossRef] [PubMed]
14. Pradas-Hernández, L.; Ariza, T.; Gómez-Urquiza, J.L.; Albendín-García, L.; De la Fuente, E.I.; Cañadas-De la Fuente, G.A. Prevalence of burnout in paediatric nurses: A systematic review and meta-analysis. *PLoS ONE* **2018**, *13*, e0195039.

15. Ramos, T.M.; Rennó, H.M.S. Training in the nursing residency in Primary Care/Family Health from the perspective of the graduates. *Rev. Gaucha. Enferm.* **2018**, *39*, e20180017. [PubMed]
16. Geuens, N.; Van Bogaert, P.; Franck, E. Vulnerability to burnout within the nursing workforce—The role of personality and interpersonal behaviour. *J. Clin. Nurs.* **2017**, *26*, 4622–4633. [CrossRef] [PubMed]
17. Fang, H.; Zhao, X.; Yang, H.; Sun, P.; Li, Y.; Wu, Q. Depressive symptoms and workplace-violence-related risk factors among otorhinolaryngology nurses and physicians in Northern China: A cross-sectional study. *BMJ. Open.* **2018**, *8*, e019514. [CrossRef] [PubMed]
18. Molina-Praena, J.; Ramírez-Baena, L.; Gómez-Urquiza, J.L.; Cañadas, G.R.; De la Fuente, E.I.; Cañadas-De la Fuente, G.A. Levels of burnout and risk factors in medical area nurses: A meta-analytic study. *Int. J. Environ. Res. Public Health* **2018**, *15*, 2800. [CrossRef] [PubMed]
19. Gómez-Urquiza, J.; Monsalve-Reyes, C.; San Luis-Costas, C.; Fernández-Castillo, R.; Aguayo-Estremera, R.; Cañadas-De la Fuente, G.A. Factores de riesgo y niveles de burnout en enfermeras de atención primaria: Una revisión sistemática [Risk factors and burnout levels in Primary Care nurses: A systematic review]. *Aten. Prim.* **2017**, *49*, 77–85. [CrossRef]
20. Seisdedos, N. *MBI. Inventario "Burnout" de Maslach: Manual*; TEA: Madrid, Spain, 1997.
21. Costa, P.T., Jr.; McCrae, R.R. *The Revised NEO Personality Inventory (NEO-PI-R) and NEO-Five-Factor Inventory (NEO-FFI) Professional Manual*; Psychological Assessment Resources: Odessa, FL, USA, 1992.
22. Costa, P.; McCrae, R. *Inventario de Personalidad NEO Revisado*; TEA: Madrid, Spain, 1999.
23. Lozano, L.; García-Cueto, E.; Lozano, L.M. *Cuestionario Educativo Clínico de Ansiedad y Depresión*; TEA: Madrid, Spain, 2007.
24. Ley Orgánica de Protección de Datos de carácter personal (LOPD): *Ley orgánica* 15. Madrid, Spain. 1999.
25. Golembiewski, R.T.; Munzenrider, R.; Carter, D. Phases of progressive burnout and their work-site covariants. *J. Appl. Behav. Sci.* **1983**, *19*, 461–482. [CrossRef]
26. Cañadas-De la Fuente, G.A.; Albendín-García, L.; De la Fuente, E.I.; San Luis, C.; Gómez-Urquiza, J.L.; Cañadas, G.R. Síndrome de burnout en profesionales de enfermería que realizan jornada física complementaria en servicios de cuidados críticos y urgencias [Burnout in Nursing Professionals Performing Overtime Workdays in Emergency and Critical Care Departments. Spain]. *Rev. Esp. Salud. Publica.* **2016**, *90*, e1–e9.
27. Gómez-Urquiza, J.L.; Vargas, C.; De la Fuente, E.I.; Fernández-Castillo, R.; Cañadas-De la Fuente, G.A. Age as a risk factor for burnout syndrome in nursing professionals: A meta-analytic study. *Res. Nurs. Health* **2017**, *40*, 99–110. [CrossRef] [PubMed]
28. Cañadas-De la Fuente, G.A.; Ortega, E.; Ramírez-Baena, L.; De la Fuente-Solana, E.I.; Vargas, C.; Gómez-Urquiza, J.L. Gender, marital status, and children as risk factors for burnout in nurses: A meta-analytic study. *Int. J. Environ. Res. Public Health* **2018**, *15*, 2102. [CrossRef] [PubMed]
29. Kim, L.Y.; Rose, D.E.; Soban, L.M.; Stockdale, S.E.; Meredith, L.S.; Rubenstein, L.V. Primary care tasks associated with provider burnout: Findings from a veterans health administration survey. *J. Gen. Intern. Med.* **2018**, *33*, 50–56. [CrossRef]
30. Monsalve-Reyes, C.S.; San Luis-Costas, C.; Gómez-Urquiza, J.L.; Albendín-García, L.; Aguayo, R.; Cañadas-De la Fuente, G.A. Burnout syndrome and its prevalence in primary care nursing: A systematic review and meta-analysis. *BMC. Fam. Pract.* **2018**, *19*, 59. [CrossRef] [PubMed]
31. Grigorescu, S.; Cazan, A.M.; Grigorescu, O.D.; Rogozea, L.M. The role of the personality traits and work characteristics in the prediction of the burnout syndrome among nurses-a new approach within predictive, preventive, and personalized medicine concept. *EPMA J.* **2018**, *9*, 355–365. [CrossRef] [PubMed]
32. Barr, P. The five-factor model of personality, work stress and professional quality of life in neonatal intensive care unit nurses. *J. Adv. Nurs.* **2018**, *74*, 1349–1358. [CrossRef]
33. Da Silva, A.T.; Peres, M.F.; Lopes, C.S.; Schraiber, L.B.; Susser, E.; Menezes, P.R. Violence at work and depressive symptoms in primary health care teams: A cross-sectional study in Brazil. *Soc. Psychiatry. Psychiatr. Epidemiol.* **2015**, *50*, 1347–1355. [CrossRef]
34. Duhoux, A.; Menear, M.; Charron, M.; Lavoie-Tremblay, M.; Alderson, M. Interventions to promote or improve the mental health of primary care nurses: A systematic review. *J. Nurs. Manag.* **2017**, *25*, 597–607. [CrossRef]
35. Kennedy, B.; Curtis, K.; Waters, D. The personality of emergency nurses: Is it unique? *Australas. Emerg. Nurs. J.* **2014**, *17*, 139–145. [CrossRef]

36. Hegney, D.G.; Craigie, M.; Hemsworth, D.; Osseiran-Moisson, R.; Aoun, S.; Drury, V. Compassion satisfaction, compassion fatigue, anxiety, depression and stress in registered nurses in Australia: Study 1 results. *J. Nurs. Manag.* **2014**, *22*, 506–518. [CrossRef] [PubMed]
37. Mudallal, R.H.; Othman, W.M.; Al Hassan, N.F. Nurses' burnout: The influence of leader empowering behaviors, work Conditions, and demographic traits. *Inquiry* **2017**, *54*, 46958017724944. [CrossRef] [PubMed]
38. Ang, S.Y.; Dhaliwal, S.S.; Ayre, T.C.; Uthaman, T.; Fong, K.Y.; Della, P. Demographics and personality factors associated with burnout among nurses in a Singapore Tertiary Hospital. *Biomed. Res. Int.* **2016**, *2016*, 6960184. [CrossRef] [PubMed]
39. Pérula-de Torres, L.A.; Atalaya, J.C.V.; García-Campayo, J.; Roldán-Villalobos, A.; Magallón-Botaya, R.; Bartolomé-Moreno, C.; Moreno, C.M. Collaborative group of the MINDUUDD study. Controlled clinical trial comparing the effectiveness of a mindfulness and self-compassion 4-session programme versus an 8-session programme to reduce work stress and burnout in family and community medicine physicians and nurses: MINDUUDD study protocol. *BMC. Fam. Pract.* **2019**, *20*, 24.
40. Velando-Soriano, A.; Ortega-Campos, E.; Gómez-Urquiza, J.L.; Ramírez-Baena, L.; De la Fuente, E.I.; Cañadas-De la Fuente, G.A. Impact of social support in preventing burnout syndrome in nurses: A systematic review. *Jpn. J. Nurs. Sci.* in press.

4

Nursing Students' Experiences of Clinical Practices in Emergency and Intensive Care Units

María González-García [1,2,3], Alberto Lana [2,3,*], Paula Zurrón-Madera [2,3,4], Yolanda Valcárcel-Álvarez [1,2,3] and Ana Fernández-Feito [2,3]

1 Health Care Service of Asturias, Central University Hospital of Asturias, Avda. Roma, s/n, 33011 Oviedo, Spain; maguig87@hotmail.com (M.G.-G.); yolanda.valcarcel@sespa.es (Y.V.-Á.)
2 Department of Medicine, School of Medicine and Health Sciences, University of Oviedo, Avda. Julián Clavería, s/n, 33006 Oviedo, Spain; zurronpaula@uniovi.es (P.Z.-M.); fernandezfana@uniovi.es (A.F.-F.)
3 Healthcare Research Area, Health Research Institute of Asturias (ISPA), Avda. Roma, s/n, 33011 Oviedo, Spain
4 Mental Health Center of La Corredoria, Health Care Service of Asturias (Spain), C. Alfredo Blanco, s/n, 33011 Oviedo, Spain
* Correspondence: lanaalberto@uniovi.es

Abstract: Clinical practices are key environments for skill acquisition during the education of nursing students, where it is important to encourage reflective learning. This study sought to explore the experience of final year nursing students during their clinical placement in emergency and intensive care units and to identify whether differences exist between female and male students. Using qualitative methodology, a documentary analysis of 28 reflective learning journals was carried out at a public university in Northern Spain. Four themes were identified: "an intense emotional experience", "the importance of attitudes over and above techniques", "identifying with nurses who dominate their environment and are close to the patient in complex and dehumanized units" and "how to improve care in critically ill patients and how to support their families". The female students displayed a more emotional and reflective experience, with a strong focus on patient care, whereas male students identified more with individual aspects of learning and the organization and quality of the units. Both male and female students experienced intense emotions, improved their learning in complex environments and acquired attitudes linked to the humanization of care. However, the experience of these clinical rotations was different between female and male students.

Keywords: clinical placements; emergency hospital service; intensive care units; nursing care; nursing education research; nursing students; nursing

1. Introduction

During undergraduate nursing studies, the acquisition of competencies, in a broad sense, is essential. In addition to theoretical and practical learning and the development of nursing attitudes, it is important to establish transversal competencies, such as leadership, communication, or interpersonal skills, as well as competencies for adequate personal and professional development. To achieve these transversal competencies, it is important to encourage reflection [1].

Clinical practices are an essential element of learning for nursing students [2,3], as they enable the application of theoretical knowledge in a real environment, the training of technical skills through interaction with patients and health workers and the development of nursing attitudes [4]. In addition, this is an ideal opportunity for students to reflect on their learning. Emergency departments and intensive care units (ICU) are clinical environments that encourage competence development; however, they also pose a challenge for students and teachers. These units are very complex, with high pressure to care for serious patients, which can negatively influence the students' experience [5]. Careful planning, with guidance and follow-up by an instructor, are central elements in their development [6].

2. Background

Significant learning is not possible without reflection [7]. The reflective analysis of lived experiences or problems faced during professional practice can serve as a stimulus for learning [8]. A reflective attitude can be even more useful than technical mastery when dealing with changing situations in professional practice. During nursing training, reflective learning can take place through a reflective learning journal (RLJ). The RLJ is a written document in which students carefully analyze their thoughts, actions or interactions with others over a period of time [3,7]. Several studies have documented the usefulness of RLJs in enhancing the learning experience during clinical practice [9–11], stimulating professional development [12] and even personal development in the process of becoming a nurse [13–15]. In this way, RLJ can be used as an additional tool for teachers to assess students' acquisition of nursing competencies during clinical education but also to learn about students' personal experiences, including their coping strategies, thoughts, emotions and feelings [4,7,13].

Addressing emotions during clinical practice is very important [3,10,13]. When students are asked to keep an RLJ, they are voicing emotions experienced during clinical placements that are usually relegated to the context of individual students [10]. In addition, writing and reflecting on their feelings and emotions can also be therapeutic for students, since it allows them to stop and externalize their experiences [9,16], which increases their confidence in their ability to face future difficulties [13,17] and increases their capacity to empathize with patients and their families [18,19].

In addition, RLJs provide a "snapshot" of the daily reality on the clinical level (e.g., characteristics of services, type of patients, quality of nursing care, etc.) and the teaching process (e.g., student–nurse interaction, clinical practice schedules, etc.). Knowing the day to day life of emergency department and ICU from the perspective of students can be an enriching way to identify areas of improvement in these two nursing dimensions: clinical practice and teaching activity.

There is some prior research on the experience of students during the first year of clinical practice training [2,3,17,19,20]; however, there are fewer approaches to the experience of clinical placements in senior year students and in complex care settings, even though these may be more representative of how students will cope with the impending start of their professional development. In addition, we were unable to find any papers that compared clinical practice experiences by gender. Only a few studies include the student's gender in the verbatim, without establishing a comparative analysis [9]. This is relevant because previous research has documented differences between male and female nursing students in relation to professional values [21], personal values [22], career choice and post-graduation outcomes [23]. In addition, socially constructed traditional gender norms can determine expected behaviors and attitudes in both male and female students in the context of a traditionally female profession [24]. During clinical practice, and through the RLJ, it is possible to observe whether there are differences in the preference or rejection of some activities based on gender—for example, whether men feel more attracted to management and coordination aspects or whether women identify more with the humanization of care, empathy with patients, etc., both of which are situations that are dictated by gender roles.

The aim of our study was to explore the experience of final year nursing students during their clinical practices in emergency department and ICU and to examine how this experience is interpreted by both female and male students.

3. Materials and Methods

3.1. Design

A qualitative study using documentary analysis of RLJs written by nursing students in their senior year during their clinical practices.

3.2. Participants and Setting

In Spain, the Degree in Nursing is a four-year university degree with 240 credits (in accordance with the European Credit Transfer and Accumulation System, ECTS). During the final year, students at the University of Oviedo (Spain) take a specific course on clinical practices in the emergency department and ICU (12 ECTS credits). All students must perform at least two clinical rotations, one in the emergency department and another in ICU, to complete 230 h of training. In addition, students must submit a clinical case study and an RLJ of the subject, which accounts for 10% of the final grade. During the 2017/2018 academic year, 78 students studied this course at the University of Oviedo (Spain). Twenty-eight RLJs were selected from the students (15 from women and 13 from men) who obtained the highest grades in the January 2018 evaluation.

Clinical practices took place in the emergency department and ICU of six public hospitals. The center where the largest number of students performed clinical practices ($n = 20$) was a level 3 public university hospital (1000 beds), where around 300 patients are seen daily in the emergency department and which has 75 ICU boxes. The remaining hospitals that received students were level 2 (<500 beds).

3.3. Research Team

The research team consisted of five nurses (four women and one man) from the University of Oviedo. The principal investigator had two years' experience in critical care. She was a doctor, associate professor in nursing and the head of the clinical practicum subject. Three of the nurses had professional experience in emergency department and ICU and teaching experience in the Degree of Nursing. One researcher was also the teacher of the "Research in Nursing" subject at the University of Oviedo. The students knew the researchers through their participation in other subjects during the nursing degree.

3.4. Instruments

In this course, students are required to complete a compulsory portfolio on clinical practices. The portfolio consists of two sections. The first was a descriptive section with administrative and clinical data on the clinical practices, including data on the hospital and the practice unit, type of pathologies and nursing activities performed. The second was a reflective part (RLJ) on the contributions of the placements to their learning, on the level of satisfaction with the clinical practicum and suggestions for improvement. Specifically, students are strongly required to reflect on the following competencies achieved in three areas (knowledge, skills and attitude): (1) providing nursing care to critically ill patients; (2) correctly performing the most common techniques in emergency department and ICU; (3) respecting ethical values related to privacy, confidentiality and respect for patients; (4) meeting the information and communication needs of patients and families. This is delivered by email at the end of students' clinical practice training in a text document of unlimited length. At the beginning of the course, there is a two-hour face-to-face information session at the university on how to perform the RLJ, emphasizing its reflective nature, which must be more than just a description of the activities performed. Students were asked to engage in a reflective exercise concerning their daily actions [8] and to only record in their RLJ those aspects that were most relevant. They were given instructions on how to record each reflection, including the actions taken, the context, their emotions and how they could improve. In addition, several examples were provided. They were also encouraged to reflect on how the same activity could be done differently depending on the unit and the nurse carrying it out—for example, communication with a sedated patient.

3.5. Data Analysis

According to the methodology proposed by other authors [25,26], a three-phase content analysis of the RLJs was carried out. In the first phase, the texts were prepared for analysis. Within each journal, the sections "Identification of contributions to learning", "Description of the competencies acquired (knowledge, skills and attitudes)" and "Suggestions for improvement" were selected. In the second phase, the information was organized and the actual content analysis was carried out [27]. The meaning units identified in the reports were assigned codes. The codes were then grouped and gathered into subcategories and categories. Finally, the main themes that summarized the students' experience were formulated. According to the format of the RLJ, a previous thematic category, "knowledge, skills and attitudes competencies", was used as a starting point; however, the remaining topics emerged after the documentary analysis. In the third "reporting" phase, the results were presented. The complete analysis process was presented (codes, subcategories, categories and themes) as well as the description or storyline of the results.

The analyses were carried out without the use of software. The analyses were conducted independently by two researchers and, after pooling the analyses, they were triangulated with the participation of another researcher from the group.

3.6. Ethical Considerations

All students provided informed consent to the use of their journal for research purposes. Each participant was assigned a code to maintain anonymity, which was identified using "W" for women and "M" for men. Participation in this study had no influence on the grade assigned in their evaluation since this investigation was initiated months after the students completed the course. Our study was exempt from ethics committee approval, although it was conducted in accordance with the ethical standards set out in the original Declaration of Helsinki and its subsequent amendments.

4. Results

4.1. Experience of Nursing Students in Emergency Department and Intensive Care Units

Overall, the student experience reflected in the RLJs was positive in terms of learning, although a high emotional burden related to attendance at these units was noted. Most students perceived a high degree of coordination in these units and the importance of nurse/medical collaboration.

During the analysis, four themes were identified from the students' reflection on the competencies (Figure 1). The first referred to the student's feelings of undergoing "an intense emotional experience" and the second referred to the skills and attitudes achieved "the importance of attitudes over and above techniques." The third theme was related to nursing professionals and some characteristics of clinical practice units "to identify with nurses who dominate their environment and are close to the patient in complex and dehumanized units". Finally, the fourth theme referred to patients and their families: "how to improve care for critically ill patients and support their families."

4.1.1. Intense Emotional Experience

For all the students, these clinical placements involved intense emotions. Prior to the clinical practices, negative emotions predominated, as the previous confrontation of female and male students was characterized by fear, pressure, emotional block, etc. However, during the clinical training, they experienced emotional ambivalence. Thus, they experienced positive feelings, especially linked to the patient's favorable evolution and identification with the nursing profession. Concurrently, they also experienced negative emotions, associated with facing the care of patients in very serious clinical situations and death, causing them to reflect on life (Table 1).

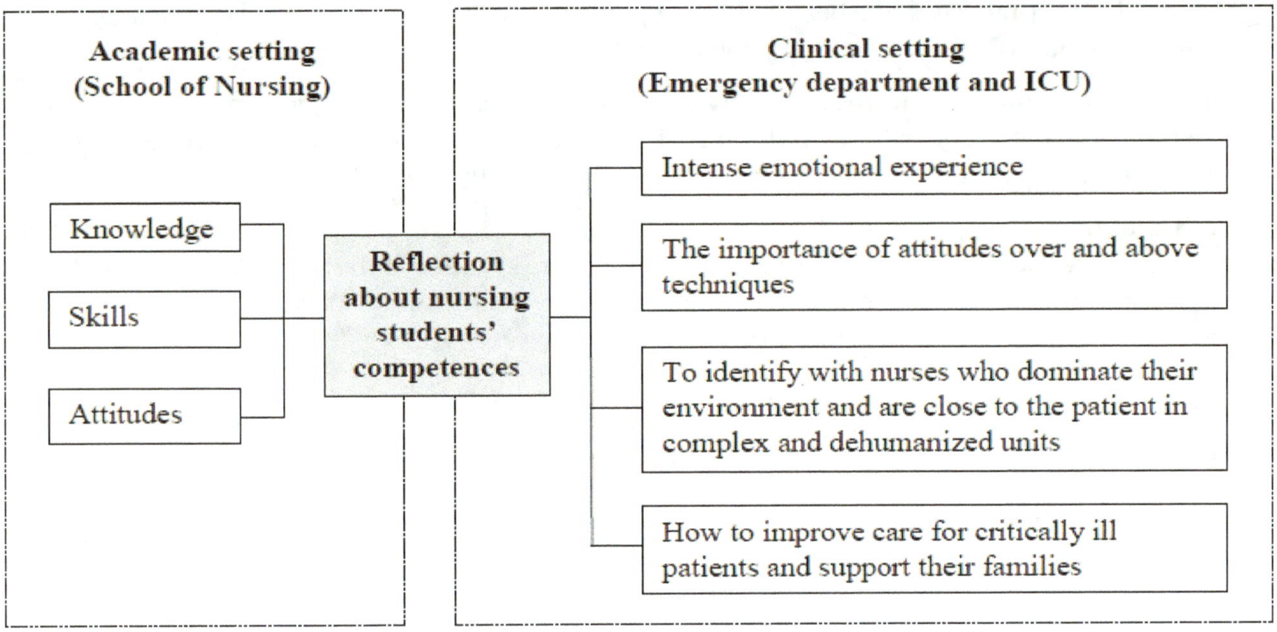

Figure 1. Experience of nursing students in emergency department and ICU during clinical practices.

Table 1. Main categories, sub-categories and codes about the theme "intense emotional experience".

Main Codes	Sub-Categories	Categories
Fear of the unknown Pressure Nervousness Emotional blockage	Previous expectations	
Identification of severe young patients Tough experience Fatigue Impotence of not being able to communicate Feeling lucky	Intense experience	Feelings
Insecurity in complex patients Fear of making mistakes Helplessness lack of time Helplessness poor patient evolution Satisfaction for good patient progress Gratification humanizing care Progressive safety/self-monitoring	Emotions during clinical practices	
Feeling like a nurse Professional and personal enrichment Awareness of the importance of the nursing profession Satisfaction with correct performance of techniques Gratification of professional collaboration	Identification with the nursing profession	
Feeling overwhelmed Fine line life/death Inexperience in facing death	Difficulty coping with death	Thoughts
Irreversible change in a second Valuing what matters Temporality of human life	Reflecting on life	

As for the previous expectations, there were no great differences between girls and boys, in both groups, and feelings of fear, pressure, being "frozen" or blocked, etc. predominated. During the clinical practices, positive feelings of satisfaction and personal growth were expressed.

"These clinical practices have been a turning point in my career as I have been able to grow as a person and as a future nursing professional." W4

"In this clinical module I have shown myself how right I have been in choosing a profession like this, how close one is to the patient and how much chance one has of, with very little, improving the condition of the patient and his or her family." M10

Both the female and male students showed progressive confidence as the clinical practicum progressed, facing these with greater ease and feeling more satisfied if the patients progressed well.

Some acknowledged their difficulty in coping with death, either because of inexperience or because they felt overwhelmed by the situation.

4.1.2. Importance of Attitudes over and above Techniques

The acquired competencies were articulated in three areas: knowledge, skills and attitudes (Table 2).

Table 2. Main categories, sub-categories and codes about the theme "importance of attitudes over and above techniques".

Main Codes	Sub-Categories	Categories
Identify situations of risk Prioritizing by triage	How to act	Knowledge
New and specific knowledge Distribution of work/tasks according to professional profile Integrating theoretical knowledge Getting to know other cultures	Expanding knowledge	
Performing new techniques Specific techniques Refinement of already known techniques Care linked to infection prevention Rapid action Performing under pressure	Technical skills	Skills
Only one aspect of care Relative importance Observation	Emphasis on techniques	
Responsibility Autonomy Confidentiality Teamwork Accepting errors Adapting to a changing environment Keeping calm Humanizing care	Acquired attitudes	Attitudes
Empathy Guaranteeing privacy Paying attention to patient's emotions Importance of talking and listening Respect	Regaining human values	

In terms of theoretical knowledge, some categories common to both sexes were learning how to handle critically ill patients or how to prioritize emergency care through triage. They also recognized learning new and specific knowledge, required in these units.

Regarding the competencies linked to skills or abilities, all mentioned the handling of devices and the refinement of new techniques as well as the improvement of other already known techniques. They also learned to act quickly, adjusting to the urgency of the moment.

Attitude-related competencies were extensively analyzed as they constituted a very large section within the RLJs. Two themes were appreciated: firstly, in relation to their personal experience as students where the acquired responsibility or autonomy stands out; secondly, almost all referred to learning related to the humanization of care, based on respect for the patient, empathy and accompaniment.

> "I have learned that many times there is no need to speak or, rather, "fill the silences" with words, we should simply be there, giving company and human touch if necessary." W12

> "When the intubated patients were thirsty I would dip a gauze in water and place it between their lips and they would thank me. I also, for example, put the radio on for a patient because it's quite tedious for everyone, I suppose, to be in bed all day without any entertainment." M12

In addition, students mentioned acquiring cultural competencies in dealing with people with social problems and patients from other countries/ethnicities.

> "On the other hand, I have been in contact with people who are drug addicts as a result of a serious social problem and with a major underlying mental illness." W4

> "Respecting the patients' beliefs and cultures, always seeking their integration in the hospital." M7

4.1.3. Identifying with Nurses Who Dominate Their Environment and Are Close to the Patient in Complex and Dehumanized Units

The perceptions of nursing professionals in the context of the emergency department and ICU are presented in Table 3. All the students appreciated the warm welcome to the units, the involvement of the nurses who taught them and their "willingness to teach".

Table 3. Main categories, sub-categories and codes about the theme "identify with nurses who dominate their environment and are close to the patient in complex and dehumanized units".

Main Codes	Sub-Categories	Categories
A warm welcome Motivation for teaching Integration of students into the team	Attitude of nurses towards students	Attitude of the nurses
Control of complex environment Autonomy/initiative Not overwhelmed Acting calmly in emergencies High pressure to provide care	Nursing activity work environment	Nurses' Actions
Reassuring attitude Informational role Close ties to the patient and family	Attending to patients	
Identifying nurses who are humane Learning by imitation of good practice Identifying each professional's style	Professional Identification: I want to be	Nurses as models
Contempt towards patients Poor education	Professional rejection: I don't want to be	
Highly technical services High complexity High care pressure (emergencies) Depersonalized services	Complex and dehumanized services	Characteristics of services
Paying attention to pain Listening more to patients Quieter and less noisy environment Improving communication Emotional support Improve use of the emergency service Limiting mobile phone use	As it should be	

> "I've discovered a part of nursing that's exciting and that, if there's one thing professionals have in this service, it's passion and drive." W1

In addition, the students were grateful for the nurses' attitudes.

> "On a day-to-day basis in the special services, doubts and learning opportunities arose in which the nurses were always willing to help and explain things to me." M6

Both female and male students identified the emergency department and ICU as highly technical and labor-intensive environments. They also appreciated that nurses in these units worked more independently and autonomously than their colleagues in other units, e.g., inpatient units, and that they fulfill an important role in informing and reassuring patients:

> "They are in control of the complexity of the situation at all times, always preventing it from overwhelming them." W3

> "Nurses are not only the professionals who know how to inject, administer medication or put a bandage on. The most important thing is to know how to listen and be close to their patients, who at certain times only need someone close by, to feel their support and understanding." M7

4.1.4. How to Improve Care in Critically Ill Patients and How to Support the Families

Both female and male students recognized that patients in these units presented very specific pathologies, which involved advanced practice care. They also understood the importance of informing and explaining the techniques to the patients in advance, as a measure to reassure them and avoid conflicts, especially due to long waits in the emergency department (Table 4). In this overall context, the students identified a certain depersonalization in patient care and proposed a more humane treatment, with simple verbal and non-verbal communication actions, such as calling each patient by their name or holding their hand.

Table 4. Main categories, sub-categories and codes about the theme "how to improve care for critically ill patients and support their families".

Main Codes	Sub-Categories	Categories
Highly complex patients Severity	Patient characteristics	Negative patient experience
Concerned Nervous	Negative emotions	
Informing appropriately Favorable environment Conveying reassurance Making the effort to listen	Professional care	Necessary actions with patients
Humanization Facilitate rest and comfort Guaranteeing privacy	Humanized care	
Offering trust and support Reassuring Providing information Stressful situation	Support for families	Actions with families
Interaction with professionals/students Facilitating a pleasant environment Strong emotional impact	Visit	

Regarding the families, all stressed the importance of adequately addressing their needs, creating a climate of trust and support, as they are under great pressure. The information that they receive plays an important role in this relationship as it can help to reassure them (Table 4). Both female and male students identified the importance of visiting times and how students and professionals should act during these encounters.

> "Always showing them that we are there and that they can trust us to take care of their relatives." W3

> "From my point of view I think it is important that the moment of family visits be as comfortable as possible for the relatives and the patient." M1

Lastly, several male and female students stressed the importance of reinforcing training on humanization in care before the start of the placements.

4.2. Differences in the Experiences of Clinical Practices in Critical Services by Gender

Female students reflected on a much more intense and negative emotional experience, linked to the environment of critical care practices with critically ill patients or by identification with young patients. Personal gratification after providing emotional care to patients was also common, as was concern for ensuring the best care:

> "I have realized that if you treat them with affection and try to help them in any way you can, not only are they very grateful to you, but you also go home with a good feeling, and knowing that your work has served a purpose." W10

> "Since we also usually have to make decisions or act very quickly which sometimes made me nervous because it can lead to confusion very easily." W13

However, for male students, perceived satisfaction was related to the identification of emergency department and ICU as an employment option.

> "I must admit that it was the rotation that I enjoyed by far the most, especially in the area of emergencies, so I am seriously considering continuing to study to work in this type of care area in the future." M2

> "The student's autonomy has to take a step forward in order to prepare for the professional world." M8

In relation to competencies, the majority of female students stated that the techniques were not the most important aspect but rather the provision of basic care, such as those related to comfort, rest or pain relief.

> "Anyone with training can channel a venous line or perform an electrocardiogram. As a nurse, you are there to support that person, reassure them, and accompany them in their distress. Sometimes the best cure is a smile, a hand on the shoulder or an "I'm there for you."" W15

> "Here, I learned how to take care of a patient, to keep an eye on him all the time, to wash him, to comb his hair, to take care of his nails... things that are less technical and more humane." W8

However, the male students gave importance to specific knowledge, such as how to change shifts properly or how to adapt to changing environments. The importance of teamwork was mentioned by virtually all male students.

> "I see it as very important to be able to give shift changes in a proper manner. I have paid a lot of attention to those who, in my opinion, perform good shift changes and I have tried to assimilate this way of working." M3

> "Teamwork, the willingness to always help one's partner is one of the attitudes that I have encouraged during the rotation, there is no "so-and-so's patient", we are all there for everyone and we help each other with everything." M10

In terms of identifying with the nurses and the environment in these units, several female students reflected on attitudes that caused them to feel rejection and that they did not want to imitate.

> "I have learned how I do not want to work in terms of how some health professionals describe and treat patients, not respecting their privacy, making value judgments and talking about patients in a derogatory way." W7

Finally, in relation to patients, the female students outlined the negative feelings perceived in patients with great detail (e.g., fear, nervousness, stress, worry) and the importance of ensuring intimacy.

> "People who are conscious, in addition to their illness, are afraid and isolated and alone." W7

> "From my point of view and according to what I have been able to learn while I was there, we can and must guarantee assistance, always respecting the patient's physical and emotional intimacy." W3

5. Discussion

According to the results of our study, for the nursing students, clinical practice in the emergency department and ICU implied an intense emotional experience, demanding the importance of attitudes towards the techniques. The profile of the nurses highlighted their human nature and their role as a reference for students in these complex units with high care demands. They also identified the need to adequately inform and support critical patients and their families. Differences were detected between female and male students regarding the experience during this clinical training.

RLJs have been a useful tool for learning more about the experience of nursing students in complex units. Some authors [3,8] had already reflected on the usefulness of the journal as a method for venting and expressing feelings and for stimulating personal growth during the process of becoming a nurse [13,28]. Moreover, writing can be considered a therapeutic tool, in the same way as it is for patients admitted to ICU [29], and it can be useful for nursing students facing stressful situations such the emergency department and ICU [30,31].

The expectation surrounding these placements was very similar to that described by other authors: nervousness and worry before facing a new post, the need to apply knowledge and techniques previously explained in theory and progressive confidence and security over time [32]. In our case, this transition could be affected by the complexity and severity of the patients in specific services, which could accentuate the expression of negative feelings, which became evident during a very intense emotional experience [3,17,28].

The students expressed the same feelings that the patients displayed: nerves, fear, freezing up in urgent situations, etc. [32,33], as if they were acting as a mirror reflecting the same negative emotional reaction, whereas the nurses assumed a reassuring and controlling role in the situation, as identified by both male and female students.

Student autonomy in complex services is limited [5], thus generating greater dependence on the nursing preceptor and greater observation of his/her clinical performance. The students in our study, as in other reports [34], have felt supported by the nurses during their clinical practices, who have integrated them into the team. During the process of becoming a nurse, which is more complex than simply having practical knowledge or skills [19,35], it is very important for students to have models and feel supported and accompanied during the mentoring process. The importance of this mentoring should be emphasized, not only through the nurse preceptors in the practice units but also on behalf of the university faculty, accompanying the students throughout the process, especially during the senior year [13]. To achieve this objective, it could be very useful to integrate this reflexive student learning into the creation of an environment of mutual trust and growth between teacher and student [10,12]. It is also important to consider the working conditions in these units, where high care loads and staff shortages can make it difficult for nurses to teach [36].

Both through the attitudes learned and the nursing care observed in the units, the humanization of care was essential. The students assigned great importance to respecting patients and the need to attend to their feelings and demonstrate empathy. Indeed, developing an empathic attitude is one of the fundamental pillars of the relationship between health professionals and patients/families [37]. Sensitivity to patient suffering was increased in our study since they were in a hostile environment, where patients were vulnerable, separated from their families and almost entirely dependent on the health professional, from making a rapid and effective diagnosis in the emergency unit to covering a human being's basic needs in the ICU. Most of the plans for the ICU integrate the elements proposed by students, which is positive since it shows a growing awareness among future nursing professionals to improve the environment in these units [38].

In general, our results coincide with research conducted in Spain on RLJs as an assessment tool during the learning process of nursing students [11]. Many of the journals included reflections on the techniques but also frequently addressed patient and family related care, interactions with the team and the nurse preceptor and even death. Moreover, this study mentions very interesting aspects, such as the importance of providing clear guidelines for the implementation of these journals, the figure of the teacher as a guide in the process of reflection within the framework of a relationship of trust and the importance of assigning importance to the evaluation, in the understanding that, if it is proposed as a voluntary activity, students generally fail to participate.

In our study, a different experience was found among female and male students. The female students described their negative feelings in more detail during the clinical training and showed a more reflective attitude. This reality could be related to a greater ease of expressing emotions among the women, whereas the men may have had similar experiences or thoughts, although they may have ultimately decided not to include them in the journal or not to delve into the experience.

Regarding the competences achieved, female students focused more on the humanization of care whereas male students more frequently mentioned aspects linked to their individual learning or organizational aspects in these units. This different approach by gender coincides with the results observed in nurses working in the ICU [39]. Further research is necessary to better understand these differences and to assess whether students may be imitating or reproducing the model identified by the nurse preceptors.

Female students were also more concerned about poor patient progression or fear of making mistakes, which is consistent with the study by Fernandez-Feito et al., [21] where female students considered it more important to seek help when they could not meet patient needs.

5.1. Implications for Clinical Practice

Enhancing the use of these reflective tools can contribute to a better understanding of the experience of nursing students during their clinical placements and encourage personal and professional growth, which is difficult to achieve through theoretical training. In addition, it would be important to encourage male students to share their experience and their personal feelings. After being aware of this experience, it would be appropriate to design interventions to reduce the associated emotional impact and provide the students with strategies (e.g., coping styles) to reduce anxiety or negative feelings.

In turn, teachers and nurse preceptors play a key role in accompanying the student in the process of "becoming" a nurse, and, in this process, creating and sharing a reflective narrative (student–preceptor–teacher) can be very helpful.

5.2. Limitations

In our study, the RLJ represented a percentage of the final grade. It would be very interesting to comment on the narratives with the students in a session not only aimed at modifying the assigned grade but also analyzing the overall experience in these services, as a group. The differences found according to gender should be interpreted with caution since the analysis was not performed blinded to the students' genders, which may have biased the interpretation of the results. The results obtained were not subjected to the process of triangulation with other techniques, such as individual interviews or focus groups with students; this will be addressed in future research.

6. Conclusions

For nursing students, clinical practices in emergency department and ICU represent an intense emotional experience that allows them to improve their learning and cope with complex environments. In addition to acquiring new knowledge and refining already learned techniques, these clinical practices allow students to acquire attitudes clearly linked to the humanization of care. Female and male students experienced these clinical rotations from different viewpoints. Female students were more emotionally and reflectively focused on patient care, whereas male students identified more with individual aspects of learning and the organization and quality of the units.

Author Contributions: Conceptualization, M.G.-G. and A.F.-F.; methodology, M.G.-G., A.L. and A.F.-F.; formal analysis, M.G.-G., Y.V.-Á. and A.F.-F.; data collection, P.Z.-M., Y.V.-Á. and A.F.-F.; writing—original draft preparation, M.G-G., A.L., Y.V.-Á., P.Z.-M. and A.F.-F.; writing—review and editing, A.L. and A.F.-F. All authors have read and agreed to the published version of the manuscript.

Acknowledgments: We would like to thank all the senior nursing students for their reflections and the nurse preceptors at the emergency department and ICU for their contribution to the training of these students.

References

1. Kajander-Unkuri, S.; Salminen, L.; Saarikoski, M.; Suhonen, R.; Leino-Kilpi, H. Competence Areas of Nursing Students in Europe. *Nurse Educ. Today* **2013**, *33*, 625–632. [CrossRef]
2. Levett-Jones, T.; Pitt, V.; Courtney-Pratt, H.; Harbrow, G.; Rossiter, R. What are the primary concerns of nursing students as they prepare for and contemplate their first clinical placement experience? *Nurse Educ. Pract.* **2015**, *15*, 304–309. [CrossRef] [PubMed]
3. Mlinar Reljić, N.; Pajnkihar, M.; Fekonja, Z. Self-reflection during first clinical practice: The experiences of nursing students. *Nurse Educ. Today* **2019**, *72*, 61–66. [CrossRef] [PubMed]
4. Mahlanze, H.T.; Sibiya, M.N. Perceptions of student nurses on the writing of reflective journals as a means for personal, professional and clinical learning development. *Health SA Gesondheid.* **2017**, *22*, 79–86. [CrossRef]
5. Vatansever, N.; Akansel, N. Intensive Care Unit Experience of Nursing Students during their Clinical Placements: A Qualitative Study. *Int. J. Caring Sci.* **2016**, *9*, 1040–1048.
6. Bongar, M.V.V.; Pangan, F.C.; Macindo, J.R.B. Characteristics of a critical care clinical placement programme affecting critical care nursing competency of baccalaureate nursing students: A structural equation modelling. *J. Clin. Nurs.* **2019**, *28*, 1760–1770. [CrossRef]
7. Fernández-Peña, R.; Fuentes-Pumarola, C.; Malagón-Aguilera, M.C.; Bonmatí-Tomàs, A.; Bosch-Farré, C.; Ballester-Ferrando, D. The evaluation of reflective learning from the nursing student's point of view: A mixed method approach. *Nurse Educ. Today* **2016**, *44*, 59–65. [CrossRef]
8. Schön, D.A. *La Formación de Profesionales Reflexivos: Hacia un Nuevo Diseño de la Formación y el Aprendizaje en las Profesiones*; Ediciones Paidós: Madrid, Spain, 1992.
9. Bagnato, S.; Valerio, D.; Lorenza, G. The reflective journal: A tool for enhancing experience- based learning in nursing students in clinical practice. *J. Nurs. Educ. Pract.* **2013**, *3*, 102–111. [CrossRef]
10. Ruiz-López, M.; Rodríguez-García, M.; Villanueva, P.G.; Márquez-Cava, M.; García-Mateos, M.; Ruiz-Ruiz, B.; Herrera-Sánchez, E. The use of reflective journaling as a learning strategy during the clinical rotations of students from the faculty of health sciences: An action-research study. *Nurse Educ. Today* **2015**, *35*, e26–e31. [CrossRef]
11. San Rafael Gutiérrez, S. El Diario de Prácticas Clínicas Como Herramienta de Evaluación de los Procesos de Enseñanza Aprendizaje de los Alumnos de Enfermería. Ph.D. Thesis, Universidad de Alicante, Alicante, Spain, 2016.
12. Dahl, H.; Eriksen, K.Å. Students' and teachers' experiences of participating in the reflection process "THiNK". *Nurse Educ. Today* **2016**, *36*, 401–406. [CrossRef]

13. Bjerkvik, L.K.; Hilli, Y. Reflective writing in undergraduate clinical nursing education: A literature review. *Nurse Educ. Pract.* **2019**, *35*, 32–41. [CrossRef] [PubMed]
14. Rodriguez García, M.; Ruiz López, M.; González Sanz, P.; Fernandez Trinidad, M.; De Blas Gómez, I. Experiencias y vivencias del estudiante de 4° de enfermería en el practicum. *Cult. Cuid.* **2014**, *18*, 25–33. [CrossRef]
15. García-Carpintero Blas, E.; Siles-González, J.; Martínez-Roche, E. Percepciones de los estudiantes sobre sus vivencias en las prácticas clínicas. *Enferm. Univ.* **2019**, *16*, 259–268.
16. Naber, J.; Markley, L. A guide to nursing students' written reflections for students and educators. *Nurse Educ. Pract.* **2017**, *25*, 1–4. [CrossRef] [PubMed]
17. Sun, F.K.; Long, A.; Tseng, Y.S.; Huang, H.M.; You, J.H.; Chiang, C.Y. Undergraduate student nurses' lived experiences of anxiety during their first clinical practicum: A phenomenological study. *Nurse Educ. Today* **2016**, *37*, 21–26. [CrossRef]
18. Reis, S.P.; Wald, H.S.; Monroe, A.D.; Borkan, J.M. Begin the BEGAN (The Brown Educational Guide to the Analysis of Narrative)—A framework for enhancing educational impact of faculty feedback to students' reflective writing. *Patient Educ. Couns.* **2010**, *80*, 253–259. [CrossRef]
19. Teskereci, G.; Boz, İ. "I try to act like a nurse": A phenomenological qualitative study. *Nurse Educ. Pract.* **2019**, *37*, 39–44. [CrossRef]
20. Westin, L.; Sundler, A.J.; Berglund, M. Students' experiences of learning in relation to didactic strategies during the first year of a nursing programme: A qualitative study. *BMC Med. Educ.* **2015**, *15*, 1–8. [CrossRef]
21. Fernández-Feito, A.; Basurto Hoyuelos, S.; Palmeiro Longo, M.G.D.V. Differences in professional values between nurses and nursing students: A gender perspective. *Int. Nurs. Rev.* **2019**, *66*, 577–589. [CrossRef]
22. Luciani, M.; Rampoldi, G.; Ardenghi, S.; Bani, M.; Merati, S.; Ausili, D.; Strepparava, M.G.; Di Mauro, S. Personal values among undergraduate nursing students: A cross-sectional study. *Nurs. Ethics* **2020**. [CrossRef]
23. Hoffart, N.; McCoy, T.P.; Lewallen, L.P.; Thorpe, S. Differences in Gender-related Profile Characteristics, Perceptions, and Outcomes of Accelerated Second Degree Nursing Students. *J. Prof. Nurs.* **2019**, *35*, 93–100. [CrossRef] [PubMed]
24. McDonald, J. Conforming to and Resisting Dominant Gender Norms: How Male and Female Nursing Students Do and Undo Gender. *Gend. Work Organ.* **2013**, *20*, 561–579. [CrossRef]
25. Elo, S.; Kyngäs, H. The qualitative content analysis process. *J. Adv. Nurs.* **2008**, *62*, 107–115. [CrossRef] [PubMed]
26. Vaismoradi, M.; Turunen, H.; Bondas, T. Content analysis and thematic analysis: Implications for conducting a qualitative descriptive study. *Nurs. Health Sci.* **2013**, *15*, 398–405. [CrossRef]
27. Graneheim, U.H.; Lundman, B. Qualitative content analysis in nursing research: Concepts, procedures and measures to achieve trustworthiness. *Nurse Educ. Today* **2004**, *24*, 105–112. [CrossRef]
28. Siles González, J.; Solano Ruiz, M.C.; Noreña Peña, A.; Gabán Gutiérrez, A.; Gil Estevan, M.D.; Martínez Sabater, A.; Núñez del Castillo, M.; Ferrer Hernández, M.E.; Rocamora Salort, F.; Fernández Molina, M.A.; et al. *XII Jornadas de Redes de Investigación en Docencia Universitaria: El reconocimiento Docente: Innovar e Investigar con Criterios de Calidad*; Percepción de los alumnos de enfermería de las unidades especiales a través de sus diarios; Universidad de Alicante: Alicante, Spain, 2014; pp. 510–525.
29. Nydahl, P.; Fischill, M.; Deffner, T.; Neudeck, V.; Heindl, P. Diaries for intensive care unit patients reduce the risk for psychological sequelae: Systematic literature review and meta-analysis. *Med. Klin. Intensivmed. Notfmed.* **2019**, *114*, 68–76. [CrossRef]
30. Walton, J.A.; Lindsay, N.; Hales, C.; Rook, H. Glimpses into the transition world: New graduate nurses' written reflections. *Nurse Educ. Today* **2018**, *60*, 62–66. [CrossRef]
31. Alteren, J. Narratives in student nurses' knowledge development: A hermeneutical research study. *Nurse Educ. Today* **2019**, *76*, 51–55. [CrossRef]
32. Alonso-Ovies, Á.; La Calle, G.H. Icu: A branch of hell? *Intensive Care Med.* **2016**, *42*, 591–592. [CrossRef]
33. Johnson, C.C.; Suchyta, M.R.; Darowski, E.S.; Collar, E.M.; Kiehl, A.L.; Van, J.; Jackson, J.C.; Hopkins, R.O. Psychological Sequelae in Family Caregivers of Critically Ill Intensive Care Unit Patients. A Systematic Review. *Ann. Am. Thorac. Soc.* **2019**, *16*, 894–909. [CrossRef]

34. Álvarez Teruel, J.D.; Tortosa Ybánez, M.T.; Pellín Buades, N. *Investigación y Propuestas Innovadoras de Redes Universidad de Alicante Para la Mejora Docente*; El diario de prácticas clínicas en la unidad de cuidados intensivos; Universidad de Alicante: Alicante, Spain, 2015; pp. 1665–1676.
35. Sandvik, A.H.; Eriksson, K.; Hilli, Y. Becoming a caring nurse—A Nordic study on students' learning and development in clinical education. *Nurse Educ. Pract.* **2014**, *14*, 286–292. [CrossRef]
36. Rodríguez García, M.C. Percepción de los estudiantes del Grado en Enfermería sobre su entorno de prácticas clínicas: Un estudio fenomenológico. *Enferm. Clin.* **2019**, *29*, 264–270. [CrossRef] [PubMed]
37. Moreto, G.; González Blasco, P.; Piñero, A. Reflections on dehumanisation in medical education: Empathy, emotions, and possible pedagogical resources for the emotional education of the medical student. *Educ. Med.* **2018**, *19*, 172–177. [CrossRef]
38. Rojas, V. Humanización de los cuidados intensivos. *Rev. Méd. Clín. Condes* **2019**, *30*, 120–125. [CrossRef]
39. Via Clavero, G.; Sanjuán Naváis, M.; Martínez Mesas, M.; Pena Alfaro, M.; Utrilla Antolín, C.; Zarragoikoetxea Jáuregui, I. Identidad de género y cuidados intensivos: Influencia de la masculinidad y la feminidad en la percepción de los cuidados enfermeros. *Enferm. Intensiva* **2010**, *21*, 104–112. [CrossRef] [PubMed]

5

Mishel's Model of Uncertainity Describing Categories and Subcategories in Fibromyalgia Patients

Ana Fernandez-Araque [1,*], Julia Gomez-Castro [1], Andrea Giaquinta-Aranda [1,2], Zoraida Verde [3] and Clara Torres-Ortega [1,4]

1 Department of Nursing, Faculty of Health Sciences, University of Valladolid, 42004 Soria, Spain; juliamaria.gomez@uva.es (J.G.-C.); agaranda1993@hotmail.com (A.G.-A.); clara.torres@enf.uva.es (C.T.-O.)
2 Haemodialysis Service, Santa Bárbara Hospital, 42005 Soria; Spain
3 Department of Biochemistry, Molecular Biology and Physiology, University of Valladolid, 42004 Soria, Spain; zoraida.verde@uva.es
4 Emergency Service of the Hospital Santa Bárbara, 42005 Soria, Spain
* Correspondence: anamaria.fernandez@uva.es

Abstract: The aim of this review was to demonstrate the presence of categories and subcategories of Mishel's model in the experiences of patients with fibromyalgia by reviewing qualitative studies. Uncertainty is defined as the inability to determine the meaning of disease-related events. A scoping review of qualitative studies was carried out. Twenty articles were included, with sample sizes ranging from 3 to 58 patients. Articles from different countries and continents were included. Three categories of the model and eight subcategories could be shown to be present in the experiences of fibromyalgia patients through the scoping review. The first category, concerning antecedents of uncertainty in patients with fibromyalgia, is constituted by the difficulty in coping with symptoms, uncertainty about the diagnosis and uncertainty about the complexity of the treatment. The second concerns the cognitive process of anxiety, stress, emotional disorder and social stigma. The third category refers to coping with the disease, through the management of social and family support and the relationship with health care professionals.

Keywords: fibromyalgia; stigma; illness uncertainty; scoping review; qualitative research

1. Introduction

Uncertainty characterizes the nature of fibromyalgia syndrome (FMS). FMS is associated with psychiatric comorbidity and coping problems [1,2]. FMS is a chronic pain condition, which has a global mean prevalence of 2.7 % [3,4]. FMS is a chronic musculoskeletal disease which affects physical, mental and sexual health [5]. FMS affects 2.4% of the Spanish population [4]. The Committee of the American College of Rheumatology (ACR) formulated a construct of fibromyalgia 30 years ago in an attempt to rectify a situation of diagnostic confusion faced by patients presenting with widespread pain [6].

Fibromyalgia is a complex syndrome. Evidence-based interdisciplinary guidelines have suggested a comprehensive clinical assessment to avoid this diagnostic conundrum [7]. At diagnosis, most individuals have been experiencing symptoms and have been in the health care system for at least 5 to 8 years [8]. The profound symptomatic impact of FMS may be exacerbated by the perceived inauthenticity [9,10]. Its unpredictable course raises concerns about when and how symptoms will appear or progress, with uncertainty being one of the most characteristic emotions of this disease [11]. All this can have a negative emotional, psychological and socioeconomic impact, both on the patient and on the family [12]. Emphasis in FMS research has shifted over the past decade and in the last year [13].

The concept of uncertainty has been used in many disciplines including nursing, medicine, and health communication with slightly differing definitions, extensions, and applications. Nurses provide information that helps patients develop meaning from the illness experience by providing structure. Nurses help patients to manage chronic uncertainty by assisting with patients' reappraisal of uncertainty from stressful to hopeful in addition to providing relevant information [14,15].

The Uncertainty in Illness Theory and its reconceptualization are models derived from and for nursing practice [16]. Uncertainty in illness is defined as a cognitive state resulting from insufficient cues with which to form a cognitive schema or meaning of a situation or event. Mishel proposes that managing uncertainty is critical to adaptation during illness, and his theory explains how individuals cognitively process illness-associated events and construct meaning from them [17]. This theory is based on Warburton's information processing theories, the study of Budner's personality and is influenced in turn by the ideas of Lazarus and Folkman that relate uncertainty with stress and coping [18]. However, Mishel added uncertainty as a stressor in the context of the disease, which is valuable for nurses. This allows us to assess aspects categorized into complex diseases that the individual has to face [19]. The concepts of the theory are organized around three categories using what is known as Mishel's model of uncertainty in disease [16,17]: firstly, the antecedents of uncertainty refer to the form, composition and structure of the stimuli that the person perceives before some prominent subcategories such as difficulty coping with symptoms, uncertainty regarding diagnosis and uncertainty about the complexity of treatment; the second category is the cognitive appraisal of uncertainty, which can vary from person to person and depends on two main subcategories—uncertainty as a danger, and anxiety, stress expression, emotional disorder and stigma [20]; the final subcategory involves coping with uncertainty through social and family support, through health professionals and through support with peers [21].

Uncertainty affects almost every aspect of a person's life. In response to the confusion and disorder caused by a state of continuous uncertainty, the system has no choice but to change to survive. Ideally, under conditions of chronic uncertainty, the person should gradually move from a negative assessment of uncertainty to the adoption of a new way of seeing life that accepts this as part of its reality. This occurs through the cognitive assessment of uncertainty and coping with the uncertainty relating to the disease [22,23].

Therefore, we consider it relevant to show how the three basic categories of Mishel's model for uncertainty about the disease may be present in qualitative studies carried out in patients with fibromyalgia due to its high potential for uncertainty and high emotional demands. Although the studies analyzed in this article are not based on this model, we intend to demonstrate the presence of these categories and be able to detect them, and to show professionals how and where to act, based on the experiences of the patients themselves through the review of qualitative studies. This makes it possible to determine at which moment of the disease process are nursing interventions most time-effective and beneficial for the positive adaptation of the person to their experience of fibromyalgia [24].

The aim of this review was to demonstrate the presence of categories and subcategories of Mishel's model in the experiences of patients with FMS by reviewing qualitative studies.

2. Materials and Methods

A scoping review was carried out, considering qualitative studies with methodological rigor. We selected original articles that explored the experiences of patients with fibromyalgia in order to detect the existence of the three categories present in Mishel's theory of uncertainty about the disease.

2.1. Search

The inclusion criteria for the selection of studies were qualitative designs on adult patients diagnosed with fibromyalgia syndrome, with individual or group intervention methods and verbal accounts of experiences, regardless of the use of the Mishel model as a theoretical framework. Studies selected were conducted within the last ten years, in any language, with free or private access; as we used the library database of the University of Valladolid, this provided us access to articles without free access.

Different search sources and databases were used, such as SCOPUS, CINAHL and PubMed. In the same way, we used descriptors from MESH, CINAHL/MeSH, subject. Headings and DeCS (for the Spanish Language) were employed, in addition to non-standardized terms. The English terms that we used were fibromyalgia, uncertainty, coping, and Mishel. The search was conducted from October 2019 to January 2020, including publications until 2020. We used the following search string for Scopu: fibromyalgia AND uncertainty AND Mishel. For the PubMed database, we used fibromyalgia OR fibro * [tiab] O fibromyalgia AND coping [tiab] O uncertainty [tiab] Mishel O experiences and qualitative investigation [mh]. For the CINAHL Boolean/Phrase, we used the terms fibromyalgia, uncertainty, and Mishel.

2.2. Critical Evaluation

First, we carried out a selection by the title and the abstract of the articles. Then, we discarded repeated articles and those that had no relation to our objective. The articles that we considered relevant, after reading the full text, were evaluated through a peer review. The model used to evaluate the methodological quality of the articles analyzed was the CASPe program for qualitative studies [25], eliminating those that did not meet the minimum established methodological criteria (Table S1). The assessment points included in this guide are "present", "doubtful" and "not registered". Therefore, some eligibility criteria were proposed: of the nine questions, when an article presented three negative responses or two negative responses and a doubtful one, this article was excluded for the review of this study. In total, three articles were excluded, which guarantied the methodological quality of this review.

2.3. Data Extraction

Subsequently, two authors performed an in-depth reading and extracted the data shown in Table 1. The first extraction consisted of obtaining the following data from each article, for a first analysis: relevant data (author/s, publication date and country); setting context design/model; aim of this study; age range; sample; gender of participants, method of data collection, type of interview.

For the review of the participants' experiences, the same two authors also proceeded to look for the existence in the discourses of aspects related to uncertainty about the disease itself—called antecedents of uncertainty—with a cognitive appraisal of uncertainty and coping with uncertainty.

The presence of the three categories of the Mishel model allowed us to go one step further by searching for subcategories within each category, which was intended to show real evidence in the verbal accounts of FMS patients with greater emphasis and clarity. Supplementary file 1 shows this review.

2.4. Process Followed to Determine the Categories and Subcategories of Uncertainty

We proceeded with two steps to extract and show the presence in the verbal accounts and experiences of patients with FMS of the categories and possible subcategories in each study: (1) we identified statements, responses, individual or group aspects related to uncertainty, cognitive processes and coping with the disease in each study and their coincidence or not with the rest of the studies reviewed; (2) after having identified the categories, we carried out a second in-depth reading that allowed us to obtain subcategories and classify them according to the Mishel model [19].

Table 1. Summary of studies included in the review.

Authors, Publication Date and Setting	Context	Design/Theory	Age Range	N/Sample Characteristic	Method of Data Collection	Type of Interview
Alameda et al., 2019 (Madrid, Spain) [26]	Community	Phenomenological	36–74	13/12 W-1 M	Life Story Interview	Individual
Boulton.,2018 (Canada, U.K.) [27]	Community	Narrative analysis	21–69	31/25 W-6 M	In-depth interviews	Individual
Briones et al., 2016 (Valencia, Spain) [28]	Association	Descriptive-exploratory	24–61	13/13 W	In-depth interviews	Individual
Briones et al., 2014 (Valencia, Spain) [29]	Primary care	Descriptive-exploratory	24–61	16/13 W-3 M	Semi-structured interview	Individual
Cedraschi et al.,2013 (Geneva, Switzerland) [22]	Primary care	Interpretative	33–76	56/56 W	Semi-structured interview	Individual
Cooper et al., 2017 (Johannesburg, South Africa) [30]	Community	Descriptive-exploratory	23–59	15/15 W	In-depth interviews and focal group	Individual and group
Escudero-Carretero et al., 2010 (Spain) [8]	Primary care	Interpretative	33–62	21/20 W-1 M	Focal group	Group
Humphrey et al., 2010 (EEUU, Germany, France) [31]	Primary care	Grounded Theory	25–79	40/20/5 M-15 W (EEUU) 10/5 M-5 W(Germany) 10/2 M-8 W (France)	Semi-structured interview	Individual
Juuso et al., 2011 (Sweden) [32]	Community	Phenomenological	38–64	13/13 W	Interview (Unspecified)	Individual
Matarın et al., 2017 (Spain) [33]	Association	Qualitative study with methodology using Gadamer's philosophical hermeneutics was carried out.	22–56	13/13 W	Focus group and semi-structured interviews	Individual and group
Miranda et al., 2016 (Brazil) [34]	Primary care	Grounded Theory		11/Unspecified	Semi-structured interviews Group dynamics and participant observation	Individual and group
Montesó-Curto et al., 2018 (Catalonia, Spain) [35]	Primary care	Phenomenological	53–69	44/43 W-1 M	Group Problem-Solving Therapy.	Group
Olive et al., 2013 (Cataluña, Spain) [36]	Community	Ethnographic narrative	49–56	3/2 W-1 M	Participant observation and In-depth interviews	Individual
Oliveira et al., 2019 (Río de Janeiro, Brasil) [37]	Community	Interpretative	33–73	12 W	Observation of group dynamics and semi-structured interview	Individual and group
Romero -Alcalá et al., 2019 (Spain, Chile) [38]	Association	Phenomenological and Gadamerian hermeneutics and the Roy adaptation theory	37–53	35 W and their partner	In-depth interviews and focal group	Individual and group
Sallinen et al., 2019 (Oslo, Norway) [39]	Community	Descriptive- exploratory		5/5 M	Life story interviews	Individual
Sorense et al., 2017 (Norway) [40]	Hospital	Hermeneutic analysis	12–19	Unspecified	In-depth interviews	Individual
Taylor et al., 2016 (Virginia, EEUU) [23]	Community	Interpretative	18–64	20/19 W- 1 M and 20 control	Semi-structured interview	Individual
Triviño Martínez et al., 2016 (Alicante, España) [11]	Community	Phenomenological	45–65	14/14 W	Semi-structured interview	Individual
Wuytack et al., 2011 (Gante, Belgium) [41]	Hospital	Exploratory through Husserl's concept of transcendental subjectivity	36–66	6/6 W	Semi-structured interview	Individual

FMS: fibromyalgia; W: woman, M: men.

3. Results

Our search strategy resulted in a total of 20 final references after the selection process, as observed in Figure 1.

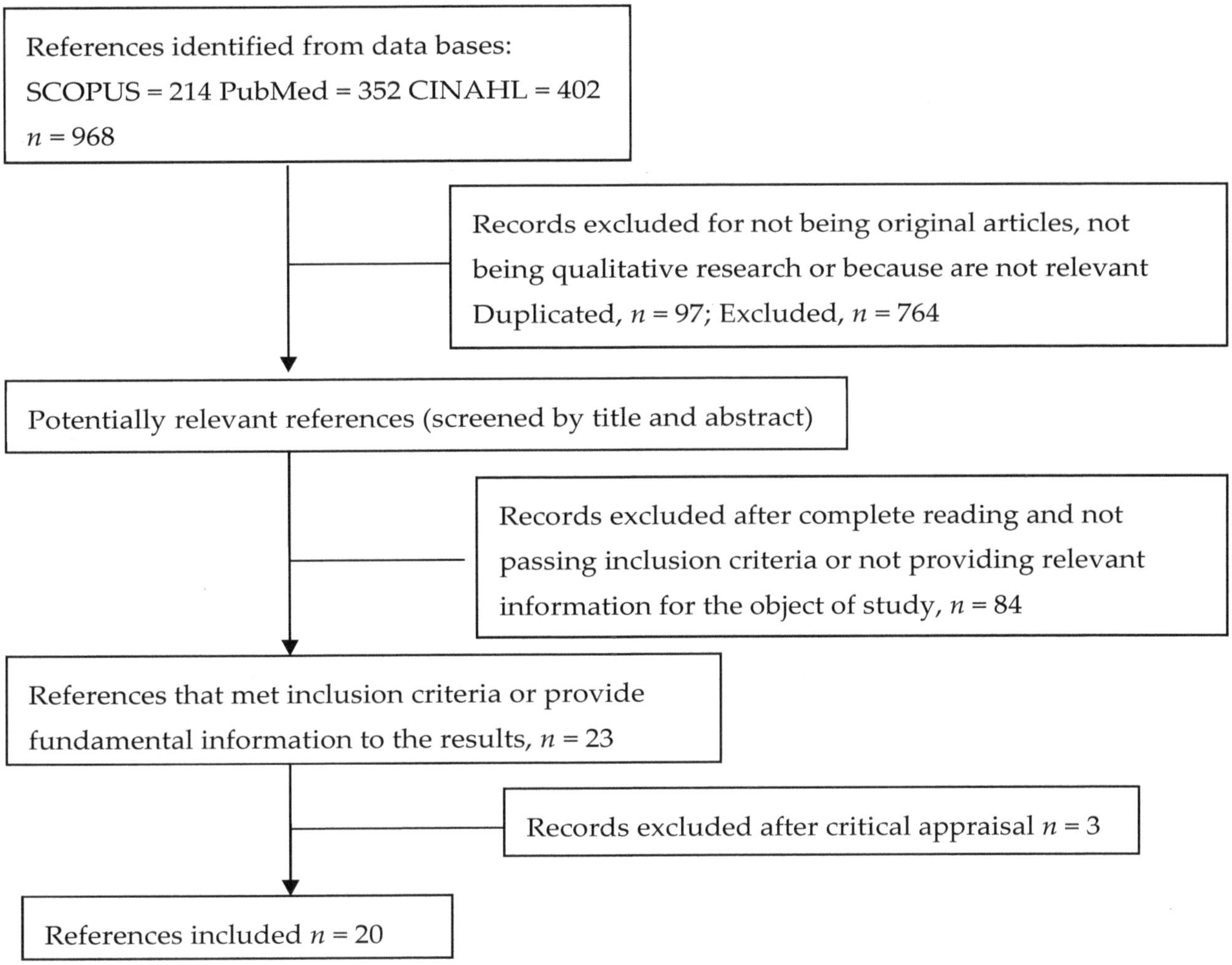

Figure 1. Flowchart of the study selection process.

Of the 20 studies that met the inclusion criteria, the sample sizes ranged from 3 to 58 participants. In all studies, the age range was 18 years old and over; the oldest subject was 90 years old. The predominant sex in the studies was female. In total, 45% of the studies reviewed were carried out with women only. Patients were from Canada, the United States, the United Kingdom, Spain, Germany, France, Belgium, Switzerland, Sweden, South Africa, Brazil and Chile (Table 1).

A review of the literature allowed us to identify the existence of categories related to the Mishel model on uncertainty regarding the disease and secondly to group the experiences of fibromyalgia patients by subcategories, obtaining eight relevant subcategories present in the discourses reviewed in the different studies (Table 2, Table S2).

In the first category—antecedents of uncertainty—we integrate the results related to the difficulty in coping with the symptoms, uncertainty about the diagnosis and uncertainty about the complexity of the treatment. The second category of Mishel's theory is cognitive assessment, which includes anxiety, stress, emotional disorder, and social stigma. The last category refers to coping with uncertainty about the disease. In this case, the subcategories detected in the different discourses and experiences of patients with FMS exhibited a reduction in uncertainty through effective coping due to the existence of subcategories related to the relationship between management and control by health professionals regarding the disease, as well as the support of the family and of peers (Table 2, Table S3).

Table 2. Categories and subcategories of Mishel's model of uncertainty in fibromyalgia syndrome identified in the experiences of patients with different qualitative studies.

Categories	**1. Antecedents of Uncertainty**			**2. Cognitive Appraisal**		**3. Coping with Uncertainty**		
Subcategories:	1.1. Difficulty with symptoms	1.2. Uncertainty regarding diagnosis	1.3. About complexity of treatment	2.1. As a danger Anxiety, stress expression, emotional disorder	2.2. Stigma	3.1. Coping with social and family support	3.2. Through health professionals	3.3. Through support with peers (e.g., associations)
Alameda et al., 2019 [26]	✓	✓	✓	✓			✓	
Boulton, et al., 2018 [27]	✓	✓					✓	
Briones et al., 2016 [28]		✓	✓	✓	✓		✓	
Briones et al., 2014 [29]		✓		✓	✓	✓	✓	
Cedraschi et al., 2013 [22]	✓		✓	✓	✓		✓	✓
Cooper et al., 2017 [30]	✓	✓		✓				
Escudero-C.et al., 2010 [8]	✓	✓		✓		✓	✓	
Humphrey et al., 2010 [31]	✓	✓						
Juuso et al., 2011 [32]	✓	✓		✓	✓	✓	✓	✓
Matarín et al., 2017 [33]	✓					✓	✓	✓
Miranda et al., 2016 [34]	✓						✓	
Montesó-Curtó et al., 2018 [35]	✓	✓		✓	✓	✓	✓	✓
Olive et al., 2013 [36]	✓	✓	✓	✓		✓	✓	✓
Oliveira JPR et al., 2019 [37]	✓	✓		✓	✓	✓	✓	✓
Romero-Aet al., 2019 [38]						✓	✓	
Sallimen et al., 2019 [39]		✓	✓		✓	✓	✓	
Sorense et al., 2017 [40]	✓		✓	✓		✓		✓
Taylor et al., 2016 [23]	✓	✓		✓	✓	✓		
Triviño Martínez et al., 2016 [11]								
Wuytack et al., 2011 [41]		✓				✓		

3.1. *Antecedents of Uncertainty*

3.1.1. Difficulty Coping with Symptoms

In total, 75% of the studies reviewed in our article agree that the unpredictable and changing nature of symptoms leads to a negative evaluation of physical symptoms. The most prominent factors are generalized chronic pain, fatigue, sleep disorders, memory problems, and the feeling of bloating. All these symptoms influence the perceived difficulty to cope with the disease and therefore to adapt to the disease [8,31,33,36]. As a result of the review within this category, we obtained a subcategory—difficulty in coping with symptoms—due to their severity and variability as a stressful factor in the disease process [16,22,28,30,37,40,42] which must be thoroughly evaluated to reduce uncertainty.

3.1.2. Uncertainty Regarding Diagnosis

Diagnosis occurs a last resort because there is no conclusive proven evidence of the disease, so it is considered an invisible disease [27,28]. From the time a patient begins contacting healthcare professionals until diagnosis, an average of approximately 7 years elapses [28,36,41]. During this time, patients are in a situation of uncertainty [40]. In total, 76.16% of the reviewed studies show—in the experiences of FMS patients—the need for a firm diagnosis as a turning point to develop coping strategies in the health–disease process and reduce anxiety. Therefore, it is the second subcategory identified in our results.

3.1.3. Uncertainty about Complexity of Treatment

This third subcategory—the complexity of the treatment of this syndrome—identified appears in the verbal accounts and experiences of 33.33% of the selected studies [27,28,33]. Patients with the highest degree of uncertainty about prognosis were those with the worst adherence to treatment [36]. Most of the participants in the different studies (Table 2) stated that health professionals lack information on the use of the various medications prescribed [40]; patients manifested unpleasant side effects of medications, which occasionally led them to avoid their use [23,28]. These patients then look for other therapy options such as non-pharmacological treatment and moderate physical exercise.

3.2. *Cognitive Appraisal*

In regard to the category of cognitive assessment, the presence of two subcategories is highlighted: the perception of danger by the presence of stress, anxiety and emotional disorders, and the cognitive perception and experience caused by the stigma of the disease [22,29,30,33,36,38,41].

3.2.1. Uncertainty as a Danger: Anxiety, Stress and Emotional Disorder

This disease is linked to psychopathology, stress, anxiety and depression. Chronic pain as a routine produces a great deal of suffering and limitations [37], and people affected by FMS feel imprisoned by pain [40]. Another method which some people use to try to confront the diagnosis is to approach religion or spirituality [16], which emerges as an emotional support. Faith in some superior being fills these people with motivation, relief, self-improvement, and strength.

Therefore, stressful and emotional factors may lead to a sense of danger that may constitute another subcategory drawn from the experiences of patients suffering from this disease. Depending on the individuals' own experiences, education and internal resources, the cognitive assessment of danger will differ from one patient to another.

3.2.2. Stigma

This subcategory was found in 38% of the selected articles (Table 2). Social stigma is the feeling of prejudice against people with FMS. On one hand, there is a stigma of the mental illness that surrounds this pathology; on the other hand, patients may feel morally offended by the supposed faking of their symptoms, when no obvious signs of illness are found [27,30,33]. Feeling believed by society and supported is a reinforcement of the mechanism of adaptation to FMS [40,41]. Many fibromyalgia patients, in addition to suffering discrimination and prejudice from others, also suffer from these feelings towards themselves.

Furthermore, we discovered another flaw within the social stigma, which we can label as a gender stigma: gender stigma appears as FMS mainly affects women, and there is a stereotype of a "woman who complains" [29]. In total, 14% of the articles analyzed identify gender self-stigma as the inability to fulfil feminine tasks imposed by society, which creates a feeling of remorse in women [29,35,36]. In men, fatigue is seen worse than in women, thus generating a feeling of helplessness and loss of virility [32].

3.3. *Coping with Uncertainty*

Coping strategies are the thoughts and behaviors that the person often uses to respond to stressful situations and lessen the perceived threat of experiencing chronic illness [19,20,41]. As a result of our review, we have identified important repetitions in the verbal accounts of the experiences of FMS patients that need to be reduced though effective coping mechanisms.

3.3.1. Coping with Social and Family Support

This subcategory was found in the review by means of three main verbal accounts: social support, family and work repercussion. In 16 of the articles included in this review (Table 2), the importance of sufferers having effective social relationships in their lives is expressed, because these relationships help them to overcome negative situations related to the disease. Pain and relapses can lead to the impossibility of making plans and social isolation, because patients cannot perform the same activities as before the disease [23]. In order not to be judged by people close to them, some patients avoid talking about the disease and the feelings that it entails, therefore avoiding the problem and developing a maladaptation to the situation [41].

Another aspect that many studies show is the great impact on work that the disease produces [32,35,37,40,42]. In environments where there is no public health system, patients may depend on parents or partners to pay for medical bills, leaving those without family support unprotected [31]. It is important to highlight among these results that people try to maintain personal and work roles, using energy dosing strategies to improve their self-concept [39]. The relationship with partners is especially affected because the physical discomfort of these patients leads to a negative mood. On the other hand, the disease involves a change in affectivity and sexual life that is not always well accepted in a couple [29,33,38].

3.3.2. Coping through Health Professionals

One of the subcategories identified and the one that most concerns us is that related to health professionals. This factor was highlighted by more than half of the studies analyzed (Table 2); it was found that a patient's lack of confidence in healthcare professionals is one of the factors that increases uncertainty. The relationship with healthcare professionals is controversial since there are those who believe in the disease and those who do not [25].

Participants demand credibility from healthcare professionals from the first moment they attend the consultation. Empathy is demanded, along with a comprehensive approach, taking into account expectations and the psychological dimension [22,30]. Most often, patients report that their doctors told them the name of their illness, but they were not informed about its possible physical and mental consequences, nor the possible treatments or therapies [27]. This discourse shows us a subcategory that requires the evaluation of our work as health professionals.

3.3.3. Coping through Peer Support (e.g., Associations)

In total, 38% of articles showed that patient associations can play an important role in finding information, especially when the health system is fragile. Patient associations provide peer support, relief, and shared experiences with others in the same situation. For this reason, in our results, this subcategory was detected as an element to contribute to adequate adaptation and an effective method of coping with FMS [40].

4. Discussion

The results of this review show the presence of the three main categories of Mishel's model about uncertainty in adults who suffer from FMS, which was the goal of our study, which was carried out through the revision of the verbal accounts of patients and their experiences in the 20 studies selected. The review included studies from different countries.

This theory has been applied to many chronic diseases, but few studies have been carried out in people with fibromyalgia [11]. However, the identification of uncertainty as a stressor and the ability to establish cognitive processes against stigma and coping through the use and availability of family resources, peers and healthcare professionals can be useful for comprehensive patient care. Furthermore, this can help us to evaluate and help patients to effectively deal with all the aspects related to uncertainty cause by their disease.

Assessing patients with FMS by these categories will allow us to understand the nature of the uncertainty for each patient individually and will help us to determine how to handle the uncertainty of patients with this disease as these are the most relevant aspects of their disease which concern the patients and interfere with the way they are coping with it [23].

The studies do not show differences in uncertainty regarding fibromyalgia between men and women, perhaps due to the lack of studies in men; only one study with men in this review met criteria for inclusion [39], and in those studies that involved men and women, there were a greater proportion of women than men, as can be seen in Table 1 [8,23,35]. Although one author concluded that FMS has a greater impact in men and it causes them to seek medical retirement earlier than women, this has not been proven with a significant sample size or in a qualitative study [43].

In regard of patient's age, the core sample were adults and mainly of intermediate age, which is similar to other studies showing the prevalence of FMS [42]. Patients of working age experience greater uncertainty.

We can affirm the existence of the first category of the Mishel model in the reviewed studies. The perception of patients with FMS, on the basis of initial experience, even before knowing the diagnosis, is similar [4,6,10,34,35,37,43,44], highlighting the difficulties that they have to understand the symptoms, their uncertainty with regard to the diagnosis and uncertainty about the complexity of treatment. It is important to consider the importance of the history of uncertainty in chronic diseases [15,45].

In half of the reviewed studies, we observed that patients mentioned feelings of uncertainty because of the symptoms, because of the pain and diagnosis complexity and because of the lack of adequate treatment [8,27,28,31–34,37,38,41]. Patients with more pain, who suffer more frequent relapses, have less resistance to stressors related to the disease, and therefore more uncertainty and consequently a worse adaptation [42,43]. All this provokes chronicity and hopelessness [22]. Being diagnosed with fibromyalgia caused mixed feelings in many of the participants [46], although it was a relief for them to have a name for their pain [8,27,30,47]. When patients find a meaning for their disease experience, they reduce their uncertainty or value the knowledge as providing a second chance. This indicates the need to act at this stage and to assess the subcategories of the diagnosis, the symptoms and the treatment, as well as to give information to the patients as nursing professionals and to be in closer contact with the patients, meeting their requirements and supporting them as necessary.

Other authors such as Boulton et al. [28] and Cedraschi et al. [22] warn that diagnosis does not suffice to reduce uncertainty due to the little knowledge that exists about the evolution of the disease and the prognosis; the feeling of the lack of knowledge of the disease and its treatment floods the affected people with despair. The diagnosis is a relief, although it is sometimes difficult to live with chronicity. The subcategory of the complexity of the treatment showed that those patients with the greatest degree of uncertainty about their prognosis were those with the worst adherence to treatment [36]. This is another important factor that nurses should understand about FMS patients.

The category of cognitive assessment was reflected in patients with FMS when they reported their experiences of fear and threat [36]. In total, 66% of the patients in the studies analyzed show feelings of vulnerability and fear without really accepting their new health–disease condition. This disease is linked to psychopathology, stress, anxiety and depression. Chronic pain as a routine produces a great deal of suffering and limitations [37], and people affected by FMS feel imprisoned by pain [40]. Another way in which some people try to confront the diagnosis is to approach religion or spirituality [16], which emerges as an emotional support. Faith in some superior being fills these people with motivation, relief, self-improvement, and strength.

Patients use different strategies to cope with the disease, which are family support, peer support, associations and support groups. Health professionals represent a main source of support.

In relation to health professionals, study participants value their credibility from the outset, including their comprehensive and individualized attention. They seek a good level of communication and understanding by professionals, and they need support in the search for effective solutions, considering this therapeutic support in itself [27,30,35]. Therefore, the coordination of different professionals is essential to understand the treatment prescribed, so multidisciplinary sessions would be necessary [27,38]. Multidisciplinary intervention allows the implementation of solutions for self-care, active listening, and reflection, leading to awareness and autonomy [38]. Health education in self-care, support and understanding empowers a person with FMS [32]. According to the search of Alameda et al. [27], the ultimate goal of nursing is to determine the vulnerability caused by the exclusion of these people.

Family members may also experience uncertainty about the illness of one of their relatives; if this occurs, care can be affected. Nurses should address the concerns of caregivers and provide information about the disease [42]. The stability of women improves with the physical and moral support of the partner and family [29].

Therefore, the three subcategories that have been detailed in Table 2 are present frequently in the discourses of the experiences of FMS patients, and these coincide with the most important aspects to assess in chronic and complex diseases [46]. This revision gives credence to these aspects in improving the management of uncertainty.

For some patients, beating FMS means being happy in difficult circumstances and finding small pleasures in daily life [41]. For others, it means clinging to fragments of their previous lives, whether through work or by continuing to pay attention to aspects of daily life. Taking this into consideration, we must continue to carry out studies and reviews that produce a benefit for a better nursing assessment and performance in these patients.

This review is not exempt from limitations. Even though the sources used in the search are pertinent, they might not give a full account of all the relevant studies in this subject. We must bear in mind that, although the databases used to search for the studies are relevant, not all the available studies were collected; therefore, there may be some missing relevant research in this area. We avoided the use of excessive databases to limit the number of repeated articles found; however, a large number of duplicate documents were discarded.

Finally, it would have been interesting to include studies with a more balanced sample of male and female patients and to have been able to review and analyze a gender comparison with more scientific evidence, as well as to have been able to identify possible gender differences and determine actions to further reduce the level of uncertainty and to increase the patients' ability to cope with the illness.

5. Conclusions

The approach to these categories in the assessment of FMS patients can be a valuable tool for a multidisciplinary team since it allows problems to be identified and interventions to be designed which aim to reducing uncertainty and improve patients' adaptation to the disease.

Uncertainty and FMS are closely linked due to a lack of knowledge about the pathophysiological mechanisms of the disease.

People diagnosed with FMS often perceive uncertainty as a danger or threat, which leads to situations of stress, anxiety and emotional disorder. The longer the uncertainty lasts in the context of the disease, the more unstable the person's mode of functioning will be.

This review demonstrates the presence of three categories and eight subcategories based on Mishel's model of uncertainty in disease. Addressing these categories can help patients find meaning in FMS, properly manage uncertainty and accept it as a natural part of a new life that makes sense despite the disease.

Practical Implication

The key message from the study findings for nurses is that they must be alert to potential risk factors for patients with FMS.

This review shows which aspects are most relevant to assess in FMS patients to reduce their uncertainty and face their disease with the best possible professional support.

Author Contributions: Conceptualization, A.F.-A. and C.T.-O.; methodology, A.F.-A.; software, C.T.-O.; validation, A.F.-A., and A.G.-A.; formal analysis, C.T.-O.; investigation, A.F.-A.; resources, C.T.-O.; data curation, A.G.-A.; writing—original draft preparation, A.F.-A. and J.G.-C.; writing—review and editing, J.G.-C.; visualization, J.G.-C.; supervision, Z.V.; project administration, A.F.-A. All authors have read and agreed to the published version of the manuscript.

References

1. Reich, J.W.; Johnson, L.M.; Zautra, A.J.; Davis, M.C. Uncertainty of illness relationships with mental health and coping processes in fibromyalgia patients. *J. Behav. Med.* **2006**, *29*, 307–316. [CrossRef] [PubMed]
2. Galvez-Sánchez, C.M.; Montoro, C.I.; Duschek, S.; Del Paso, G.A.R. Depression and trait-anxiety mediate the influence of clinical pain on health-related quality of life in fibromyalgia. *J. Affect. Disord.* **2020**, *265*, 486–495. [CrossRef] [PubMed]
3. Ashe, S.C.; Furness, P.J.; Taylor, S.J.; Haywood-Small, S.; Lawson, K. A qualitative exploration of the experiences of living with and being treated for fibromyalgia. *Health Psychol. Open* **2017**, 4. [CrossRef] [PubMed]
4. Queiroz, L. Worldwide epidemiology of fibromyalgia. *Curr. Pain Headache Rep.* **2013**, *17*, 356. [CrossRef]
5. Levine, J.D.; Reichling, D.B. Fibromyalgia: The nerve of that disease. *J. Rheumatol.* **2005**, *32*, 29–37.
6. Long, T.C. The fibromyalgia dilemma. *J. Controv. Med. Claims* **2004**, *11*, 1–8.
7. Häuser, W.; Sarzi-Puttini, P.; Fitzcharles, M.A. Fibromyalgia syndrome: Under-, over- and misdiagnosis. *Clin. Exp. Rheumatol.* **2019**, *37*, 90–97.
8. Escudero, M.J.; García-Toyos, N.; Prieto Rodríguez, M.A.; Pérez Corral, O.; March Cerdá, J.C.; López Doblas, M. Fibromyalgia: patients' perception of their disease and the health system. Qualitative Research Study. *Reumatol. Clin.* **2010**, *6*, 16–22. [CrossRef]
9. Quintner, J.; Buchanan, D.; Cohen, M.; Taylor, A. Signification and Pain: A Semiotic Reading of Fibromyalgia. *Theor. Med. Bioeth.* **2003**, *24*, 345–354. [CrossRef]
10. Akkasilpa, S.; Goldman, D.; Magder, L.S.; Petri, M. Number of fibromyalgia tender points is associated with health status in patients with systemic lupus erythematosus. *J. Rheumatol.* **2005**, *32*, 48–50.
11. Triviño, A.; Solano, M.C.; Siles, J.; Ruiz, S. Application of an uncertainty theory for fibromyalgia. *Atten. Primaria* **2015**, *48*, 219–225.
12. Marcus, D.A.; Richards, K.L.; Chambers, J.F.; Bhowmick, A. Fibromyalgia family and relationship impact exploratory survey. *Musculoskelet. Care* **2013**, *11*, 125–134. [CrossRef] [PubMed]

13. Fitzcharles, M.A.; Yunus, M.B. The clinical concept of fibromyalgia as a changing paradigm in the past 20 years. *Pain Res. Treat.* **2012**, *2012*, 184835. [CrossRef] [PubMed]
14. Poindexter, K.H. Manejo de enfermería del síndrome de fibromialgia. *Medsurg Nurs.* **2017**, *26*, 349–352.
15. Peters, A.; McEwen, B.S.; Friston, K. Uncertainty and stress: Why it causes disease and how it is dominated by the brain. *Prog. Neurobiol.* **2017**, *156*, 164–188. [CrossRef]
16. Mishel, M. Reconceptualization of the uncertainty in illness theory. *J. Nurs. Scholarsh.* **1990**, *22*, 256–262. [CrossRef]
17. Mishel, M.H. Uncertainty in acute illness. *Annu. Rev. Nurs. Res.* **1997**, *15*, 57–80. [CrossRef]
18. Bailey, D.E., Jr.; Stewart, J.L. Uncertainty in Illness Theory. In *Nursing Theorists and Their Work*, 8th ed.; Alligood, M.R., Ed.; Elsevier Mosby: St. Louis, MO, USA, 2013; pp. 555–573.
19. Clayton, M.F.; Marleah, D.; Merle, M. Middle Range Theory for Nursing. In *Theories of Uncertainty in Illness*; Springer Publishing Company: New York, NY, USA, 2018; ISBN 978-0-8261-5991-5 49-88.
20. Kroencke, D.C. Coping with Multiple Sclerosis: The Impact of Uncertainty on Illness. Master's Thesis, University of Catalunya, Tarragona, Spain, 1999.
21. Malin, K.; Littlejohn, G.O. Personality and fibromyalgia syndrome. *Open Rheumatol. J.* **2012**, *6*, 273. [CrossRef]
22. Cedraschi, E.; Girard, C.; Luthy, M.; Kossovsky, J.; Desmeules, A.F. Primary attributions in women suffering fibromyalgia emphasize the perception of a disruptive onset for a long-lasting pain problem. *J. Psichosom. Res.* **2013**, *74*, 265–269. [CrossRef]
23. Taylor, A.G.; Adelstein, K.E.; Fischer-White, T.G.; Murugesan, M.; Anderson, J.G. Perspectives on Living with Fibromyalgia. *Glob. Qual. Nurs. Res.* **2016**, 3. [CrossRef]
24. Cano, A.; González, T.; Cabello, J. Template to help you understand a qualitative study. In *CASPe Guidelines for Critical Reading of Medical Literature*; University of Alicante: Alicante, Spain, 2010.
25. Anema, C.; Johnson, M.; Zeller, J.M.; Fogg, L.; Zetterlund, J. Spiritual well-being in individuals with fibromyalgia syndrome: Relationships with symptom pattern variability, uncertainty, and psychosocial adaptation. *Res. Theory Nurs. Pract.* **2020**, *223*, 8–22. [CrossRef] [PubMed]
26. Alameda Cuesta, A.; Pazos Garciandía, Á.; Oter Quintana, C.; Losa Iglesias, M.E. Fibromyalgia, Chronic Fatigue Syndrome, and Multiple Chemical Sensitivity: Illness Experiences. *Clin. Nurs. Res.* **2019**. [CrossRef] [PubMed]
27. Boulton, T. Nothing and Everything: Fibromyalgia as a Diagnosis of Exclusion and Inclusion. *Qual. Health Res.* **2018**, *29*, 809–819. [CrossRef] [PubMed]
28. Briones-Vozmediano, B.; Tula, E.; Vives Cases, C.; Goicolea, I. "I'm not the woman I was": Women's perceptions of the effects of fibromyalgia on private life. *Health Care Women Int.* **2016**, *37*, 836–854. [CrossRef] [PubMed]
29. Briones-Vozmediano, E.; Ronda-Perez, E.; Vives-Cases, C. Perceptions of patients with fibromyalgia on the impact of the disease in the workplace. *Aten Primaria* **2014**, *47*, 205–212. [CrossRef]
30. Cooper, S.; Gilbert, L. An exploratory study of the experience of fibromyalgia diagnosis in South Africa. *Health* **2017**, *21*, 337–353. [CrossRef]
31. Humphrey, L.; Arbuckle, R.; Mease, P.; Williams, D.A.; Samsoe, B.D.; Gilbert, C. Fatigue in fibromyalgia: A conceptual model informed by patient interviews. *BMC Musculoskelet. Disord.* **2010**, *11*, 216. [CrossRef]
32. Juuso, P.; Skär, L.; Olsson, M.; Söderberg, S. Living with a double burden: Meanings of pain for women with fibromyalgia. *Int. J. Qual. Stud. Health Well-Being* **2011**, *6*. [CrossRef]
33. Matarín, T.M.; Fernández-Sola, C.; Hernández-Padilla, J.M.; Correa Casado, M.; Antequera Raynal, L.H.; Granero-Molina, J. Perceptions about the sexuality of women with fibromyalgia syndrome: A phenomenological study. *J. Adv. Nurs.* **2017**, *73*, 1646–1656. [CrossRef]
34. Miranda, N.A.C.G.; Berardinelli, L.M.M.; Saboia, V.M.; Brito, I.S.; Santos, R.S. Interdisciplinary care praxis in groups of people living with fibromyalgia. *Rev. Bras. Enferm.* **2016**, *69*, 1115–1123. [CrossRef]
35. Montesó-Curto, P.; García-Martinez, M.; Romaguera, S.; Mateu, M.L.; Cubí-Guillén, M.T.; Sarrió-Colas, L.; Panisello-Chavarria, M.L. Problems and solutions for patients with fibromyalgia: Building new helping relationships. *J. Adv. Nurs.* **2018**, *74*, 339–349. [CrossRef]
36. Olivé Ferrer, M.C.; Isla Pera, M.P. Experience of fibromyalgia. *Rev. Enferm.* **2013**, *36*, 48.
37. Oliveira, J.; Pereira Ramos, B.; Marcia Migueis, L.; Cavaliere, M.L.A.; Celi Alves, R.; Costa, L.P.D.; Barbosa, J.S.O. The routines of women with fibromyalgia and an interdisciplinary challenge to promote

self-care. *Rev. Gaúcha Enferm.* **2019**, *40*, e20180411. Available online: http://www.scielo.br/scielo.php?script=sci_arttext&pid=S1983-14472019000100431&lng=en (accessed on 15 December 2019).
38. Romero-Alcalá, P.; Hernández-Padilla, J.M.; Fernández-Sola, C.; del Rosario Coín-Pérez-Carrasco, M.; Ramos-Rodríguez, C.; Ruiz-Fernández, M.D.; Granero-Molina, J. Sexuality in male partners of women with fibromyalgia syndrome: A qualitative study. *PLoS ONE* **2019**, 14. [CrossRef] [PubMed]
39. Sallinen, M.; Mengshoel, A.M.; Solbrække, K. "I can't have it; I am a man. A young man!"—Men, fibromyalgia and masculinity in a Nordic context. *Int. J. Qual. Stud. Health Well-Being* **2019**, *14*, 1. [CrossRef] [PubMed]
40. Sorense, K.; Christianensen, B. Adolescents' experience of complex persistent pain. *Scand. J. Pain* **2017**, *15*, 106–112. [CrossRef] [PubMed]
41. Wuytack, F.; Miller, P. The lived experience of fibromyalgia in female patients, a phenomenological study. *Chiropr. Man. Ther.* **2011**, *19*, 22. [CrossRef]
42. Mas, A.J.; Carmona, L.; Valverde, M.; Ribas, B. Prevalence and impact of fibromyalgia on function and quality of life in individuals from the general population: Results from a nationwide study in Spain. *Clin. Exp. Rheumatol.* **2008**, *26*, 519.
43. Perez, I.R.; Linares, M.U.; Perez, M.B.; Brown, J.P.; Labry Lima, A.O.; Torres, E.H. Differences in characteristics sociodemographic, clinical and psychological men and women diagnosed with fibromyalgia. *Span. Clin. Mag.* **2007**, *207*, 433–439.
44. Clauw, D.J.; D'Arcy, Y.; Gebke, K.; Semel, D.; Pauer, L.; Kim, D. Jones Normalizing fibromyalgia as a chronic illness. *Postgrad. Med.* **2018**, *130*, 9–18. [CrossRef]
45. Råheim, M.; Håland, W. Lived experience of chronic pain and fibromyalgia: Women's stories from daily life. *Qual. Health Res.* **2006**, *16*, 741–761. [CrossRef]
46. Mannerkorpi, K.; Palstam, A.; Gard, G. Factors promoting sustainable work in women with fibromyalgia. *Disabil. Rehabil.* **2013**, *35*, 1622–1629.
47. Menzies, V. CE: Fibromyalgia Syndrome Current Considerations in Symptom Management. *Am. J. Nurs.* **2016**, *116*, 24–32. [CrossRef] [PubMed]

6

Satisfaction with Social Support Received from Social Relationships in Cases of Chronic Pain: The Influence of Personal Network Characteristics in Terms of Structure, Composition and Functional Content

Rosario Fernández-Peña [1,*], José Luis Molina [2] and Oliver Valero [3]

1 Department of Nursing, University of Cantabria (Spain), SALBIS Research Group, Nursing Research Group IDIVAL, 39008 Santander, Spain

2 Department of Social and Cultural Anthropology, GRAFO, Universitat Autònoma de Barcelona, 08193 Barcelona, Spain; joseluis.molina@uab.cat

3 Servei d'Estadística Aplicada, Universitat Autònoma de Barcelona, 08193 Barcelona, Spain; oliver.valero@uab.cat

* Correspondence: roser.fernandez@unican.es

Abstract: The worldwide burden of chronic illnesses, constitutes a major public health concern and a serious challenge for health systems. In addition to the strategies of self-management support developed by nursing and health organizations, an individual's personal network represents a major resource of social support in the long-term. Adopting a cross-sectional design based on personal network analysis methods, the main aim of this study is to explore the relationship between satisfaction with the social support received by individuals suffering chronic pain and the structure, composition, and functional content in social support of their personal networks. We collected personal and support network data from 30 people with chronic pain (20 person's contacts (alters) for each individual (ego), 600 relationships in total). Additionally, we examined the level of satisfaction with social support in each of the 600 relationships. Bivariate and multivariate tests were performed to analyze the satisfaction with the social support received. Using cluster analysis, we established a typology of the 600 relationships under study. Results showed that higher satisfaction was associated with a balance between degree centrality and betweenness (i.e., measures of network cohesion and network modularity, respectively). Finally, new lines of research are proposed in order to broaden our understanding of this subject.

Keywords: social support; patient satisfaction; chronic disease; chronic pain

---

1. Introduction

Chronic illness constitutes a critical public health challenge that affects both social and economic development worldwide. Chronic illness also represents a major challenge for health services. Data from the WHO reveals that noncommunicable diseases (NCDs) cause 41 million deaths annually, equivalent to 71% of all deaths globally [1].

The steady increase in the prevalence of chronic illnesses is due, in part, to the progressive aging of the population, together with an increased life expectancy. Thus, people with several illnesses or chronic conditions live longer than in the past [2]. Faced with this scenario, health services are undergoing a reorganizational shift from a model centered on illness and treatment, to one centered on the individual and their particular chronic conditions. Both institutional and personal environments are also very important to chronic illness patients, comprising sources of support outside the more formal health and/or social systems.

A key element of the models developed to face chronicity is self-management. This concept emphasizes the patient's role in managing health and has been defined as an 'individual's ability to manage the symptoms, treatment, physical, and psychosocial consequences and lifestyle changes inherent in living with a chronic condition' [3]. This is a changing construct, which reflects the different types of support needed throughout the progression of the illness, mediated by such factors as the stage of the illness, its stability over time, the symptoms, and the physical limitations, among others [4]. However, as proposed by Morris et al. [5], the notion of self-management is questionable, as an individual construct, namely because many practices concerning the management of illnesses involve the support and/or negotiation of roles within the framework of relationships. Therefore, in essence, chronic illnesses are not restricted to the individual, rather they are 'embedded in family, community, and societal conditions that shape and influence—and may constrain—the choices people make, or can make' [6]. Based on this change in paradigm, the Innovate Care for Chronic Conditions (ICCC) of the WHO, propose a framework for health systems to improve the management of chronic conditions. This framework proposes the following micro, meso, and macro levels of health care systems: The level of interaction with the patient (micro), the organization of healthcare at the community level (meso), and the level of politics (macro). Each level dynamically interacts and influences the other two over time, via feedback loops [7]. According to the ICCC framework, optimal outcomes are achieved when a partnership exists between health care teams, community partners, and patients and their families [8], i.e., when individual self-management is embedded in the social systems of support that make it possible. Furthermore, certain aspects of the community are highly relevant, such as associations for patients and their families, making caregivers increasingly influential [9].

Along these lines, different dedicated programs and interventions have been developed by health organizations to improve self-management, including assessments based on the perspectives of both patients and health professionals [10–12]. Likewise, other programs have used a community approach, focusing on supporting the self-management of chronic illness on behalf of the individual's social networks [5,13–17]. However, these latter approaches do not provide tie-level measures of the social environments in which self-management may be developed. In addition, they use the terms 'social support' and 'social networks' interchangeably, conflating two related but unidentical social phenomena. Social support has been defined as 'support accessible to an individual through social ties to other individuals, groups, and the larger community' [18]. Instead, social networks have been described as 'the direct and indirect ties linking a group of individuals over certain definable criteria, such as kinship, friendship, and acquaintances.' Therefore, social networks provide a structural framework in which support may, or may not, be accessible to the individual [19]. We aim to contribute to the research in this field by providing detailed social tie-level information about the social environment of individuals in situations of chronic pain on one hand, and information about the content of the relationship on the other without prejudging the existence of social support.

Furthermore, in the study of social support, three differentiated aspects of social ties are distinguished: (1) the existence or number of relationships as a reflection of social integration, (2) the formal structure of the same or social networks, and the functional content, in this case, social support (3) and the influence of the structure of social relationships on functional content in social support [20,21].

Social network analysis (SNA) is a research method that examines the interactions between individuals, groups, and organizations, which has been applied in a variety of research areas. In the context of health, this approach has led to academic literature which has significantly increased in recent decades, prioritizing the role of social structure, including the areas of community and primary health, care and nursing research [22–26], identifying new challenges and providing opportunities for innovative research.

Social support has been studied in several contexts, one of which is informal caregiving [27,28]. Compared to other approaches in social support research, personal network analysis (PNA), also labeled as egocentric network analysis in the literature [29], is based on the ensemble of relationships that surround an individual (ego) across social settings (i.e., family, work colleagues, neighbors, ...), as well as the relationships between the person's contacts (alters) [30,31]. This enables the simultaneous study of micro phenomena (interactions) and meso phenomena (the social networks and institutions that the individual belongs to on a community level) [32]. Previous research has noted the effects of personal networks on individual outcomes based on theoretical frameworks, such as the social capital and the social influence through diffusion and social support, with the latter being one of the most studied areas based both on this approach and on different disciplines [33]. From this perspective, a PNA, constitutes an excellent approach to the study of social support in the context of informal care in chronic illness, since this can be used to measure the structure and composition of personal networks and the functional content of social support. This enables the possibility of differentiating the personal network from the support network (comprising both support providers and non-providers), as well as relating these personal network characteristics, including the structural variables, with other variables of interest. Whereas, in general, social support studies evaluate the quality, or the quantity, of a person's social ties, studies based on PNA regard these ties as being potentially of interest [34]. This is based on the importance of the relationships between the interacting units [30]. Therefore, the structural variables of these relationships are commonly included in the analysis.

In the study of social support, one dimension of interest is the quality or sense of satisfaction. This dimension reflects the discrepancy among the interactions between real and desired (or necessary) support. The relevance of this distinction is that satisfaction with social support provides a better explanation of the quality of life and health outcomes when compared with the mere provision or number of support providers [35,36]. Regarding the assessment of satisfaction, although it has been used in some instruments intended to evaluate social support [37], there is a gap in the literature regarding the role of the personal networks' characteristics in the quality or satisfaction with social support. Thus, this study focuses on the quality of social support received from personal networks in the context of chronic pain. This dimension has seldom been researched [36,38] despite being a highly relevant health problem due to its prevalence, complexity, and the consequences for both the individual and the social environment in which it is embedded [39,40]. Our approach provides a rich set of measures at the tie level that allows us to measure with detail personal networks' structure, composition, and functional content of social support along with its perceived quality. Just having this type of detailed information, it is possible to suggest ways to improve the effective self-management of individuals in chronic pain situations.

2. Materials and Methods

This research is part of a larger study aimed at examining social support and quality of life in the context of chronic pain [41]. In a prior publication, the descriptive results of this larger study were presented using a mixed approach [42], showing that different types of personal networks were associated with self-reported quality of life, which scored below the populational mean in all dimensions considered.

2.1. Design

A descriptive, cross-sectional study using personal network analysis.

2.2. Sample Description

The inclusion criteria of participants were people over the age of 18 diagnosed with chronic pain, and receiving care at Marques de Valdecilla University Hospital Pain Unit of Santander (Spain), without mental or cognitive decline and who agreed to participate voluntarily in the study. Convenience sampling was used to select participants: An equal number of men and women (15 in each case) that met the inclusion criteria and were recommended by professionals working at the pain management unit among their patients. All voluntary participants were briefed about the goals and methods of the research and signed an informed consent form (see Section 2.6 below). All of them agreed to be interviewed several times if necessary, either at the hospital or participants' homes, according to their health status and personal preferences. Nobody requested to quit the research, probably because of the positive assessment of both the attention and feedback about their personal networks they received during the interviews. Fieldwork and data analysis were conducted between July 2014 and July 2015. The personal networks of the 30 cases amounted to a total of 600 personal relationships (20 relationships per ego).

2.3. Variables

The data collection included participant variables (ego), their contacts (alter) and details regarding their personal network (see [41,42] for further information regarding the variables):

(a) Sociodemographic data (ego characteristics): sex, age, civil status, level of studies, and work situation.
(b) Variables regarding the composition of the personal network (alter characteristics): Age, sex, type of tie with ego, place of residence, and proximity.
(c) Social support (function): type (emotional, instrumental, informational, and combinations of the same), satisfaction, reciprocity, variation over time, frequency, and channel of transmission.
(d) Variables regarding the structure of the personal network: density, degree centrality (two measures; mean of the alter-alter matrix and at node level), betweenness centrality (two measures; mean of a personal network and at node level), number of components and number of isolates.

2.4. Data Collection Instruments

Personal network: EgoNet open-source software (https://sourceforge.net/projects/egonet/), was used to collect and analyze each ego's personal network data. Additionally, UCInet software [43] was used to calculate degree, and betweenness centrality for each of the 600 alters studied. Sociodemographic, pain variables, and personal network data were collected based on an ad hoc questionnaire designed in accordance with the study objectives.

2.5. Data Analysis

Bivariate linear mixed models were used to analyze the satisfaction with the social support received. These were converted into the following numerical values: very unsatisfactory = 0, quite unsatisfactory = 1, satisfactory = 2, quite satisfactory = 3, and very satisfactory = 4. Ego characteristics and structure, composition, and functional content in social support of their personal network were considered as explanatory variables. The ego was included as a random effect for the analysis of the structure and composition of alter variables. Variables with a p-value of 0.2 were included in a multivariate logistic regression model to identify which factors were related to satisfactory or very satisfactory support.

Additionally, a multiple correspondence analysis (MCA) combined with classification methods were used in order to establish typologies for the 600 relationships examined in terms of the quality of the social support received from the ego's point of view. MCA is a descriptive, exploratory technique designed to analyze multi-way contingency tables with cases as rows and categories of variables as columns [44]. Components obtained from the MCA were submitted to a cluster analysis applying Ward's hierarchical clustering method [45,46]. Results were represented in a tree dendrogram using R-squared distance. Bivariate tests were conducted between each of the explanatory variables and the profiles, using chi-square tests to describe the obtained profiles.

The statistical analysis was performed using SAS v9.4 software (SAS Institute Inc., Cary, NC, USA), and the significance level was set at $p < 0.05$.

2.6. Ethical Considerations

The Clinical Research Ethics Committee of Cantabria (Spain) provided ethical approval for this study (internal code 2014.32). All study participants received verbal and written information concerning the study objectives and procedure. Participation was voluntary, and all participants provided their signed informed consent. Furthermore, this study adhered to national and international ethical guidelines (Code of Ethics and Declaration of Helsinki) and fulfilled data confidentiality legislation (Spanish organic law 15/1999 of 13 December on the protection of personal data).

3. Results

3.1. Sociodemographic Variables

In total, 30 people participated in the study (15 women and 15 men). The mean age of participants was 54.57 years (SD 11.64, range 30–73 years). Their marital status was married or with a partner ($n = 27$); divorced ($n = 1$); and widowed ($n = 2$). Their educational level was primary education ($n = 16$), vocational education ($n = 8$), secondary education ($n = 4$), and higher education ($n = 2$). Their employment status at the time of the interview was: retired ($n = 10$), active ($n = 9$), on sick leave due to pain ($n = 6$), and homemaker ($n = 5$). The mean length of time since the onset of chronic pain was 12.2 years (SD 9.18, range 1–35 years) in men and 16.6 years (SD 12.39, range 1–39) in women.

3.2. Bivariate Analysis

The satisfaction with the social support received in the 600 personal relationships studied was distributed as follows: very satisfactory 12.3%, quite satisfactory 22%, satisfactory 26%, quite unsatisfactory 6.5%. The very unsatisfactory category was present in 33.2%, corresponding to relationships where no support was provided (see also [27] for descriptive analysis of other variables related to social support function).

3.2.1. Ego Variables

From the bivariate analysis, no statistically significant relationships were observed (p-value > 0.05) between satisfaction with social support received and the following ego variables: Age, gender, level of studies, work situation, civil status, level of pain, pain duration, and the number of cohabitants. However, the results obtained, when comparing the means of age and duration of pain variables for the ego, are notable. The quality of social support received decreased as the ego's age increased, and as the time with chronic pain increased.

Age of ego (p-value 0.174): for the categorical variable age, as age increased, satisfaction decreased (for every 10 years, satisfaction values decreased by 0.16 units):

- Participants aged between 30 and 51 years; mean satisfaction 2.01 (SD 0.19).
- Participants aged between 52 and 63 years; mean satisfaction 1.72 (SD 0.17).
- Participants aged between 65 and 73 years; mean satisfaction 1.51 (SD 0.18).

Duration of pain (p-value 0.096): using the categorical variable model and recoding the duration of pain variable, we observed that, as the duration of pain increased, satisfaction decreased:

- Duration of pain between 1 and 8 years; mean satisfaction 2.04 (SD 0.18).
- Duration of pain between 9 and 19 years; mean satisfaction 1.67 (SD 0.18).
- Duration of pain between 20 and 39 years; mean satisfaction 1.5 (SD 0.18).

3.2.2. Composition Variables

Regarding the composition variables (Table 1), the most satisfactory support was defined by an adult female alter, with whom the ego had a strong tie, who was a close family member (partner, parents, and children) and who lived geographically close.

Table 1. Satisfaction and composition variables of the personal network.

Variable	Category	Mean (SD)
Age of the alter *	≤30 years	1.36 (0.17)
	31–50 years	1.95 (0.13)
	51–60 years	1.67 (0.16)
	>60 years	1.69 (0.14)
Sex of the alter *	Women	1.91 (0.12)
	Men	1.56 (0.12)
Tie with the ego *	Partner	3.22 (0.26)
	Parents	3.03 (0.33)
	Brothers	1.75 (0.18)
	Children	2.77 (0.19)
	Other family members	1.32 (0.13)
	Friends	1.61 (0.14)
	Other ties	1.41 (0.18)
Strength of the tie *	Very close	2.83 (0.13)
	Quite close	2.19 (0.12)
	Close	1.50 (0.12)
	Not very close	0.74 (0.13)
	Not at all close	0.21 (0.20)
Place of residence of the alter compared to the ego	Same locality	1.89 (0.13)
	Same province	1.66 (0.13)
	Other province/country	1.53 (0.18)

* p-value < 0.05.

3.2.3. Structural Variables

Regarding the structural variables of the personal network (Table 2), the quality of the social support received increased as the density of the network increased. In contrast, the quality of support decreased as the number of isolates and components increased. Regarding the node, as the degree centrality of the alter increased (a measure related to the density of the network), satisfaction increased. Likewise, satisfaction increased as the betweenness centrality of the alter increased.

Table 2. Satisfaction and structure variables of the personal network and alters.

Variable	Range/Category	Mean (SD)
Density *	<40%	1.57 (0.15)
	41–60%	1.64 (0.16)
	>60%	2.28 (0.22)
Degree centrality (alter) *	0–5	1.35 (0.14)
	6–11	1.60 (0.13)
	12–19	2.35 (0.15)
Betweeness Centrality (alter) *	0	1.44 (0.13)
	0.1–1.2	1.69 (0.15)
	1.2–114.3	2.12 (0.14)
Components	1	2 (0.16)
	2	1.54 (0.20)
	3–11	1.58 (0.18)
Isolates	0	1.89 (0.14)
	1	1.63 (0.23)
	2–9	1.46 (0.22)

* p-value < 0.05.

3.2.4. Functional Social Support

Regarding the social support characteristics, of the 600 relationships examined, 401 support-providing relationships were identified (66.83%) and 199 relationships in which support was not provided (33.17%). Thus, the mean number of providers and non-providers was 13 and 7, respectively, for each ego. The functional variables concerning social support (Table 3), reveal that the personal relationships offering greater quality support from the ego's perspective were characterized by offering various types of support (multiplexity). This was provided face-to-face or combined with daily telephone calls, which could become more frequent over time and occurred in reciprocal support relationships.

Table 3. Satisfaction and social support variables.

Variable	Category	Mean (SE)
Social support variables in provider relationships (n = 401)		
Type *	Emotional	2.37 (0.07)
	Emotional and instrumental	3.18 (0.10)
	Emotional, instrumental and informational	3.62 (0.18)
	Other types of support	2.55 (0.14)
Frequency *	Daily	3.26 (0.09)
	Weekly	2.57 (0.08)
	Biweekly	2.42 (0.12)
	Monthly	1.94 (0.11)
	>2 months	1.83 (0.15)
Transmission channel *	Face-to-face	2.70 (0.09)
	By telephone	2.22 (0.13)
	Face-to-face and by telephone	2.74 (0.10)
	Internet/Telephone + internet	2.16 (0.28)
Variation of support *	Increases	3.22 (0.18)
	No variation	1.47 (0.12)
	Decreases	1.73 (0.19)
Reciprocity *	Yes	1.97 (0.10)
	No	0.99 (0.14)

SE = Standard Error.* p-value < 0.05.

3.3. *Multivariate Logistic Regression Model*

From the multivariate logistic regression model, we obtained that the variables which were related to the satisfactory or very satisfactory support were: Age of the ego (the level of satisfaction with the social support received decreased as the age of the ego increased), sex of the alter (women offered more satisfactory support compared to men), tie with the ego (close family members, friends, and neighbors provide more satisfactory support), reciprocal relationships in the support and relationships in which the ego has a very strong tie.

3.4. *Cluster Analysis*

In order to explore the 600 relationships examined in terms of the quality of the social support received a multiple correspondence analysis was performed. Variables included in the analysis were the sex of the alter, tie with the ego, type of support, satisfaction, frequency, transmission channel, reciprocity, and proximity. We obtained 11 factors that accounted for 75% of the total variability. Applying a classification algorithm to these factors, three clusters were obtained, which comprise the totality of the 600 studied relationships. The satisfaction profiles presented the following distribution: Profile 1 (237 relationships), represented by a majority of satisfactory relations with the social support received; Profile 2 (164 relationships), represented by a majority of very and quite satisfactory relationships considering the social support received, and Profile 3 (199 relationships), represented in its totality by very unsatisfactory relationships, and corresponding to the non-providers of social support present in the personal networks studied.

Table 4 displays the distribution of egos among the three profiles according to age. In consonance with the results of the bivariate analysis presented above and which revealed a decrease of satisfaction as the age of the ego increases, the relationships containing cluster 3 and valued as being very unsatisfactory with the social support received corresponded with egos over the age of 65 in almost 50% of cases.

Table 4. Age of ego and relationships according to the three profiles (%).

Category	Profile 1	Profile 2	Profile 3
30–49 years	38.4	31.1	19.1
50–64 years	35.9	37.2	37.2
65 and over	25.7	31.7	43.7
Total	100	100	100

Graphically, these relations are grouped, forming three profiles, as shown in the following dendrogram (Figure 1). The horizontal axis represents individuals that are grouped by horizontal lines at a height that represent the distance between the two linked clusters.

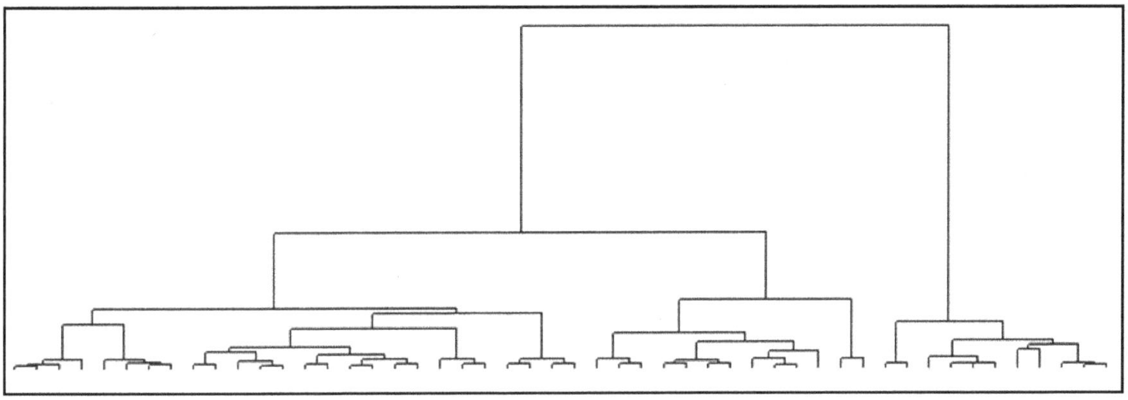

Figure 1. Dendrogram of the hierarchical cluster analysis.

3.4.1. Composition Variables

Table 5 presents the distribution of the personal network composition variables across the three profiles (bivariate tests between the explanatory variables and the profiles). The social support that was deemed more satisfactory was provided by (a) women, (b) close family members (followed by the friends), (c) middle-aged people, (d) those with whom the ego has a strong tie, (e) reciprocal support relationships, and (f) people living geographically close to the ego. Although to a lesser degree, there was a presence of more unsatisfactory relations with non-providers in the case of close adult family members.

For the analysis of the family roles, we have considered: (a) close family members: partner, parents, siblings, and children; (b) family members: Aunts/uncles, grandchildren, cousins, grandparents, nephews/nieces, and brothers/sisters-in-law, and (c) other family members: family roles not included in (a) and (b). The variable 'proximity' was examined based on five categories, which were recoded into two categories: A = strong tie: very close, quite close, and close, and (b) weak tie: not very close and not close at all.

Table 5. Composition variables of the personal network according to the three profiles (%).

Variable	Category	Profile 1	Profile 2	Profile 3
Age of the alter *	<20	2.1	7.3	15.1
	20–39	21.5	24.4	19.6
	40–59	45.6	45.2	32.7
	>60	30.8	23.1	32.6
Sex of the alter *	Male	45.1	41.5	57.8
	Female	54.9	58.5	42.2
Relationship with ego *	Close family members	17.3	59.8	14.1
	Family members	24.9	7.9	24.1
	Other family member	4.2	9.1	17.6
	Friends	35.9	17.1	32.2
	Neighbors	8.4	3	6.5
	Work and professional colleagues	9.3	3	5.5
Strength of the tie *	Strong tie	77.2	100	49.2
	Weak tie	22.8	0	50.8
Place of residence of the alter compared to the ego *	Same location	35	58	43.2
	Same province	43	32.9	40.2
	Other province	17.4	8.5	12.6
	Other province/country	4.6	0.6	4

* p-value < 0.05.

3.4.2. Structural Variables

Table 6 presents the multivariate analysis findings considering the importance that structural measures have on the personal network for the quality of the support, in consonance with the results of the bivariate analysis presented above. In this manner, the personal network providing the most highly-valued level of satisfaction combined both a degree centrality and high density with a high betweenness centrality, both of which were above the overall mean. Likewise, the findings reveal a tendency for satisfaction levels to decrease in networks that were more fragmented, with less cohesion or with a greater number of isolates and components.

Table 6. Structural variables of the personal network. Profile and global means.

Variable	Profile 1	Profile 2	Profile 3	Global Mean
Density	0.44	0.53	0.41	0.45
Degree Centrality [(a)]	7.08	12.44	7.25	8.60
Betweeness Centrality [(a)]	2.41	8.53	2.10	3.98
Components	2.41	2.11	3.03	2.53
Isolates	0.91	0.74	1.62	1.10

[(a)] Alters' centrality measures

3.4.3. Functional Social Support

Regarding the specific characteristics of the social support provided (Table 7), the greatest quality was associated with the combination of different types of support, especially emotional and instrumental support. Likewise, the frequency of the provision of support and face-to-face contact or combined with the provision of telephone support represents the most satisfactory support relationships.

Below, we display the graphs of two study participants with different levels of satisfaction with the social support received. The most satisfactory support network (Figure 2) corresponds to a woman aged 40 years who had chronic pain for 14 years, whereas the graph that illustrates the least satisfactory support network (Figure 3) is that of a man aged 66 years who had experienced chronic pain for 35 years. Table 8 shows the legend of graphs, and Table 9 displays the quantitative results of the differences in these three personal network dimensions examined, as well as the quality of social support.

Table 7. Social support variables in the three profiles (%).

Variable	Category	Profile 1	Profile 2	Profile 3
Type *	Emotional	83.5	34.8	0
	Instrumental	5.1	2.4	0
	Informative	2.1	0	0
	All three types of support	0.4	12.8	0
	Emotional and instrumental	3.4	46.3	0
	Emotional and informative	3.4	3.7	0
	Instrumental and informative	0.4	0	0
	Professional	1.7	0	0
	None	0	0	100
Frequency *	Daily	7.6	63.4	0.5
	Weekly	39.2	31.7	0.5
	Biweekly	17.3	3.7	0
	Monthly	23.6	0.6	0
	Every 2 or 3 months	6.3	0.6	0
	Every 3 months or more	5.9	0	99
Channel of transmission *	Face-to-face	43.5	54.3	0
	By telephone	24.1	3.7	0
	Internet	3	0.6	0
	Face-to-face and by telephone	27.8	41.5	0
	Telephone and internet	1.7	0	0
	No support	0	0	100
Variation *	Has not varied	70.5	61	92
	More support	13.1	31.1	0
	Less support	16.5	7.9	8
Reciprocity *	Yes	78.9	93.3	59.3

* p-value < 0.05.

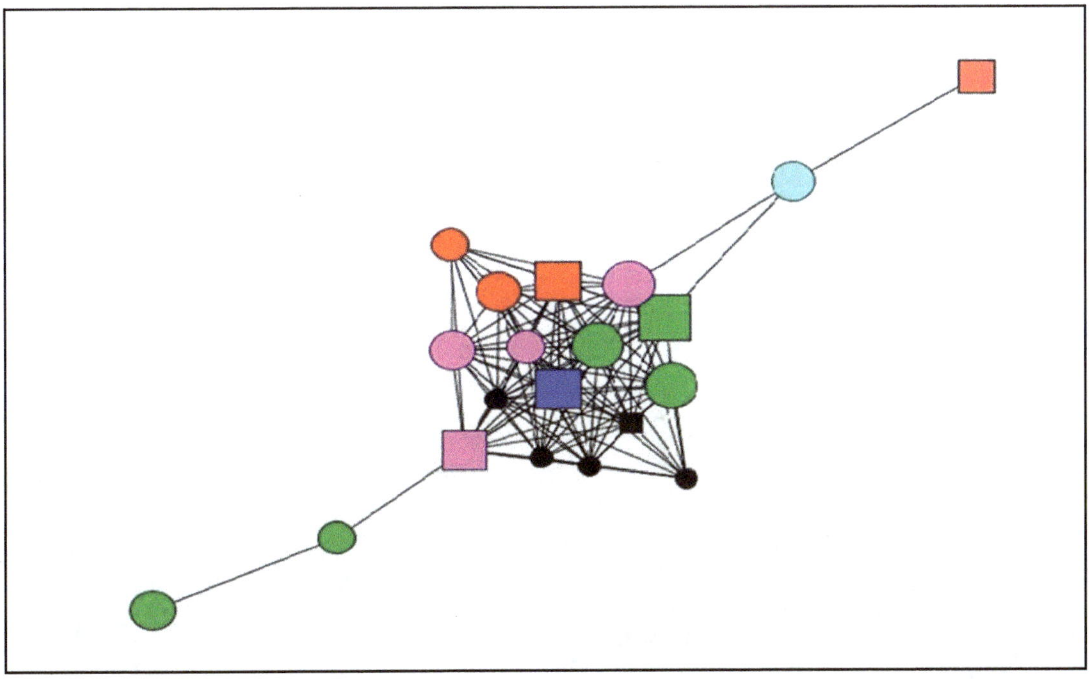

Figure 2. Graph Case 1. Woman (40 years old), living with chronic pain for 14 years.

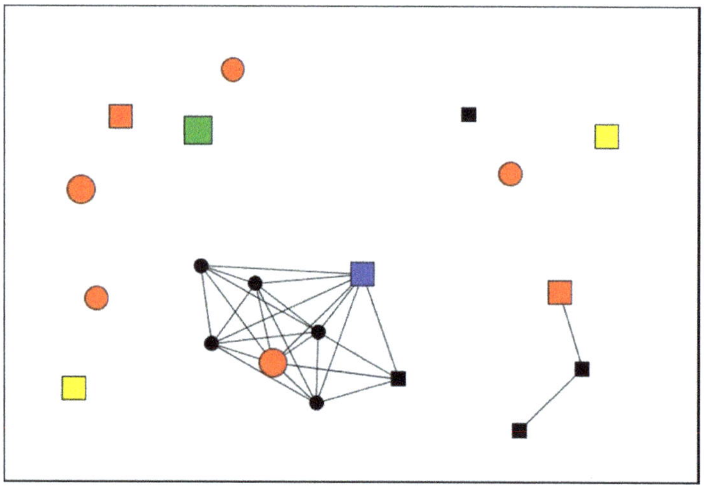

Figure 3. Graph Case 28. Man (66 years old), living with chronic pain for 35 years.

Table 8. Legend of graphs.

Node Shape: Sex	Node Size: Satisfaction	Node Colour: Type of Social Support
Circle: Women Square: Men	Large: More satisfaction Small: Less satisfaction	Red: Emotional Dark blue: Instrumental Pink: Emotional and instrumental Yellow: Informational Green: All types Black: Non-providers Light blue: Emotional and informational Orange: Professional

Table 9. Descriptive analysis of social support at the ego level.

		Case 01	Case 28
Satisfaction (%)	Very satisfactory	20	0
	Quite satisfactory	35	15
	Satisfactory	20	40
	Quite unsatisfactory	0	0
	Very unsatisfactory	25	45
Structure	Density	0.605	0.137
	Degree Centrality (mean)	11.5	2.6
	Betweenness Centrality (mean)	5.7	0.25
	Components	1	11
	Isolates	0	9
Composition (%)	Sex of the alters		
	Women (vs. men)	70	50
	Strength of the tie		
	Strong tie (vs. weak)	80	90
	Place of residence of alters		
	Same locality as ego	80	15
	Reciprocity		
	Yes	45	90
Social support (%)	Type of support		
	All three types	25	5
	Emotional and instrumental	20	0
	Non-providers	25	45
	Variation of support		
	Increases	55	15
	Frequency of support		
	Daily	25	5
	2 or 3 times per week	10	0
	Transmission channel		
	Face-to-face	65	45
	Face-to-face and telephone	10	10

In addition to the differences of age and time since onset of pain in each of the two cases presented, the comparison of these two networks reveals differences affecting the structure, composition, and content of the social support as well as the satisfaction with the social support received by each of the two participants.

4. Discussion

This study aimed to examine the structure, composition, and functional content of social support in the context of personal networks, in relation to satisfaction from the ego perspective. It is important to consider these conditions in order to assess social support as a relational element that is contained and transmitted within social relations [20].

4.1. Composition Variables

The most highly-valued social support was provided by middle-aged female alters, with whom the ego maintained a close relationship and who lived geographically close to the ego. These characteristics highlight the importance of the age of the alter on the ability to offer support (children and older people as non-providers) or the geographical proximity of the alter, which is considered key, especially for the provision of instrumental or tangible support [47–49]. Regarding the type of tie with the ego, our results add to the existing literature, which underlines the significant role of the family and friends in the provision of social support [50]. Nonetheless, it is necessary to consider that, although family roles represent 76.8% of the most satisfactory relationships, they also represent 55.8% of the total number of relationships in the profile identified as the most unsatisfied with the social support received. Therefore, when considering social support in the framework of social relationships, it should be appreciated that not all aspects of so-called close relationships are positive [20,51]. Negative interactions, together with social loss and loneliness, constitute adverse aspects of social interactions [52], which can be detrimental to a person's health by influencing the sense of wellbeing, life stress, less supportive networks, and psychological distress [53–55]. Likewise, specifically in cases of chronic pain, it is also necessary to consider the impact of pain and the resultant effects on a person's social and family relationships [39,40,56], including effects on their partners [57–60]. Therefore, these findings suggest the need for contextual and longitudinal assessments of support in long-term conditions, as these factors affect both the receiver, as well as the provider of support and the relationship dynamics.

4.2. Structural Variables

Our results have shown that quality in the provision of social support is related to certain levels of density as well as with a relatively high betweenness centrality. Nonetheless, none of these explain separately the maximum level of satisfaction. Therefore, the results suggest that the ideal support network should strive for a certain balance between a dense center and a periphery that may act as a bridge with other more diverse relationships.

From a sociological point of view, social structures affect and are affected by human behavior [61]. In the field of health, several studies have underlined the role that the network structure plays in different health outcomes, such as the effect of the same on health-related behaviors [62–64] in the transmission of sexually transmitted diseases [65,66] in mental health [67] or the relation between network structure and health status [68]. Likewise, some studies have found certain benefits derived from having a network with different social domains and with a diverse typology of alters, as these can act as facilitators of other resources offering different types of support [69,70]. Therefore, an alter with a high betweenness, as shown by our results, represents a quality support resource for ego, which can benefit from these indirect relationships. Conversely, some studies have found that density is not automatically related to social support [71,72] and that networks with low density are more adaptive and offer greater support according to determined contexts [73]. We contend that this idea of *balance* among density and intermediation in the structure of the personal network is important when evaluating social support. For the case of chronic pain, a dense network may guarantee the availability of emotional support in which strong ties mainly are represented by kin and close relationships. However, the same relationships over time may lead to a redundancy of the already-known support resources, and alters with a high betweenness might enable access to new support resources (information, contacts, etc.) of great value for ego. Although certain levels of density are necessary for achieving a feeling of safety, something necessary in a healthy personal context, the effectiveness of the network in relation to social support is based on ties that allow access to diverse resources with alternative ways of thinking and acting [74,75], and that the person may use as 'social capital' assets [76]. Therefore, in certain contexts, density and intermediation offer different advantages and may, in fact, be complementary [77].

4.3. Functional Social Support

Concerning the types of support provided, emotional support was most highly-valued, followed by the combination of emotional and instrumental support, reinforcing the importance of a multiplexity or diversity of resources [34]. Thus, in the context of chronic pain, emotional support may guarantee a feeling of accompaniment, understanding, and empathy for the other person's situation, as well as constituting a coping resource, enhancing the ability to adapt to the situation and acting as a facilitator of self-management. Furthermore, in the case of chronic pain, having the instrumental support of others is necessary because of the impairments associated with the performance of basic activities of daily living such as, for example, mobilization, hygiene, or personal grooming. Our findings support previous research [78–80] showing that relationships characterized by reciprocal support are those that are most highly-valued, highlighting the importance of this characteristic in relationships involving health aspects. In addition, increasing and frequent face-to-face support is a characteristic of the most highly-valued support relationships. It is important to note that these findings may be related to caregiver burden as a consequence of caring for people with chronic illnesses in the long term [81–83].

According to previous studies [84], and highlighting the importance of the dynamic nature of personal relationships throughout the life cycle, our findings reveal that satisfaction with the social support received decreases as the age of the ego increases and as the time since the onset of pain increases. This aspect is highly relevant in chronic illness and, more specifically, in the case of chronic pain, mainly because of: (a) the increased prevalence of this disorder in aging populations [39,56], (b) the changes in personal networks at the ego-alter level, i.e., the alters that are lost and are added to the personal network over time, and (c) changes in the characteristics of the relationships as a consequence of life events (e.g., marriage, divorce, chronic illness, retirement, etc.) that may affect the content in social support [85–87].

Personal contexts, namely the characteristics of relationships and personal networks, are key elements that help us understand the complexity of satisfaction with social support for self-management in chronic illnesses.

Future research with a longitudinal design is recommended, focused on the study of variations in social support over time in individuals with chronic pain. Lastly, comparative studies involving personal network research may reveal possible differences in structure, composition, and content in the social support of personal networks according to the age of the ego, as well as providing further information on the support networks of older people.

5. Conclusions

The satisfaction with the informal care received by people with chronic pain, via their personal network resources, is different according to personal characteristics, such as age, pain, the amount of time since the onset of chronic pain, as well as characteristics related to their personal network. Person-centered care implies considering the different social and relational contexts in which people live their lives. Support for self-management in situations of chronic illness includes the support provided by primary care nursing professionals and health organizations via different strategies, as well as the support from the social and personal environment surrounding the person and, therefore, both can be considered as being complementary. From the point of view of the support provided by the personal network, we have shown that a balance between degree centrality and betweenness (an indicator of the existence of various social circles connected through the ego) is needed in order to achieve higher satisfaction with the support received. This finding may help to enhance the self-management capabilities of this type of patient by introducing small adjustments to their personal network structures. In this vein, cases in which insufficient or inappropriate social support are detected in an individual's personal environment could benefit from the implementation of strategies, based on specially designed network interventions, with the aim of guaranteeing the continuity and appropriateness of care and support over time.

Author Contributions: R.F.-P. and J.L.M. conceived of the study and designed the research. O.V. analyzed the data. R.F.-P. and J.L.M. wrote the initial manuscript. All authors have read and agreed to the published version of the manuscript.

Acknowledgments: We thank all the people who agreed to take part in the study for their availability and kindness even in times of illness. We also thank the health professionals at the Marqués de Valdecilla University Hospital Pain Unit for their valuable assistance during field work.

References

1. WHO Noncommunicable Diseases. Available online: https://www.who.int/news-room/fact-sheets/detail/noncommunicable-diseases (accessed on 2 April 2020).
2. Wagner, E.H.; Austin, B.T.; Davis, C.; Hindmarsh, M.; Schaefer, J.; Bonomi, A. Improving chronic illness care: Translating evidence into action. *Health Aff.* **2001**, *20*, 64–78. [CrossRef] [PubMed]
3. Barlow, J.; Wright, C.; Sheasby, J.; Turner, A.; Hainsworth, J. Self-management approaches for people with chronic conditions: A review. *Patient Educ. Couns.* **2002**, *48*, 177–187. [CrossRef]
4. Van Houtum, L.; Rijken, M.; Heijmans, M.; Groenewegen, P. Self-management support needs of patients with chronic illness: Do needs for support differ according to the course of illness? *Patient Educ. Couns.* **2013**, *93*, 626–632. [CrossRef] [PubMed]
5. Morris, R.L.; Kennedy, A.; Sanders, C. Evolving 'self'-management: Exploring the role of social network typologies on individual long-term condition management. *Heal. Expect.* **2015**, *19*, 1044–1061. [CrossRef]
6. Kendall, P.R.W. *Investing in Prevention:Improving Health and Creating Sustainability*; Bristish Columbia: Vancouver, Canada, 2010.
7. World Health Organization. *Innovative Care for Chronic Conditions: Building Blocks for Action*; WHO: Geneva, Switzerland, 2002.
8. Epping-Jordan, J.E. Integrated approaches to prevention and control of chronic conditions. *Kidney Int.* **2005**, *68*, 86–88. [CrossRef]
9. Nuño, R.; Coleman, K.; Bengoa, R.; Sauto, R. Integrated care for chronic conditions: The contribution of the ICCC Framework. *Health Policy* **2012**, *105*, 55–64. [CrossRef]
10. Barlow, J.H.; Brancroft, G.V.; Turner, A.P. Self-management training for people with chronic disease: A shared learning experience. *J. Health Psychol.* **2005**, *10*, 863–872. [CrossRef]
11. Davies, F.; Wood, F.; Bullock, A.; Wallace, C.; Edwards, A. Interventions to improve the self-management support health professionals provide for people with progressive neurological conditions: Protocol for a realist synthesis. *BMJ Open* **2017**, *7*, e014575. [CrossRef]
12. Nøst, T.H.; Steinsbekk, A.; Bratås, O.; Grønning, K. Expectations, effect and experiences of an easily accessible self-management intervention for people with chronic pain: Study protocol for a randomised controlled trial with embedded qualitative study. *Trials* **2016**, *17*, 325.
13. Crotty, M.M.; Henderson, J.; Ward, P.R.; Fuller, J.; Rogers, A.; Kralik, D.; Gregory, S. Analysis of social networks supporting the self-management of type 2 diabetes for people with mental illness. *BMC Health Serv. Res.* **2015**, *15*, 257. [CrossRef]
14. Gallant, M.P. The influence of social support on chronic illness self-management: A review and directions for research. *Heal. Educ. Behav.* **2003**, *30*, 170–195. [CrossRef] [PubMed]

15. Vassilev, I.; Rogers, A.; Blickem, C.; Brooks, H.; Kapadia, D.; Kennedy, A.; Sanders, C.; Kirk, S.; Reeves, D. Social networks, the "Work" and work force of chronic illness self-management: A survey analysis of personal communities. *PLoS ONE* **2013**, *8*, e59723. [CrossRef] [PubMed]
16. Koetsenruijter, J.; Van Lieshout, J.; Vassilev, I.; Portillo, M.C.; Serrano, M.; Knutsen, I.; Roukova, P.; Lionis, C.; Todorova, E.; Foss, C.; et al. Social support systems as determinants of self-management and quality of life of people with diabetes across Europe: Study protocol for an observational study. *Health Qual. Life Outcomes* **2014**, *12*, 29. [CrossRef] [PubMed]
17. Reeves, D.; Blickem, C.; Vassilev, I.; Brooks, H.; Kennedy, A.; Richardson, G.; Rogers, A. The contribution of social networks to the health and self-management of patients with long-term conditions: A longitudinal study. *PLoS ONE* **2014**, *9*, e98340. [CrossRef] [PubMed]
18. Lin, N.; Ensel, W.; Simeone, R.; Kuo, W. Social support, stressful life events, and illness: A model and an empirical test. *J. Heal. Soc. Behav.* **1979**, *20*, 108–119. [CrossRef]
19. Lin, N.; Dean, A.; Ensel, W.M. Social support scales: A methodological note. *Schizophr. Bull.* **1981**, *7*, 73–89. [CrossRef]
20. House, J.S. Social support and social structure. *Sociol. Forum* **1987**, *2*, 135–146. [CrossRef]
21. House, J.S.; Landis, K.R.; Umberson, D. Social relationships and health. *Science* **1988**, *241*, 540–545. [CrossRef]
22. Rn, D.C.B.; Rn, F.P.; Benton, D.C.; Pérez-Raya, F.; Fernández-Fernández, M.P.; González-Jurado, M.A. A systematic review of nurse-related social network analysis studies. *Int. Nurs. Rev.* **2014**, *62*, 321–339.
23. Bae, S.H.; Nikolaev, A.N.; Seo, J.; Castner, J. Health care provider social network analysis: A systematic review. *Nurs. Outlook* **2015**, *63*, 566–584. [CrossRef]
24. Scherlowski, H.; Guimaraes de Araújo, M.; Andrade, J.; Feijó, T.; Souza, V.; dos Santos, R. Social network analysis in primary health care: An integrative review. *Integr. Rev.* **2018**, *31*, 108–115.
25. Hawe, P.; Webster, C.; Shiell, A. A glossary of terms for navigating the field of social network analysis. *J. Epidemiol. Community Health* **2004**, *58*, 971–975. [CrossRef] [PubMed]
26. Parnell, J.M.; Robinson, J.C. Social network analysis: Presenting an underutilised method for nursing research. *J. Adv. Nurs.* **2018**, *74*, 1310–1318. [CrossRef] [PubMed]
27. Del-Pino-Casado, R.; Frías-Osuna, A.; Palomino-Moral, P.; Ruzafa-Martínez, M.; Ramos-Morcillo, A. Social support and subjective burden in caregivers of adults and older adults: A meta-analysis. *PLoS ONE* **2018**, *13*, e0189874. [CrossRef] [PubMed]
28. Rodríguez-Madrid, M.N.; del Río-Lozano, M.; Fernandez-Peña, R.; Jiménez-Pernett, J.; García-Mochón, L.; Lupiañez-Castillo, A.; García-Calvente, M.M. Gender differences in social support received by informal caregivers: A personal network analysis approach. *Int. J. Environ. Res. Public Health* **2019**, *16*, 91. [CrossRef] [PubMed]
29. Perry, B.; Pescosolido, B.; Borgatti, S. *Egocentric Network Analysis: Foundations, Methods, and Models*; Cambridge University Press: Cambridge, UK, 2018.
30. McCarty, C. Structure in personal networks. *J. Soc. Struct.* **2002**, *3*, 20.
31. Hâncean, M.; Molina, J.L.; Lubbers, M.J. Recent advancements, developments and applications of personal network analysis. *Int. Rev. Soc. Res.* **2016**, *6*, 137–145. [CrossRef]
32. Molina, J.L. El estudio de las redes personales: Contribuciones, métodos y perspectiva. *Empiria Rev. Metodol. Cienc. Soc.* **2005**, *10*, 71–105.
33. McCarty, C.; Lubbers, M.J.; Vacca, R.; Molina, J.L. How personal networks have been used so far. In *Conducting Personal Network Research. A Practical Guide*; The Guilford Press: New York, NY, USA, 2019; p. 270.
34. Smith, K.; Christakis, N. Social networks and health. *Annu. Rev. Sociol.* **2008**, *34*, 405–418. [CrossRef]
35. Doeglas, D.; Suurmeijer, T.; Briançon, S.; Moum, T.; Krol, B.; Bjelle, A.; Sanderman, R.; Van der Heuvel, W. An international study on measuring social support: Interactions and satisfaction. *Soc. Sci. Med.* **1996**, *43*, 1389–1397. [CrossRef]
36. Franks, H.M.; Cronan, T.A.; Oliver, K. Social support in women with fibromyalgia: Is quality more important than quantity? *J. Community Psychol.* **2004**, *32*, 425–438. [CrossRef]
37. Tardy, C. Social support measurement. *Am. J. Community Psychol.* **1985**, *13*, 187–202. [CrossRef]
38. Bernardes, S.F.; Forgeron, P.; Fournier, K.; Reszel, J. Beyond solicitousness: A comprehensive review on informal pain-related social support. *Pain* **2017**, *158*, 2066–2076. [CrossRef] [PubMed]
39. Breivik, H.; Collett, B.; Ventafridda, V.; Cohen, R.; Gallacher, D. Survey of chronic pain in Europe: Prevalence, impact on daily life, and treatment. *Eur. J. Pain* **2006**, *10*, 287–333. [CrossRef]

40. Dueñas, M.; Ojeda, B.; Salazar, A.; Mico, J.A.; Failde, I. A review of chronic pain impact on patients, their social environment and the health care system. *J. Pain Res.* **2016**, *9*, 457–467. [CrossRef]
41. Fernández Peña, R. El Estudio del Apoyo Social y la Calidad de Vida Desde las Redes Personales: El Caso del Dolor Crónico. Ph.D. Thesis, Universidad Autónoma de Barcelona, Barcelona, Spain, 2015.
42. Fernández-Peña, R.; Molina, J.L.; Valero, O. Personal network analysis in the study of social support: The case of chronic pain. *Int. J. Environ. Res. Public Health* **2018**, *15*, 2695.
43. Borgatti, S.P.; Everett, M.G. *Analyzing Social Networks*; Sage Publications: London, UK, 2013.
44. Greenacre, M. *Correspondence Analysis in Practice*, 2nd ed.; Chapman & Hall: London, UK, 2007.
45. Ward, J.H., Jr. Hierarchical grouping to optimize an objective function. *J. Am. Stat. Assoc.* **1963**, *58*, 236–244. [CrossRef]
46. Hartigan, J.A. *Clustering Algorithms*; Wiley & Sons: New York, NY, USA, 1975.
47. Weiner, A.S.B.; Hannum, J.W. Differences in the quantity of social support between geographically close and long-distance friendships. *J. Soc. Pers. Relat.* **2012**, *30*, 662–672. [CrossRef]
48. Fernández, M. Social support networks in Spain: The factors that determine models of choice. *Int. Sociol.* **2012**, *27*, 384–402.
49. Mok, D.; Wellman, B. Did distance matter before the Internet? Interpersonal contact and support in the 1970s. *Soc. Netw.* **2007**, *29*, 430–461. [CrossRef]
50. Tomini, F.; Tomini, S.M.; Groot, W. Understanding the value of social networks in life satisfaction of elderly people: A comparative study of 16 European countries using SHARE data. *BMC Geriatr.* **2016**, *16*, 203. [CrossRef] [PubMed]
51. Antonucci, T.C.; Akiyama, H.; Lansford, J.E. Negative effects of close social relations. *Fam. Relat.* **1998**, *47*, 379–384. [CrossRef]
52. Cohen, S.; Janicki-Deverts, D. Can we improve our physical health by altering our social networks? *Perspect. Psychol. Sci.* **2009**, *4*, 375–378. [CrossRef] [PubMed]
53. Rook, K.S. The negative side of social interaction: Impact on psychological well-being. *J. Pers. Soc. Psychol.* **1984**, *46*, 1097–1108. [CrossRef] [PubMed]
54. Rook, K.S. Exposure and reactivity to negative social exchanges: A preliminary investigation using daily diary data. *J. Gerontol.* **2003**, *58*, 100–111. [CrossRef] [PubMed]
55. Newsom, J.T.; Rook, K.S.; Nishishiba, M.; Sorkin, D.H.; Mahan, T.L. Understanding the relative importance of positive and negative social exchanges: Examining specific domains and appraisals. *J. Gerontol.* **2005**, *60*, 304–312. [CrossRef]
56. Català, E.; Reig, E.; Artés, M.; Aliaga, L.; López, J.S.; Segú, J.L. Prevalence of pain in the Spanish population: Telephone survey in 5000 homes. *Eur. J. Pain* **2002**, *6*, 133–140. [CrossRef]
57. Geisser, M.E.; Cano, A.; Leonard, M. Factors associated with marital satisfaction and mood among spouses of persons with chronic back pain. *J. Pain* **2005**, *6*, 518–525. [CrossRef]
58. Leonard, M.T.; Cano, A.; Johansen, A.B. Chronic pain in a couples context: A review and integration of theoretical models and empirical evidence. *J. Pain* **2006**, *7*, 377–390. [CrossRef]
59. Cano, A.; Leonard, M. Integrative behavioral couple therapy for chronic pain: Promoting behavior change and emotional acceptance. *J. Clin. Psychol.* **2006**, *62*, 1409–1418. [CrossRef]
60. Roy, R. What happens to spouses? In *Social Relations and Chronic Pain*; Kluwer Academic Publishers: New York, NY, USA, 2002; pp. 57–70. ISBN 0306471973.
61. Entwisle, B.; Faust, K.; Rindfuss, R.R.R.; Kaneda, T. Networks and contexts: Variation in the structure of social ties. *Am. J. Sociol.* **2007**, *112*, 1495–1533. [CrossRef]
62. Jolly, A.; Muth, S.; Wylie, J.; Potterat, J. Sexual networks and sexually transmitted infections: A tale of two cities. *J. Urban Heal.* **2001**, *78*, 433–446. [CrossRef] [PubMed]
63. Smith, A.M.A.; Grierson, J.; Wain, D.; Pitts, M.; Pattison, P. Associations between the sexual behaviour of men who have sex with men and the structure and composition of their social networks. *Sex. Transm. Infect.* **2004**, *80*, 455–458. [CrossRef] [PubMed]
64. Birkett, M.; Kuhns, L.; Latkin, C.; Muth, S.; Mustanski, B. The sexual networks of racially diverse young men who have sex with men. *Arch. Sex. Behav.* **2015**, *44*, 1787–1797. [CrossRef] [PubMed]
65. Morris, M. Sexual networks and HIV in four african populations: The use of standardized behavioral surveys with biological markers. In *Network Epidemiology: A Handbook for Survey Design and Data Collection*; Oxford University Press on Demand: Oxford, UK, 2004; pp. 58–84. ISBN 9780199269013.

66. Bearman, P.S.; Moody, J.; Stovel, K. Chains of affection: The structure of adolescent romantic and sexual networks. *Am. J. Sociol.* **2004**, *110*, 44–91. [CrossRef]
67. Hansen, L.R.; Pedersen, S.B.; Overgaard, C.; Torp-Pedersen, C.; Ullits, L.R. Associations between the structural and functional aspects of social relations and poor mental health: A cross-sectional register study. *BMC Public Health* **2017**, *17*, 860. [CrossRef]
68. Haas, S.A.; Schaefer, D.R.; Kornienko, O. Health and the structure of adolescent social networks. *J. Health Soc. Behav.* **2010**, *51*, 424–439. [CrossRef]
69. Agneessens, F.; Waege, H.; Lievens, J. Diversity in social support by role relations: A typology. *Soc. Netw.* **2006**, *28*, 427–441. [CrossRef]
70. Platt, J.; Keyes, K.M.; Koenen, K.C. Size of the social network versus quality of social support: Which is more protective against PTSD? *Soc. Psychiatry Psychiatr. Epidemiol.* **2014**, *49*, 1279–1286. [CrossRef]
71. Stokes, J.P. Predicting satisfaction with social support form social network structure. *Am. J. Community Psychol.* **1983**, *11*, 141–152. [CrossRef]
72. Ashida, S.; Heaney, C.A. Differential associations of social support and social connectedness with structural features of social networks and the health status of older adults. *J. Aging Health* **2008**, *20*, 872–893. [CrossRef] [PubMed]
73. Hirsch, B.J. Natural support systems and coping with major life changes. *Am. J. Community Psychol.* **1980**, *8*, 159–172. [CrossRef]
74. Burt, R.S. Structural holes and good ideas. *Am. J. Sociol.* **2004**, *110*, 349–399. [CrossRef]
75. Wellman, B.; Wortley, S. Different strokes from different folks: Community ties and social support. *Am. J. Sociol.* **1990**, *96*, 558–588. [CrossRef]
76. Coleman, J.S. Social capital in the creation of human capital. *Am. J. Sociol.* **1988**, *94*, S95–S120. [CrossRef]
77. Putnam, R.D. Bowling alone: America's declining social capital. In *Culture and Politics*; Palgrave Macmillan: New York, NY, USA, 2000; pp. 223–234.
78. Chandola, T.; Marmot, M.; Siegrist, J. Failed reciprocity in close social relationships and health: Findings from the Whitehall II study. *J. Psychosom. Res.* **2007**, *63*, 403–411. [CrossRef]
79. Knowlton, A.R.; Yang, C.; Bohnert, A.; Wissow, L.; Chander, G.; Arnsten, J.A. Informal care and reciprocity of support are associated with HAART adherence among men in baltimore. *AIDS Behav.* **2011**, *15*, 1429–1436. [CrossRef]
80. Mercken, L.; Candel, M.; Willems, P.; De Vries, H. Disentangling social selection and social influence effects on adolescent smoking: The importance of reciprocity in friendships. *Addiction* **2007**, *102*, 1483–1492. [CrossRef]
81. Adelman, R.D.; Tmanova, L.; Delgado, D.; Dion, S.; Lachs, M.S. Caregiver burden: A clinical review. *J. Am. Med. Assoc.* **2014**, *311*, 1052–1059. [CrossRef]
82. Jones, S.L.; Hadjistavropoulos, H.D.; Janzen, J.A.; Hadjistavropoulos, T. The relation of pain and caregiver burden in informal order adult caregivers. *Pain Med.* **2011**, *12*, 51–58. [CrossRef]
83. Rodakowski, J.; Skidmore, E.R.; Rogers, J.C.; Schulz, R. Role of social support in predicting caregiver burden. *Arch. Phys. Med. Rehabil.* **2012**, *93*, 2229–2236. [CrossRef] [PubMed]
84. Shaw, B.A.; Krause, N.; Liang, J.; Bennett, J. Tracking changes in social relations throughout late life. *J. Gerontol.* **2007**, *62*, 90–99. [CrossRef] [PubMed]
85. Feld, S.L.L.; Suitor, J.J.J.; Gartner, J.G.; Hoegh, J.G.; Gartner, J.G. Describing changes in personal networks over time. *Field Methods* **2007**, *19*, 218–236. [CrossRef]
86. Mollenhorst, G.; Volker, B.; Flap, H. Changes in personal relationships: How social contexts affect the emergence and discontinuation of relationships. *Soc. Netw.* **2014**, *37*, 65–80. [CrossRef]
87. Fischer, C.S.; Beresford, L. Changes in support networks in late middle age: The extension of gender and educational differences. *J. Gerontol. Ser. B Psychol. Sci. Soc. Sci.* **2015**, *70*, 123–131. [CrossRef] [PubMed]

7

Association between Health Problems and Turnover Intention in Shift Work Nurses: Health Problem Clustering

Jison Ki [1], Jaegeum Ryu [2], Jihyun Baek [2], Iksoo Huh [1,2] and Smi Choi-Kwon [1,2,*]

1 College of Nursing, Seoul National University, 103, Daehak-ro, Jongno-gu, Seoul 03080, Korea; candy8@snu.ac.kr (J.K.); huhixoo@gmail.com (I.H.)

2 The Research Institute of Nursing Science, Seoul National University, 103, Daehak-ro, Jongno-gu, Seoul 03080, Korea; jgryu21@gmail.com (J.R.); jihyunoctober@gmail.com (J.B.)

* Correspondence: smi@snu.ac.kr

Abstract: Shift work nurses experience multiple health problems due to irregular shifts and heavy job demands. However, the comorbidity patterns of nurses' health problems and the association between health problems and turnover intention have rarely been studied. This study aimed to identify and cluster shift work nurses' health problems and to reveal the associations between health problems and turnover intention. In this cross-sectional study, we analyzed data from 500 nurses who worked at two tertiary hospitals in Seoul, South Korea. Data, including turnover intention and nine types of health issues, were collected between March 2018 and April 2019. Hierarchical clustering and multiple ordinal logistic regressions were used for the data analysis. Among the participants, 22.2% expressed turnover intention and the mean number of health problems was 4.5 (range 0–9). Using multiple ordinal logistic regressions analysis, it was shown that sleep disturbance, depression, fatigue, a gastrointestinal disorder, and leg or foot discomfort as a single health problem significantly increased turnover intention. After clustering the health problems, four clusters were identified and only the neuropsychological cluster—sleep disturbance, fatigue, and depression—significantly increased turnover intention. We propose that health problems within the neuropsychological cluster must receive close attention and be addressed simultaneously to decrease nurse's turnover intentions.

Keywords: nurses; turnover intention; hierarchical clustering; fatigue; sleep

1. Introduction

Nurses often work irregular shifts and bear high physical and psychological job demands that may, in turn, jeopardize their health status. Specifically, shift work may cause a variety of physical and mental health problems [1]. The deterioration of nurses' health status could not only lead to a decline in their quality of life but could also affect the quality of care provided by them [2]. In addition, health problems may affect nurses' turnover, which is a serious issue worldwide [3]. The high turnover rate of nurses has led to an increase in both direct and indirect costs in the health system and could further protract the shortage of nurses that has lasted for the past several years [4]. A recent survey of Korean nurses reported that about 10% of shift work nurses cited health problems as their main reason for resigning [5].

Prior studies also show that nurses complained of two or more health problems simultaneously, which may be interrelated [2,6–8]. Musculoskeletal pain in nurses has been reported in many studies [9,10], and poor dietary habits due to irregular shift work were reported to cause gastrointestinal disorders [11,12]. Sleep disturbance, which is most frequently reported in studies of shift nurses, could lead to mood disorders, such as depression, both of which lead to chronic fatigue [13–15].

Although nurses experience various health problems, there is relatively little research on the relationships between complex health problems in nurses [2]. Moreover, few studies have investigated the relationship between concomitant health problems and turnover intention.

Because the burden may vary depending on the number and the kind of health problems shift work nurses have [16], it may be important to identify specific comorbidity patterns of nurses' health problems through clustering and determine which clusters most affect turnover intention, where a cluster-that is, a comorbid pattern of health problems—can be defined as a group of concurrent or related health problems that can be distinguished from other clusters [17].

Therefore, the purpose of this study was to first characterize shift work nurses' health problems. We then determined the pattern of symptom modalities by clustering the health problems through the hierarchical clustering method. Lastly, we identified the impact of health problem clusters on turnover intention.

2. Materials and Methods

2.1. Study Design and Participants

This cross-sectional study was part of the Shift Work Nurses' Health and Turnover (SWNHT) study, which is a prospective cohort study designed to investigate the longitudinal relationships between shift work nurses' health and turnover. It was supported by the National Research Foundation of Korea (NRF) grant funded by the Korea Ministry of Science and Information and Communications Technologies and approved by the Institutional Review Board (IRB) at two tertiary hospitals in Seoul, South Korea. Data collection was performed from March 2018 until April 2020. In the SWNHT study, we recruited 594 female nurses (294 novice nurses who had no exposure to rotating shift work, and 300 nurses with exposure to 8-hour rotating work, including night shifts, for at least 1 month) (Figure 1). Because health problems can vary according to sex [18,19] and the SWNHT study included a survey of nurses' menstrual and gynecological symptoms, the SWNHT study was limited to female nurses. Data were collected three times for novice nurses: before exposure to shift work (novice registered nurse (NRN) T0, n = 294), after six months of work (NRN T1, n = 204), and 12 months after T1 (NRN T2, n = 204). For experienced registered nurses, data were collected twice: baseline (experienced registered nurse (ERN) T1, n = 300) and 12 months after T1 (ERN T2, n = 269; see details in Section 2.2 Data Collection).

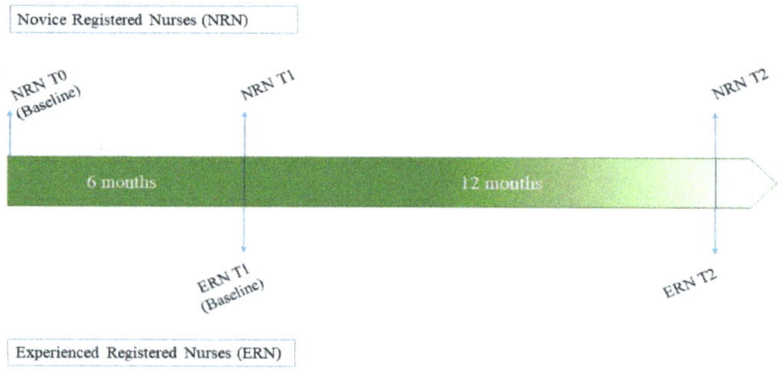

Figure 1. Schematic overview of the Shift Work Nurses' Health and Turnover (SWNHT) study.

In this study, we used data collected from October 2018 to January 2019 (NRN T1, n = 204) and from March 2018 to May 2018 (ERN T1, n = 300) to analyze the association between health problems and turnover intention among shift work nurses. In this analysis, we defined shift work as a combination of day, evening, and night shifts; therefore, we excluded four nurses, including three nurses who worked only daytime hours and one nurse who worked from midday to 8 p.m.

2.2. Data Collection

The primary purpose of the SWNHT study was to investigate health problems, presenteeism, and turnover intention in shift work nurses. To enroll novice nurses without shift work experience, we distributed and collected survey envelope packages that included survey instructions, consent forms, and a questionnaire on the third day of their work orientation before ward placement. To enroll experienced shift work nurses, we attached a recruitment notice to the ward bulletin boards, and nurses who wished to participate in the study voluntarily contacted the research team. We maximized voluntary participation by protecting confidentiality, ensuring anonymity, and no hospital-associated researchers took part in the data collection process. We collected the follow-up data through an online survey program; their response rates were 69.4% (NRN T1, NRN T2) and 89.7% (ERN T1). The SWNHT study questionnaire included questions regarding general and job-related characteristics, health-related variables (e.g., dietary habits, menstrual symptoms, exposure to blood and body fluid, sleep, fatigue, depression, physical activity, etc.), occupational stress, presenteeism, and turnover intention. To objectively verify the sleep scale data, we also obtained actigraphy data from the subjects who consented to wear the actigraphy.

2.3. *Measurements*

2.3.1. Demographic and Job-Related Characteristics

The examined demographic characteristics included age (years), education (bachelor's degree or lower/master's degree or higher), marital status (single/married), having children (yes/no), and body mass index (kg/m^2). The examined job-related characteristics included work unit (general ward, intensive care unit, delivery room, and emergency room), months of shift work experience, and the average number of night shifts per month.

2.3.2. Turnover Intention

We measured turnover intention since it is the most predictive measure of actual turnover [20]. In a longitudinal study in Europe, nurses who had turnover intentions were more likely to leave their jobs [21]. In this study, the subjects were asked to choose one of four options (strongly agree, agree, disagree, or strongly disagree) to answer the question: "I plan on staying for the next year" [22].

2.3.3. Health Problems

The nine health problems in this study were selected by two professors at a nursing college and two nurses in a research team, and were based on reviews of the literature about shift work nurses' health problems [10,18,23–27]. These were (1) upper musculoskeletal pain (including neck, shoulder, and back pain), (2) leg or foot discomfort, (3) sleep disturbance, (4) fatigue, (5) depression, (6) menstrual disorders (including dysmenorrhea and menopause symptoms), (7) gynecological disorders (including disease of the uterus or ovary), (8) headaches (including migraine, dizziness, and chronic headaches), and (9) gastrointestinal disorders (including gastric ulcer, diarrhea, constipation, and stomachache).

Among the nine health problem categories, sleep disturbance, fatigue, and depression were measured using the instruments described below. For the other six health problem categories, the subjects were asked to indicate the health problems they experienced during the last month with "yes" or "no."

Sleep Disturbance

To assess the quality of sleep, we used the Korean version of the Insomnia Severity Index (ISI), which was developed by Morin and translated by the Korean Sleep Research Society. The insomnia severity scale consists of seven questions related to sleep disorders measured on a 5-point scale (0–4 points) for each item. The score ranges from 0 to 28; higher scores indicate a lower quality of sleep. A score above 10 indicates sleep disturbance [28]. The Cronbach's alpha value of the Korean version of ISI was 0.928 in our study.

Fatigue

Fatigue was measured using the Fatigue Severity Scale (FSS). The FSS consists of nine questions about the degree of fatigue during the past week and is scored from 1 (strongly disagree) to 7 (strongly agree). A higher average score indicates higher fatigue. The criterion for fatigue is more than four points on average [29]. The Cronbach's alpha value of the FSS was 0.917 in our study.

Depression

We measured depression using the shortened Center for Epidemiological Studies Depression Scale (CES-D). The shortened CES-D consists of 10 questions about depressive feelings and thoughts during the past week and is scored from 0 (less than 1 day) to 3 (about 5–7 days). Higher total scores indicate more depressive symptoms. A total score of 10 or above indicates depression [30]. The Cronbach's alpha value of the shortened CES-D was 0.877 in our study.

2.4. Statistical Analysis

All analyses were performed using SAS version 9.4 (SAS Institute Inc., Cary, NC, USA) and R Project for Statistical Computing software version 3.4.4 (CRAN, Soule, Korea). We confirmed that there were no missing data. The descriptive statistics (frequency, percentage, mean, and standard deviation) for the demographic characteristics were analyzed. Pearson's chi-squared test, Fisher's exact test, and an analysis of variance were used to identify general characteristics associated with turnover intention. Hierarchical clustering was used to group the health problems reported by participants. Hierarchical clustering is a statistical method for grouping objects or variables according to the similarity between clusters using a bottom-up approach. In the field of nursing, this technique has been used mainly for symptom clustering of cancer patients; however, it has recently become more widely used in various studies [31]. The method used for measuring the distance between variables was the squared Euclidean distance and the linkage method used for measuring the distance between clusters was the average linkage. The number of final clusters is usually determined by the researchers by taking into account clinical suitability [32]. Multiple ordinal logistic regressions that included covariates, such as education, marital status, having children, body mass index (kg/m^2), work unit, months of shift work experience, and the number of night shifts per month, was used to investigate the association of single health problems and clusters of health problems with turnover intention. The four categories of "strongly agree," "agree," "disagree," and "strongly disagree" used for the turnover intention variable satisfied the proportional odds assumption at $p > 0.050$ with the covariates and variables of interest.

2.5. Ethical Consideration

This study was approved by the Institutional Review Board (IRB) at Seoul National University Hospital (IRB No. H-1712-094-907) and the Samsung Medical center (IRB No. 2017-12-075-002). After agreeing to participate in the study, all nurse participants signed a consent form and completed the baseline questionnaire.

3. Results

3.1. Demographic and Job-Related Characteristics

The participants were 500 female nurses working shifts, including night shifts. The nurses' mean age was 26.7 years (standard deviation (SD) = 4.20), and 19.8% were over 30 years old. There were no differences in demographic and job-related characteristics between the participants in the two tertiary hospitals. Most nurses were single (88.2%) and had no children (94.0%). The average body mass index (BMI) was 20.19 kg/m^2; 22.8% of the subjects were underweight and only one subject was obese. The shift work length was 35 months on average, which was highly correlated with age ($r = 0.92$, $p < 0.001$). Therefore, we excluded age from the covariates of the multiple ordinal logistic regressions (Table 1).

Table 1. Demographic and job-related characteristics by turnover intention (n = 500).

Variables	Categories	Total	Strong Intent to Stay	Intent to Stay	Intent to Leave	Strong Intent to Leave	χ^2 or F	p
		(n = 500, 100.0%) n (%) or M ± SD	(n = 53, 10.5%) n (%) or M ± SD	(n = 336, 67.2%) n (%) or M ± SD	(n = 99, 19.9%) n (%) or M ± SD	(n = 12, 2.4%) n (%) or M ± SD		
Age (years)		26.72 ± 4.20	28.77 ± 5.68	26.29 ± 3.87	27.08 ± 4.31	26.58 ± 2.35	5.70	0.001 *
Education	≤BSN	459 (91.8)	48 (90.6)	310 (92.3)	89 (89.9)	12 (100.0)	1.74	0.626
	≥MSN	41 (8.2)	5 (9.4)	26 (7.7)	10 (10.1)	0 (0.0)		
Marital Status	Single	441 (88.2)	42 (79.3)	303 (90.2)	85 (85.9)	11 (91.7)	6.00	0.108
	Married	59 (11.8)	11 (20.7)	33 (9.8)	14 (14.1)	1 (8.3)		
Having Children	Yes	30 (6.0)	8 (15.1)	15 (4.5)	7 (7.1)	0 (0.0)	10.14	0.030 *
	No	470 (94.0)	45 (84.9)	321 (95.5)	92 (92.9)	12 (100.0)		
Body Mass Index (kg/m^2)		20.19 ± 2.24	20.96 ± 2.36	20.19 ± 2.19	19.92 ± 2.34	18.77 ± 1.22	4.24	0.006 *
Work Unit	Ward	366 (73.2)	41 (77.4)	239 (71.1)	76 (76.8)	10 (83.3)	4.61	0.673
	ICU	109 (21.8)	8 (15.1)	79 (23.5)	20 (20.2)	2 (16.7)		
	DR, ER	25 (5.0)	4 (7.5)	18 (5.4)	3 (3.0)	0 (0.0)		
Shift Work Experience (months)		34.93 ± 42.94	58.66 ± 59.97	30.84 ± 40.01	37.03 ± 39.38	27.58 ± 27.80	6.83	<0.001 *
Average Number of Nights Per Month (days)		6.00 ± 1.26	5.62 ± 1.48	5.98 ± 1.37	6.06 ± 1.16	6.13 ± 0.78	1.45	0.228

BSN-Bachelor of Science in Nursing, MSN-Master of Science in Nursing, ICU-Intensive Care Unit, DR-delivery room, ER-emergency room; * $p < 0.05$.

One hundred and eleven nurses (22.2%) had a turnover intention and 12 nurses (2.4%) strongly intended to leave. The turnover intention was statistically higher in subjects who were younger (F = 5.70, p = 0.001), had no children (χ^2 = 10.14, p = 0.030), had a lower BMI (F = 4.24, p = 0.006), and had shorter periods of shift work (F = 6.83, $p < 0.001$).

3.2. *Prevalence and Association between Single Health Problems and Turnover Intention*

The mean number of health problems was 4.5 (range 0–9), with 95.2% (n = 476) of participants having more than two health problems. The most frequently reported health problem was upper musculoskeletal pain (82.4%), followed by leg or foot discomfort (67.8%), fatigue (65.0%), and sleep disturbance (62.4%). The associations between single health problems and turnover intention using multiple ordinal logistic regressions are provided in Table 2. Fatigue (odds ratio (OR) = 3.4, 95% confidence interval (CI) = 2.21–5.24), depression (OR = 1.79, 95% CI = 1.22–2.62), leg or foot discomfort (OR = 1.69, 95% CI = 1.12–2.56), sleep disturbance (OR = 1.61, 95% CI = 1.10–2.37), and a gastrointestinal disorder (OR = 1.51, 95% CI = 1.03–2.19) were significantly related to turnover intention.

Table 2. Association between single health problems and turnover intention using a multiple ordinal logistic regression.

Variables	Total (*n* = 500, 100.0%) *n* (%)	Adjusted [1] Odds Ratio	95% CI	*p*
Upper Musculoskeletal Pain	412 (82.4)	1.07	0.65–1.74	0.775
Leg or Foot Discomfort	339 (67.8)	1.69	1.12–2.56	0.012 *
Sleep Disturbance	312 (62.4)	1.61	1.10–2.37	0.013 *
Fatigue	325 (65.0)	3.4	2.21–5.24	<0.001 *
Depression	207 (41.4)	1.79	1.22–2.62	0.002 *
Menstrual Disorder	194 (38.8)	1.26	0.86–1.85	0.229
Gynecological Disorder	36 (7.2)	0.98	0.47–2.01	0.959
Headache	195 (39.0)	1.2	0.82–1.75	0.343
Gastrointestinal Disorder	222 (44.4)	1.51	1.03–2.19	0.031 *

[1] Adjusted for education, marital status, having children, body mass index (kg/m^2), work unit, shift work experience (months), and the number of nights per month (days) in multiple ordinal logistic regression model; * $p < 0.05$.

3.3. *Hierarchical Clustering of Health Problems*

Based on the hierarchical clustering analysis, four clusters were identified (Figure 2): the pain cluster (upper musculoskeletal pain and leg or foot discomfort), the neuropsychological cluster (depression, sleep disturbance, and fatigue), the gynecological cluster (menstrual disorder and gynecological disorder), and the gastrointestinal cluster (headache and gastrointestinal disorder).

3.4. *Prevalence and Association between Clusters of Health Problems and Turnover Intention*

As a result of our multiple ordinal logistic regression analyses, only the neuropsychological cluster (depression, sleep disturbance, and fatigue) was found to be significantly related to turnover intention. In the neuropsychological cluster, if the participant had only one health problem, it did not relate to turnover intention. If the participant experienced two (OR = 3.35, 95% CI = 1.90–5.92) or three (OR = 5.73, 95% CI = 3.17–10.33) health problems in the cluster simultaneously, the odds ratio of the turnover intention increased linearly, which was statistically significant (F = 5.84, $p < 0.001$; Table 3).

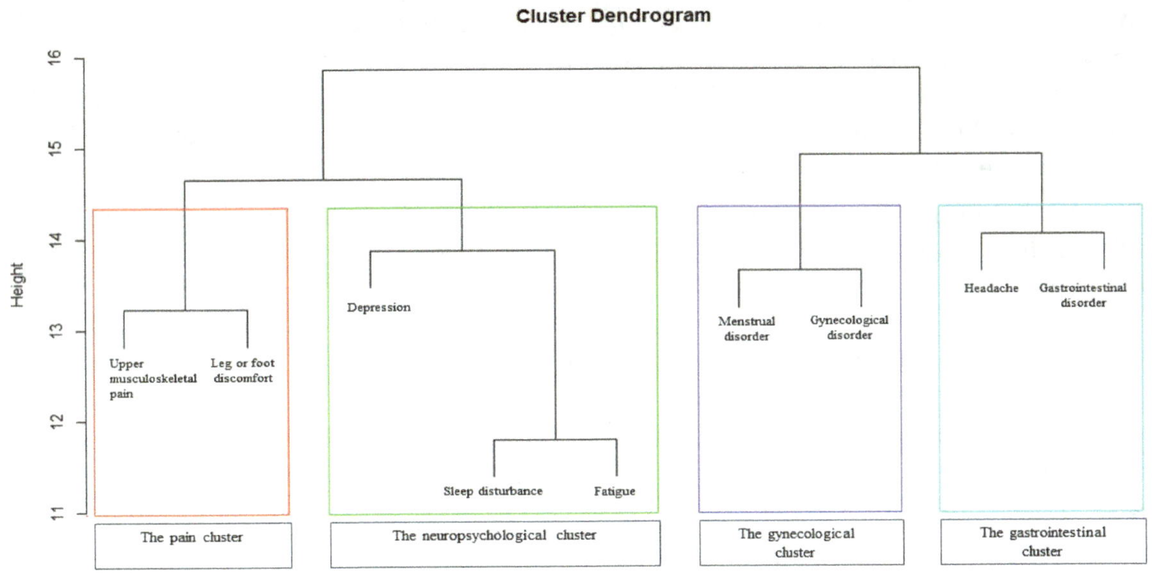

Figure 2. Dendrogram of the health problem clusters.

Table 3. Association between clusters of health problems and turnover intention using multiple ordinal logistic regressions.

Cluster	Health Problem Contents	Number	*n* (%)	Odds Ratio	Adjusted [1] 95% CI	*p*
Pain Cluster	Upper musculoskeletal pain + Leg or foot discomfort	0	37 (7.4)	1.00		
		1	175 (35.0)	0.57	0.27–1.23	0.155
		2	288 (57.6)	1.11	0.54–2.30	0.763
Neuropsychological Cluster	Sleep disturbance + Fatigue + Depression	0	99 (19.8)	1.00		
		1	97 (19.4)	1.59	0.85–2.97	0.141
		2	165 (33.0)	3.35	1.90–5.92	<0.001 *
		3	139 (27.8)	5.73	3.17–10.33	<0.001 *
Gynecological Cluster	Menstrual disorder + Gynecological disorder	0	292 (58.4)	1.00		
		1	186 (37.2)	1.22	0.83–1.81	0.298
		2	22 (4.4)	1.21	0.48–3.05	0.676
Gastrointestinal Cluster	Headache + Gastrointestinal disorder	0	193 (38.6)	1.00		
		1	197 (39.4)	1.43	0.94–2.19	0.092
		2	110 (22.0)	1.60	0.98–2.64	0.060

[1] Adjusted for education, marital status, having children, body mass index (kg/m^2), work unit, shift work experience (months), and the number of nights per month (days) in multiple ordinal logistic regression model; * $p < 0.05$.

4. Discussion

We investigated the prevalence of shift work nurses' health problems and characterized the patterns of symptom modalities by clustering health problems. We then investigated the association of single health problems and clusters of health problems with turnover intentions. We found that most shift work nurses experienced multiple health problems at the same time. We also found that having more than two health problems in the neuropsychological cluster was significantly related to turnover intention. This study was the first to attempt the clustering of nurses' health problems and explore the relationship between the clusters and turnover intention in shift work nurses.

We found that 22.2% of nurses had turnover intention. In previous studies, turnover intention varied from 4% to 54% [33–35]. The first reason for the difference in turnover intention between existing studies and our study could have been the different measurement tools used in each study. While our study asked about future plans regarding turnover, such as "I plan on staying for the next year," other studies asked how often they thought about turnover in the past [36,37]. Some studies measured turnover intention with various questions, such as whether they were seeking another job or whether they thought about leaving the nursing profession forever [33,38]. The second reason that turnover intention in our study was higher than in previous studies may be due to different hospital environments. The hospitals where our study was performed were tertiary hospitals in Seoul, which had a higher patient severity and higher nurse labor intensity than other hospitals in Korea. Third, we measured turnover intention and not actual turnover, which is reported to be higher than actual turnover rates [21]. In 2018, the annual average nurse turnover rate was 13.9% in Korea [5].

We found that fatigue was common in our subjects, highly related to turnover intention, and had the highest odds ratio (OR = 3.4, 95% CI = 2.21–5.24). Our results were consistent with a previous study that reported a positive correlation between fatigue and turnover intention [39]. Although we could not determine with certainty how long they had suffered from fatigue, it appeared that fatigue was one of the common disabling health problems that lead to turnover intention. Fatigue may exert a direct effect on turnover intention since nurses' fatigue has been reported to interfere with work efficiency and concentration and increase the risk of medical error and injury [40,41]. Although the direction of causality was not identified, nurses' fatigue was reported to be related to sleep disturbance, poor health, and depression [18,25].

Not surprisingly, we found that about 50% of nurses complained of fatigue and sleep disturbance at the same time and sleep disturbance was associated with turnover intention as a single health problem (OR = 1.61, 95% CI = 1.10–2.37). Sleep disturbance has received the most attention as a cause of turnover intention among nurses' health problems [42,43]. Irregular and insufficient sleep time due to shift work may often cause sleep disturbance, which may affect nurses' physical and mental health [1]. Another finding of interest was that about 28% of nurses had all three interrelated symptoms of fatigue, sleep disturbances, and depression; this was associated with turnover intention as a single health problem (OR = 1.79, 95% CI = 1.22–2.62). Depression in nurses is prevalent in many studies, and in one study, the prevalence of depression among nurses was almost twice as high as in other professions [26,44,45]. Depression may decrease concentration, which reduces the productivity of nursing and affects nurses' judgment, thus increasing occupational injury and turnover intention [26,43].

Our study revealed that fatigue, sleep disturbance, and depression may play important roles in increasing turnover intention as a cluster and as individual symptoms. Approximately one-third of nurses experienced all three health problems; these findings suggest fatigue, sleep disturbance, and depression in the neuropsychological cluster were correlated with each other. Despite the fact that biological and behavioral mechanisms in the development of depression, fatigue, and sleep disturbances are unknown, several studies have reported that these three health problems are related and co-occur [46,47]. Most importantly, 80% of nurses experienced one or more health problems in the neuropsychological cluster and this cluster was associated with turnover intention. Moreover, their odds ratio of turnover intention increased linearly as the number of health problems increased within this cluster. Future studies should probe the comorbidity of sleep disturbance, depression, and fatigue of shift work nurses and develop comprehensive health promotion to alleviate these three health problems.

We found that having a gastrointestinal disorder was another common health problem, which was consistent with the result of a previous study of 20,000 Korean nurses [12]. This high prevalence of gastrointestinal disorders among shift work nurses may, first, be due to disturbed circadian rhythm. The gastrointestinal system, like sleep, has a circadian rhythm, which controls bowel movement and the secretion of gastric juices [48]. Second, it might be due to irregular meal times and skipped meals [49]. Although not shown in the result, most of the nurses in our study reported eating irregularly (92.8%) and they ate breakfast twice a week, which was lower than the average number of times Korean adults eat breakfast [50]. The most common reason for skipped meals in our study was irregular work times (64.8%). Considering that having a gastrointestinal disorder was common among shift work nurses and was a single health problem that increased turnover intention, special attention needs to be paid to having regular and sufficient mealtimes as much as possible.

In our results, gastrointestinal disorders and headaches formed the gastrointestinal cluster. This connection could be explained by the association between the brain and the stomach through neural, endocrine, and immune pathways and the high prevalence of headaches in patients with a gastrointestinal disorder [51,52]. However, the gastrointestinal cluster was not related to turnover intention. It is possible that headaches, as an individual health problem, had no significant association with turnover intention, which could have decreased the effect of the cluster. Furthermore, we presume that headaches as a single health problem were not shown to be associated with turnover intention because headaches are often easily relieved by medication and may not have been as severe as a gastrointestinal disorder.

Upper musculoskeletal pain, which had the highest prevalence, formed a pain cluster with leg or foot discomfort. Nurses work most of the time in a standing position, walking an average of 8747 steps (4.1 miles) per shift [53], and high physical demands have been associated with musculoskeletal problems in nurses [54]. Additionally, multi-site musculoskeletal pain has been shown to be more common than single-site pain, especially in women [55]. Unexpectedly, this cluster was not related to turnover intention, although leg or foot discomfort was related to turnover intention. This might be because most nurses (82%) suffered upper musculoskeletal pain regardless of turnover intention and, similar to the gastrointestinal cluster, the association of the pain cluster with turnover intention was reduced by the effect of upper musculoskeletal pain. Although the pain cluster did not relate to turnover intention, given that these health problems in the pain cluster had a high prevalence and cause sickness and absence from work and decreased work productivity [24], there is a need to investigate the prevalence of musculoskeletal disorders in nurses by workplace and to provide appropriate prevention and treatment programs.

Although our study provides a new perspective on nurses' health problems, it has some limitations. First, this study relied on self-report measures of health problems, except for three health problems (sleep disturbance, depression, and fatigue). Second, we surveyed only the presence of health problems, but not the severity; however, as the participants were nurses with medical knowledge, their judgment of the presence of health problems might be more reliable than that of the general public [56], which would partially compensate for the fact that some health problems were not assessed with standardized tools. Third, we could not infer the causal relationship from the cross-sectional design of the study. The fourth significant limitation is that this study did not measure how many nurses actually leave their job; therefore, the findings of our study may not apply to actual turnover, as turnover intention does not always lead to actual turnover. Fifth, the shift work nurses who participated were all female and from two tertiary hospitals in Seoul in Korea. Therefore, the generalizability of the results is limited. Future studies on the comorbidity of sleep disturbance, depression, and fatigue in shift work nurses from various hospitals in various regions, along with the inclusion of male nurses, are recommended.

5. Conclusions

In this study, the association of single health problems and clusters of health problems with turnover intention differed. Although fatigue, sleep disturbance, depression, gastrointestinal disorders, and leg or foot discomfort were related to turnover intention as single health problems, after clustering, only the neuropsychological cluster—including fatigue, sleep disturbance, and depression—was related to turnover intention. Given that nurses had more than two health problems and turnover intention increased linearly within the neuropsychological cluster, these problems must receive close attention and be addressed to decrease the nurse turnover rate. Future studies should implement longitudinal research to determine the effect of the neuropsychological cluster on turnover.

Author Contributions: J.K. developed the concept of this manuscript, analyzed the data, and prepared this manuscript. J.R. and J.B. were responsible for the data collection and contributed to the manuscript revision. I.H. developed the study protocol and advised on the data analysis. S.C.-K. developed the study protocol and concept, and revised this manuscript to its final version. All authors have read and agreed to the published version of the manuscript.

References

1. Kecklund, G.; Axelsson, J. Health consequences of shift work and insufficient sleep. *BMJ* **2016**, *355*, i5210. [CrossRef] [PubMed]
2. Letvak, S. We cannot ignore nurses' health anymore: A synthesis of the literature on evidence-based strategies to improve nurse health. *Nurs. Adm. Q.* **2013**, *37*, 295–308. [CrossRef] [PubMed]
3. Hayward, D.; Bungay, V.; Wolff, A.C.; MacDonald, V. A qualitative study of experienced nurses' voluntary turnover: Learning from their perspectives. *J. Clin. Nurs.* **2016**, *25*, 1336–1345. [CrossRef]
4. Duffield, C.M.; Roche, M.A.; Homer, C.; Buchan, J.; Dimitrelis, S. A comparative review of nurse turnover rates and costs across countries. *J. Adv. Nurs.* **2014**, *70*, 2703–2712. [CrossRef]
5. Korea Hospital Nurse Association. *Survey on the Status of Hospital Nursing Staffing*; Korea Hospital Nurse Association: Seoul, Korea, 2018.
6. Yeom, E.Y.; Jeong, G.S.; Kim, K.A. Influencing Factors on Presenteeism of Clinical Nurses. *Korean J. Occup. Health Nurs.* **2015**, *24*, 302–312. [CrossRef]
7. Lee, Y.; Jung, M. Presenteeism and absenteeism according to health problems on nurses. *J. Korean Acad. Community Health Nurs.* **2008**, *19*, 459–468.
8. Yoshida, M.; Miki, A. Factors Related to Presenteeism in Young and Middle-aged Nurses. *J. Occup. Health* **2018**, *60*, 31–40. [CrossRef]
9. Yassi, A.; Lockhart, K. Work-relatedness of low back pain in nursing personnel: A systematic review. *Int. J. Occup. Environ. Health* **2013**, *19*, 223–244. [CrossRef]
10. Abdul Rahman, H.; Abdul-Mumin, K.; Naing, L. Psychosocial Work Stressors, Work Fatigue, and Musculoskeletal Disorders: Comparison between Emergency and Critical Care Nurses in Brunei Public Hospitals. *Asian Nurs. Res.* **2017**, *11*, 13–18. [CrossRef]
11. Wong, H.; Wong, M.C.S.; Wong, S.Y.S.; Lee, A. The association between shift duty and abnormal eating behavior among nurses working in a major hospital: A cross-sectional study. *Int. J. Nurs. Stud.* **2010**, *47*, 1021–1027. [CrossRef]
12. Kim, O.; Ahn, Y.; Lee, H.Y.; Jang, H.J.; Kim, S.; Lee, J.E.; Jung, H.; Cho, E.; Lim, J.Y.; Kim, M.J.; et al. The Korea Nurses' Health Study: A Prospective Cohort Study. *J. Women's Health* **2017**, *26*, 892–899. [CrossRef] [PubMed]
13. Zhai, L.; Zhang, H.; Zhang, D. Sleep Duration and Depression among Adults: A Meta-Analysis of Prospective Studies. *Depress. Anxiety* **2015**, *32*, 664–670. [CrossRef] [PubMed]
14. Caruso, C.C. Negative Impacts of Shiftwork and Long Work Hours. *Rehabil. Nurs.* **2014**, *39*, 16–25. [CrossRef] [PubMed]
15. Ferri, P.; Guadi, M.; Marcheselli, L.; Balduzzi, S.; Magnani, D.; Di Lorenzo, R. The impact of shift work on the psychological and physical health of nurses in a general hospital: A comparison between rotating night shifts and day shifts. *Risk Manag. Healthc. Policy* **2016**, *9*, 203–211. [CrossRef] [PubMed]
16. Kim, H.-J.; McGuire, D.B.; Tulman, L.; Barsevick, A.M. Symptom clusters: Concept analysis and clinical implications for cancer nursing. *Cancer Nurs.* **2005**, *28*, 270–282. [CrossRef]
17. Barsevick, A. Defining the Symptom Cluster: How Far Have We Come? *Semin. Oncol. Nurs.* **2016**, *32*, 334–350. [CrossRef]
18. Oyane, N.M.F.; Pallesen, S.; Moen, B.E.; Akerstedt, T.; Bjorvatn, B. Associations Between Night Work and Anxiety, Depression, Insomnia, Sleepiness and Fatigue in a Sample of Norwegian Nurses. *PLoS ONE* **2013**, *8*, e70228. [CrossRef]
19. Tuckett, A.; Henwood, T.; Oliffe, J.L.; Kolbe-Alexander, T.L.; Kim, J.R. A Comparative Study of Australian and New Zealand Male and Female Nurses' Health. *Am. J. Men's Health* **2016**, *10*, 450–458. [CrossRef]
20. Meeusen, V.C.; Van Dam, K.; Brown-Mahoney, C.; Van Zundert, A.A.; Knape, H.T. Understanding nurse anesthetists' intention to leave their job: How burnout and job satisfaction mediate the impact of personality and workplace characteristics. *Health Care Manag. Rev.* **2011**, *36*, 155–163. [CrossRef]

21. Estryn-Behar, D.; van der Heijden, B.; Fry, C.; Hasselhorn, H. Longitudinal Analysis of Personal and Work-Related Factors Associated With Turnover Among Nurses. *Nurs. Res.* **2010**, *59*, 166–177. [CrossRef]
22. Han, K.; Trinkoff, A.M.; Gurses, A.P. Work-related factors, job satisfaction and intent to leave the current job among United States nurses. *J. Clin. Nurs.* **2015**, *24*, 3224–3232. [CrossRef] [PubMed]
23. Turpin, R.S.; Ozminkowski, R.J.; Sharda, C.E.; Collins, J.J.; Berger, M.L.; Billotti, G.M.; Baase, C.M.; Olson, M.J.; Nicholson, S. Reliability and validity of the Stanford Presenteeism Scale. *J. Occup. Environ. Med.* **2004**, *46*, 1123–1133. [CrossRef] [PubMed]
24. Stolt, M.; Suhonen, R.; Virolainen, P.; Leino-Kilpi, H. Lower extremity musculoskeletal disorders in nurses: A narrative literature review. *Scand. J. Public Health* **2016**, *44*, 106–115. [CrossRef]
25. Cai, S.; Lin, H.; Hu, X.; Cai, Y.; Chen, K.; Cai, W. High fatigue and its associations with health and work related factors among female medical personnel at 54 hospitals in Zhuhai, China. *Psychol. Health Med.* **2018**, *23*, 304–316. [CrossRef] [PubMed]
26. Brandford, A.A.; Reed, D.B. Depression in registered nurses: A state of the science. *Workplace Health Saf.* **2016**, *64*, 488–511. [CrossRef]
27. Kang, W.; Jang, K.-H.; Lim, H.-M.; Ahn, J.-S.; Park, W.-J. The menstrual cycle associated with insomnia in newly employed nurses performing shift work: A 12-month follow-up study. *Int. Arch. Occup. Environ. Health* **2019**, *92*, 227–235. [CrossRef]
28. Morin, C.M.; Belleville, G.; Bélanger, L.; Ivers, H. The Insomnia Severity Index: Psychometric indicators to detect insomnia cases and evaluate treatment response. *Sleep* **2011**, *34*, 601–608. [CrossRef]
29. Krupp, L.B.; LaRocca, N.G.; Muir-Nash, J.; Steinberg, A.D. The fatigue severity scale: Application to patients with multiple sclerosis and systemic lupus erythematosus. *Arch. Neurol.* **1989**, *46*, 1121–1123. [CrossRef]
30. Radloff, L.S. The CES-D Scale: A Self-Report Depression Scale for Research in the General Population. *Appl. Psychol. Meas.* **1977**, *1*, 385–401. [CrossRef]
31. Dunn, H.; Quinn, L.; Corbridge, S.J.; Eldeirawi, K.; Kapella, M.; Collins, E.G. Cluster analysis in nursing research: An introduction, historical perspective, and future directions. *West. J. Nurs. Res.* **2018**, *40*, 1658–1676. [CrossRef]
32. Clatworthy, J.; Buick, D.; Hankins, M.; Weinman, J.; Horne, R. The use and reporting of cluster analysis in health psychology: A review. *Br. J. Health Psychol.* **2005**, *10*, 329–358. [CrossRef] [PubMed]
33. Brooks, I.; Swailes, S. Analysis of the relationship between nurse influences over flexible working and commitment to nursing. *J. Adv. Nurs.* **2002**, *38*, 117–126. [CrossRef]
34. Milisen, K.; Abraham, I.; Siebens, K.; Darras, E.; Dierckx de Casterlé, B. Work environment and workforce problems: A cross-sectional questionnaire survey of hospital nurses in Belgium. *Int. J. Nurs. Stud.* **2006**, *43*, 745–754. [CrossRef] [PubMed]
35. Jiang, F.; Zhou, H.; Rakofsky, J.; Hu, L.; Liu, T.; Wu, S.; Liu, H.; Liu, Y.; Tang, Y. Intention to leave and associated factors among psychiatric nurses in China: A nationwide cross-sectional study. *Int. J. Nurs. Stud.* **2019**, *94*, 159–165. [CrossRef] [PubMed]
36. Camerino, D.; Conway, P.M.; Estryn-Béhar, M.; Costa, G.; Hasselhorn, H.-M. Age-dependent relationships between work ability, thinking of quitting the job, and actual leaving among Italian nurses: A longitudinal study. *Int. J. Nurs. Stud.* **2008**, *45*, 1645–1659. [CrossRef]
37. Estryn-Béhar, M.; Van der Heijden, B.I.; Ogińska, H.; Camerino, D.; Le Nézet, O.; Conway, P.M.; Fry, C.; Hasselhorn, H.-M. The impact of social work environment, teamwork characteristics, burnout, and personal factors upon intent to leave among European nurses. *Med. Care* **2007**, *45*, 939–950. [CrossRef] [PubMed]
38. Chang, C.S.; Du, P.L.; Huang, I.C. Nurses' perceptions of severe acute respiratory syndrome: Relationship between commitment and intention to leave nursing. *J. Adv. Nurs.* **2006**, *54*, 171–179. [CrossRef]
39. Liu, Y.; Wu, L.M.; Chou, P.L.; Chen, M.H.; Yang, L.C.; Hsu, H.T. The influence of work-related fatigue, work conditions, and personal characteristics on intent to leave among new nurses. *J. Nurs. Scholarsh.* **2016**, *48*, 66–73. [CrossRef]
40. Richter, K.; Acker, J.; Adam, S.; Niklewski, G. Prevention of fatigue and insomnia in shift workers-a review of non-pharmacological measures. *EPMA J.* **2016**, *7*, 16. [CrossRef]
41. Ferris, J. Nursing Fatigue: An Evidence-Based Practice Review for Oncology Nurses. *Clin. J. Oncol. Nurs.* **2015**, *19*, 662–664. [CrossRef]

42. Shimizu, T.; Eto, R.; Horiguchi, I.; Obata, Y.; Feng, Q.; Nagata, S. Relationship between Turnover and Periodic Health Check-Up Data among Japanese Hospital Nurses: A Three-Year Follow-Up Study. *J. Occup. Health* **2005**, *47*, 327–333. [CrossRef] [PubMed]
43. Lai, H.; Lin, Y.; Chang, H.; Wang, S.; Liu, Y.; Lee, H.; Peng, T.; Chang, F. Intensive care unit staff nurses: Predicting factors for career decisions. *J. Clin. Nurs.* **2008**, *17*, 1886–1896. [CrossRef]
44. Hsieh, M.L.; Li, Y.M.; Chang, E.T.; Lai, H.L.; Wang, W.H.; Wang, S.C. Sleep disorder in Taiwanese nurses: A random sample survey. *Nurs. Health Sci.* **2011**, *13*, 468–474. [CrossRef] [PubMed]
45. Sun, Q.; Ji, X.; Zhou, W.; Liu, J. Sleep problems in shift nurses: A brief review and recommendations at both individual and institutional levels. *J. Nurs. Manag.* **2019**, *27*, 10–18. [CrossRef]
46. Bower, J.E.; Ganz, P.A.; Irwin, M.R.; Kwan, L.; Breen, E.C.; Cole, S.W. Inflammation and behavioral symptoms after breast cancer treatment: Do fatigue, depression, and sleep disturbance share a common underlying mechanism? *J. Clin. Oncol. Off. J. Am. Soc. Clin. Oncol.* **2011**, *29*, 3517–3522. [CrossRef]
47. Ho, S.-Y.; Rohan, K.J.; Parent, J.; Tager, F.A.; McKinley, P.S. A longitudinal study of depression, fatigue, and sleep disturbances as a symptom cluster in women with breast cancer. *J. Pain Symptom Manag.* **2015**, *49*, 707–715. [CrossRef]
48. Knutsson, A.; Bøggild, H. Gastrointestinal disorders among shift workers. *Scand. J. Work. Environ. Health* **2010**, *36*, 85–95. [CrossRef]
49. Joung Kim, Y.; Ban, D.J. Prevalence of irritable bowel syndrome, influence of lifestyle factors and bowel habits in Korean college students. *Int. J. Nurs. Stud.* **2005**, *42*, 247–254. [CrossRef]
50. Cho, S.H.; Chun, H.; Lee, H.S.; Lee, S.W.; Shim, K.W.; Lee, J.Y.; Byun, A.R.; Lee, H.Y. The Relationship between Shared Breakfast and Skipping Breakfast with Depression and General Health State in Korean Adults: The 2014 Korea National Health and Nutrition Examination Survey. *Korean J. Fam. Pract.* **2018**, *8*, 441–447. [CrossRef]
51. Lee, S.; Lee, J.; Kwon, Y.; Kim, J.; Sohn, J. Clinical Implications of Associations between Headache and Gastrointestinal Disorders: A Study Using the Hallym Smart Clinical Data Warehouse. *Front. Neurol.* **2017**, *8*, 526. [CrossRef]
52. Aamodt, A.; Stovner, L.; Hagen, K.; Zwart, J. Comorbidity of Headache and Gastrointestinal Complaints. The Head-HUNT Study. *Cephalalgia* **2008**, *28*, 144–151. [PubMed]
53. Welton, J.M.; Decker, M.; Adam, J.; Zone-Smith, L. How far do nurses walk? *Medsurg Nurs.* **2006**, *15*, 213–216. [PubMed]
54. Trinkoff, A.M.; Lipscomb, J.A.; Geiger-Brown, J.; Storr, C.L.; Brady, B.A. Perceived physical demands and reported musculoskeletal problems in registered nurses. *Am. J. Prev. Med.* **2003**, *24*, 270–275. [CrossRef]
55. Carnes, D.; Parsons, S.; Ashby, D.; Breen, A.; Foster, N.; Pincus, T.; Vogel, S.; Underwood, M. Chronic musculoskeletal pain rarely presents in a single body site: Results from a UK population study. *Rheumatology* **2007**, *46*, 1168–1170. [CrossRef]
56. Colditz, G.A.; Hankinson, S.E. The Nurses' Health Study: Lifestyle and health among women. *Nat. Rev. Cancer* **2005**, *5*, 388–396. [CrossRef]

8

Workplace Violence and its Effects on Burnout and Secondary Traumatic Stress among Mental Healthcare Nurses

Yudai Kobayashi, Misari Oe *, Tetsuya Ishida, Michiko Matsuoka, Hiromi Chiba and Naohisa Uchimura

Department of Neuropsychiatry, Kurume University School of Medicine, Asahi-machi 67, Kurume 830-0011, Japan
* Correspondence: oe_misari@kurume-u.ac.jp

Abstract: Workplace violence (WPV) in healthcare settings has drawn attention for over 20 years, yet few studies have investigated the association between WPV and psychological consequences. Here, we used a cross-sectional design to investigate (1) the 12-month prevalence of workplace violence (WPV), (2) the characteristics of WPV, and (3) the relationship between WPV and burnout/secondary traumatic stress among 599 mental healthcare nurses (including assistant nurses) from eight hospitals. Over 40% of the respondents had experienced WPV within the past 12 months. A multivariate logistic regression analysis indicated that occupation and burnout were each significantly related to WPV. Secondary traumatic stress was not related to WPV. Our results suggest that WPV may be a long-lasting and/or cumulative stressor rather than a brief, extreme horror experience and may reflect specific characteristics of psychological effects in psychiatric wards. A longitudinal study measuring the severity and frequency of WPV, work- and non-work-related stressors, risk factors, and protective factors is needed, as is the development of a program that helps reduce the psychological burden of mental healthcare nurses due to WPV.

Keywords: workplace violence; mental healthcare nurses; secondary traumatic stress; burnout; nursing license

---

1. Introduction

Workplace violence (WPV) is defined as any incident in which a person is abused, threatened, or assaulted in circumstances related to their work; this can include verbal abuse and threats as well as physical attacks [1,2]. The International Labor Organization reported that the magnitude of exposure to violence at work depends not only on a person's occupation but also upon the circumstances named "situations at risk," including those associated with working alone (e.g., small shops); working with the public (e.g., railway workers); working with valuables (e.g., financial institutions); working with people in distress (e.g., healthcare workers); working in an environment that is increasingly open to violence (e.g., school teachers); working in conditions of special vulnerability (e.g., immigrant workers); working in military and paramilitary organizations; and working in zones of conflict [3].

Workplace violence (WPV) in healthcare settings has been drawing attention for over 20 years [2,4–8] and has been reported in many places, including Europe [9], Asia [10–12], the U.S. [13], and the Middle East [14]. According to a recent review, the prevalence of WPV against healthcare workers was higher in Asian and North American countries than that in other countries [15]. Female nurses were reported to be the victims of verbal abuse more often than male nurses, and male nurses were reported to be more commonly the victims of physical abuse [7]. Most of the WPV in healthcare settings occurs in psychiatric departments, emergency services, polyclinics/waiting rooms, and geriatric units [8].

According to a review of WPV in psychiatric wards over the past 20 years, studies of WPV have examined mainly its occurrence rate, risk assessment, and risk management; fewer investigations have assessed the physical and psychological consequences of WPV [2]. WPV may cause not only physical injuries but also psychological impacts, resulting in higher rates of fear or anxiety, anger, insecurity, depression, emotional exhaustion, suicidal thoughts, post-traumatic stress symptoms, guilt, self-blame, and shame [2,8]. The consequences of WPV include decreased job satisfaction, increased intent to leave the organization, and lowered health-related quality of life [2].

WPV and its consequences among nurses in Japan have been described [10,16–20]. Of respondents to previous surveys, 33–47% of the nurses had experienced WPV during the prior 12 months [16–18]. The proportion of nurses who experienced physical aggression and verbal abuse was significantly high in psychiatric wards [16]. Another study showed that nurses who had encountered verbal abuse or violence by patients in psychiatry departments had experienced severe psychological impacts such as secondary traumatic stress and low satisfaction with family support [10]. The characteristics of WPV itself in Japan have been evaluated, but few studies have examined the psychological effects of WPV in detail.

Burnout is defined as a syndrome conceptualized as resulting from chronic workplace stress that has not been successfully managed [21]. It is characterized by three dimensions: feelings of energy depletion or exhaustion; increased mental distance from one's job or feelings of negativism or cynicism related to one's job; and reduced professional efficacy [21]. In the International Classification of Diseases, 11th revision (ICD-11), the definition is more detailed: "burnout refers specifically to phenomena in the occupational context and should not be applied experiences in other areas of life" [22]. Among healthcare workers, nurses are known to struggle with burnout symptoms the most, and this poses serious consequences for patients, other healthcare professionals, and healthcare organizations [23]. A meta-analysis on burnout in mental healthcare nurses showed that variables such as work overload, work-related stress, professional seniority, male gender, being single, and aggression at work contributed to burnout development [24]. Burnout is regarded as one of the relevant consequences of WPV [2,25]. Associations between WPV and burnout, turnover intention [26,27], and intention to leave [28] have been described.

Secondary traumatic stress (STS) is a syndrome including intrusion, avoidance, and arousal resulting from indirect traumatic exposure in a professional context [29]. A study conducted in Israel showed that psychiatric nurses reported higher levels of STS symptoms compared to community nurses [30]. Another study revealed a high correlation between work-related post-traumatic stress disorder (PTSD) symptoms (due to traumatic stressors such as WPV), STS, and burnout in psychiatric nurses [31].

We conducted the present study to investigate the prevalence of WPV and its effects on burnout and STS among mental healthcare nurses in Japan. We focused on mental healthcare nurses because there have been few investigations of the association between WPV and psychological consequences. We conducted a large-scale, multicenter study to clarify the psychological impact of WPV by using questionnaires about the respondents' well-being, psychological distress, alcohol use disorder, and anger related to harmful experiences, as well as compassion satisfaction, burnout and STS. We tested our hypothesis that mental healthcare nurses who have experienced WPV have a higher rate of burnout and higher secondary traumatic stress.

2. Participants and Methods

2.1. Study Design

This is a questionnaire-based cross-sectional study.

2.2. *Participants and Procedures*

Mental health nurses and mental health assistant nurses working at the mental health ward of a university hospital or one of seven mental health hospitals (i.e., psychiatric inpatient, outpatient, and day-treatment centers) on the island of Kyushu in Japan were recruited using the convenience (i.e., not randomized) sampling method. The inclusion criterion was age 20–79 years old. Candidates who could not understand the questionnaires in Japanese were excluded.

The researcher in charge (Y.K.) explained the purpose and methods of the research to the head nurse of the psychiatric neurology ward of A University Hospital (pseudonym) and the head of each hospital both in a letter of request and orally. After obtaining the hospital's consent to participate in the research in a letter of consent, the researcher in charge distributed a set of questionnaires to the person in charge of the target hospital (the person in charge of the facility at the head of each ward or the secretary-level depending on the hospital). The researcher in charge verbally explained the freedom of research participation, significance, the purpose of use, method of use, questionnaire items, the protection of personal information, the questionnaire handling after collection, and contact information, etc. to the person in charge at the facility. That person then verbally explained the study to the research subjects, i.e., nurses. Participants were encouraged to fill out the questionnaires when they were alone outside of work hours. The questionnaires were hand-delivered by a person in charge at each hospital, and the enclosed envelopes were sealed up to 2 weeks after distribution. The completed questionnaires were dropped into collection boxes placed temporarily at each hospital. The researcher in charge retrieved the questionnaires.

The respondents' data were collected from October 18 to November 30, 2019. The questionnaires were administered and completed anonymously. We collected sociodemographic data such as sex, age, marital status, occupation, years of experience as a registered nurse or as an assistant nurse, the type of present workplace (acute ward or others). Of 650 eligible nurses, 599 nurses and assistant nurses participated in the study (response rate, 92.2%). We did not obtain the sociodemographic information of the non-respondents.

2.3. *Measures*

2.3.1. Well-Being

The World Health Organization-Five Well-Being Index (WHO-5) is a five-item self-report questionnaire developed by the WHO; it measures the respondent's current mental well-being [32]. The total raw score, ranging from 0 to 25, is multiplied by 4 to give the final score, with 0 representing the worst imaginable well-being and 100 representing the best imaginable well-being. The Japanese version of the WHO-5 was validated by Awata et al. [33,34] and showed sufficient reliability and validity in community-dwelling elderly persons and in diabetic patients. A cutoff score of the Japanese WHO-5 version at 11/12 or 12/13 of the raw total score for detecting depression was recommended by Awata et al. for the Japanese version [33]. In the present study, we used 12/13 as the cutoff score for low well-being according to Awata's recommendation. Cronbach's alpha of the present study was 0.89.

2.3.2. Psychological Distress

The Kessler six-item scale (K6) is a self-report questionnaire measuring psychological distress; it consists of six brief questions [35]. The total score (ranging from 0 to 24) has been used as an indicator of serious mental illness or mood and anxiety disorders in the general population. The Japanese version of the K6 showed screening performance that was essentially equivalent to that of the original English version [36,37]. We adopted the 12/13 cut-off according to Kessler's recommendation [35]. The Cronbach's alpha of the present study was 0.88.

2.3.3. Alcohol Use Disorder

The Alcohol Use Disorder Identification Test (AUDIT), which was developed by the WHO for the screening of excessive drinking, is a 10-item self-report questionnaire [38]. The Japanese version of the AUDIT was validated by Kawada et al. [39] and showed satisfactory internal reliability. The score ranges from 0 to 40. In Japan, a total score ≥11 is considered indicative of alcohol abuse [40]. The Cronbach's alpha of the present study was 0.79.

2.3.4. Anger Related to Harmful Experience

The Dimensions of Anger Reaction-5 (DAR-5) is a five-item self-report questionnaire regarding the respondent's anger reaction after a harmful experience such as violence. The DAR-5 was developed and validated by Forbes et al. [41,42]. The score ranges from 5 to 25. Because the Japanese version of the DAR-5 has not been developed, we used a back-translated version provided by a principal researcher in this study. According to Forbes et al., the cutoff point of 12 was used for high risk. The Cronbach's alpha of the present study was 0.80.

2.3.5. Workplace Violence

For assessing WPV, we asked eight questions that were used in a prior study's questionnaire regarding WPV [43]; that questionnaire was derived from the "WPV in the Health Sector Country Case Studies Research Instruments Survey Questionnaires" [44] as set out by an International Labor Office/International Council of Nurses/WHO/Public Services International (ILO/ICN/WHO/PSI) project. Because there was no Japanese version for these questions, we used a back-translated version provided by a principal researcher. Among the eight questions, four were qualitative yes/no questions (the existence of violence within the past 12 months, the existence of physical injury, whether the respondent thinks that this violence was avoidable, and the presence of help-seeking behavior); one was a quantitative question (psychological influence), and the remaining three questions were qualitative multiple-choice questions (characteristics of violence, perpetrator, type of coping behaviors).

2.3.6. Burnout, Secondary Traumatic Stress, and Compassion Satisfaction

We used the ProQOL (Professional Quality of Life) scale to measure burnout and secondary traumatic stress simultaneously. As a 30-item self-report questionnaire developed by Stamm [45], the ProQOL consists of three subscales: compassion satisfaction, burnout, and secondary traumatic stress. "Compassion satisfaction" is about the pleasure that a person derives from being able to do his/her work well. Burnout and secondary traumatic stress are negative aspects of one's professional quality of life. In the ProQOL scale, burnout is indicated by exhaustion, frustration, anger, and depressive symptoms. An example of the scale's burnout subscale questions is "I feel connected to others." Secondary traumatic stress is about work-related secondary exposure to people who have experienced extremely or traumatically stressful events. The negative effects of secondary traumatic stress can include fear, sleep difficulties, intrusive images, and avoiding reminders of the person's traumatic experiences. An example of the ProQOL scale's secondary traumatic stress question is "I jump or am startled by unexpected sounds."

The Japanese version of the ProQOL was validated by Fukumori et al. [46]. According to those authors, a high risk of compassion satisfaction is indicated by a score of ≤26 points, a high risk of burnout by a score of ≥33 points, and a high risk of secondary traumatic stress by ≥28 points [46]. The Cronbach's alpha of the present study was 0.78. We considered the fact that burnout and secondary traumatic stress were clearly separated as subscales to be an advantage in the present study.

2.4. Statistical Analyses

All statistical analyses were conducted using JMP Pro for Windows, ver. 14 (SAS Institute, Cary, NC, USA). The chi-square (χ^2) test was used for testing relationships between categorical variables.

The Shapiro–Wilk test was used to check normal distributions of the continuous variables. Only the compassion satisfaction subscale of the ProQOL showed a normal distribution. In light of these results, we decided to use non-parametric analyses. The Mann–Whitney U test was used for comparisons of two independent groups. We performed a multivariate logistic regression analysis to test the association between a categorical dependent variable and a set of independent variables. All tests were two-sided and based on a 0.05 level of significance. Pairwise deletion was conducted for missing data.

2.5. Ethical Considerations

All subjects gave their informed consent for inclusion before they participated in the study. The study was conducted in accord with the Declaration of Helsinki, and the protocol was approved by the Ethical Committee of Kurume University, Japan (approval no. 19100, approved on 9 September 2019).

3. Results

3.1. Sociodemographic Characteristics of the Participants

The sociodemographic characteristics of the study participants are summarized in Table 1. Females accounted for 65.4% of the participants, and the mean age was 47.1 years. Regarding the specific nursing occupations, 66.4% of the participants were certified nurses, and 32.6% had an assistant nurse certification. Concerning marital status, 353 (58.9%) of the participants were married, 122 (20.4%) participants were single, 87 (14.5%) participants were divorced, and 30 (5.0%) participants were widowed (missing data; $n = 7$). There were 258 (43.6%) participants working at acute wards, and the others were working at chronic wards or at an outpatient division.

Table 1. Sociodemographics and comparison of the groups with and without workplace violence within the past 12 months ($n = 599$).

Variables	Total ($n = 599$)	With WPV ($n = 265$)	Without WPV ($n = 328$)	Test	Probability
	n	n (%)	n (%)	χ^2	p
Sex					
Female	390	169 (43.7)	218 (56.3)		
Male	206	95 (46.3)	110 (53.7)	0.4	0.5
Missing	3				
Occupation					
Nurse	398	197 (49.5)	201 (50.5)		
Assistant nurse	195	64 (33.5)	127 (66.5)	13.6 *	<0.01
Missing	6				
Ward					
Acute ward	258	129 (50.2)	128 (49.8)		
Others	334	134 (40.5)	197 (59.5)	5.5 *	0.02
Missing	7				
	Mean (SD)	**Mean (SD)**	**Mean (SD)**	$\lvert z \rvert$	p
Age, years	47.1 (13.2)	45.7 (11.9)	48.4 (14.0)	2.5 *	0.01
Duration as nurse, years	19.8 (13.4)	19.0 (11.9)	20.5 (14.5)	0.8	0.4
WHO-5 final score	48.2 (19.0)	45.5 (18.7)	50.3 (19.0)	2.8 *	<0.01
K6	5.4 (4.5)	6.2 (4.9)	4.7 (4.1)	3.8*	<0.01
AUDIT	3.9 (4.7)	3.9 (4.8)	3.8 (4.6)	0.4	0.7
DAR-5	7.3 (2.6)	7.9 (3.0)	6.8 (2.2)	5.2 *	<0.01
Compassion satisfaction	24.4 (8.7)	23.5 (9.0)	25.2 (8.4)	2.3*	0.02
Burnout	25.4 (6.4)	26.5 (5.8)	24.4 (6.8)	3.3*	<0.01
Secondary traumatic stress	12.0 (6.8)	13.6 (7.1)	10.6 (6.2)	5.4*	<0.01

WPV: workplace violence; WHO-5: World Health Organization-Five Well-Being Index; K6: Kessler Six-Item Scale; AUDIT: Alcohol Use Disorder Identification Test; DAR-5: Dimensions of Anger Reaction-5. * $p < 0.05$.

3.2. Prevalence of WPV within the Past 12 Months and the Characteristics of the WPV

Among these 599 mental health nurses (including assistant nurses), 265 participants (44.7%) answered that they had experienced WPV within the past 12 months. Regarding the types of violence (multiple choices were available), verbal violence was reported by 165 participants (62.3% of 265 victims); physical violence was reported by 160 participants (60.4%); and sexual violence was reported by seven participants (2.6%). Sex did not affect the percentages of the types of violence. The mean age among the nurses who experienced physical violence was significantly lower than that of the nurses who had not had this experience: (mean ± SD) 44.7 ± 12.0 vs. 48.2 ± 13.4, $|z| = 2.9$, $p < 0.01$). The percentages of verbal violence and sex violence were not significantly different among the types of working wards, but the percentage of physical violence in the participants working at acute wards (33.3%) was significantly higher than that of the participants working at other places (22.0%, $\chi^2 = 9.4$, $p < 0.01$). The percentage of sexual violence did not differ by occupation, but there was a significantly higher percentage of verbal violence among the nurses (31.1%) than among the assistant nurses (21.4%, $\chi^2 = 6.1$, $p = 0.01$), and a significantly higher percentage of physical violence among the nurses (30.8%) than among the assistant nurses (18.2%, $\chi^2 = 10.5$, $p < 0.01$).

The perpetrators of WPV were the subject of a multiple-choice question: 223 participants (84.2% of 265 victims) reported that the perpetrator was a patient, 11 participants (4.2%) described a patient's family member, 35 participants (13.2%) reported a work colleague, and 33 participants (12.5%) responded that their boss or supervisor was the perpetrator of WPV.

3.3. Mental Health Status of Nurses Who Experience WPV

The mean values and standard deviations of the mental health status results are summarized in Table 1. The number of participants who attained a low value of well-being as the WHO-5 raw score was 310 (52.6%) participants. The number of participants with high psychological distress on the K6 was 42 (7.1%). Fifty-six (10.1%) participants reported problem drinking, and 41 (7.2%) participants were at high risk of anger related to harmful experiences. The number of participants at high risk of compassion satisfaction was 332 (59.4%); that of burnout was 62 (10.9%); and that of secondary traumatic stress was 18 (3.2%).

3.4. Comparisons of the Groups with and without Workplace Violence

The results of our comparisons of mental health status between the participants with ($n = 265$) and without ($n = 328$) WPV (missing data; $n = 6$) are provided in Table 1. The χ^2 analyses revealed that there were significant differences between these two groups in occupation and type of workplace (wards). The nurses had experienced WPV more than the assistant nurses had, and the nurses who were working at acute wards had experienced WPV more compared to the nurses who worked at other wards. There was no significant difference in the experience of WPV based on marital status. The Mann–Whitney U-tests showed that there were significant differences in age, the well-being score, psychological distress, anger, and three subscales of professional quality of life. The participants who experienced WPV were younger and showed lower well-being, higher psychological distress, higher anger, lower compassion satisfaction, higher burnout, and higher secondary traumatic stress.

3.5. Risk Factors of Workplace Violence

To investigate the risk factors of WPV, we conducted a multivariate logistic regression analysis using sociodemographic characteristic variables (sex, age, years of experience, occupation, and ward type) and symptom measures (well-being, psychological distress, alcohol use, anger, (low) compassion satisfaction, burnout, and secondary traumatic stress) as listed in Table 2. Among them, occupation and burnout were each identified as a significant factor related to WPV. The odds ratio of nurses experiencing WPV compared to the assistant nurses was 2.03.

Table 2. Multivariate logistic regression analysis for workplace violence within the past 12 months.

Independent Variable	Beta	Wald	*p*	OR	95% CI
Sex, 1: male, 0: female	−0.08	0.57	0.45	0.85	0.55–1.31
Age	−0.01	0.70	0.40	0.99	0.96–1.01
Years of experience	−0.005	0.16	0.69	1.00	0.97–1.01
Occupation, 1: Nurse, 0: Assistant nurse	0.35	9.96	<0.01	2.03	1.31–3.15
Ward, 1: Acute ward, 0: other	0.09	0.72	0.39	1.19	0.80–1.78
WHO-5, 1: raw score ≤12, 0: others	0.04	0.17	0.68	1.09	0.72–1.67
K6, 1: ≥13, 0: others	0.28	1.70	0.19	1.75	0.75–4.06
AUDIT, 1: ≥11, 0: others	0.13	0.53	0.47	1.29	0.65–2.55
DAR-5, 1: ≥12, 0: others	0.29	2.09	0.15	1.78	0.81–3.90
Compassion satisfaction, 1: ≤26, 0: others	0.05	0.24	0.62	1.11	0.73–1.70
Burnout, 1: ≥33, 0: others	0.34	4.33	0.04	1.99	1.04–3.81
Secondary traumatic stress, 1: ≥28, 0: others	0.22	0.46	0.50	1.55	0.44–5.50

4. Discussion

4.1. Main Findings

The respondents' questionnaire results demonstrated that >40% of the respondents had experienced WPV within the prior 12 months. Compared to the nurses who did not experience WPV, the respondents who experienced WPV were younger and showed lower well-being scores, higher psychological distress, higher anger, lower compassion satisfaction, higher burnout, and higher secondary traumatic stress. These results revealed that WPV affects the mental health status of staff. The high prevalence of WPV observed in this study population is consistent with those of studies conducted in Japan [16] and other countries [43,47]. The effects of WPV on the present nurses' mental health status are also in line with those of previous investigations [2,8].

However, our present findings do not support our hypothesis that WPV is associated with higher burnout and higher secondary traumatic stress. In the multivariate regression analysis, only burnout was associated with WPV; secondary traumatic stress was not. The association we observed between WPV and burnout is in agreement with previous studies [25,48,49]. A cross-sectional study conducted in the Netherlands revealed that physical aggression was positively associated with the staff's burnout symptoms [48], and this association remained in the same study sample over a two-year longitudinal study [49]. The advantage of the present investigation is that we examined burnout and secondary traumatic stress using the ProQOL scale, which can avoid overlapping of symptoms. Our finding that WPV was not associated with secondary traumatic stress suggests that the psychological burden of mental healthcare nurses that is due to WPV may be recognized as a long-lasting and/or cumulative stressor rather than as a brief, extreme horror experience, and it may reflect specific characteristics of psychological effects in psychiatric wards.

Researchers in Israel investigating mental healthcare nurses reported that the association between WPV and burnout/secondary traumatic stress was observed only indirectly via general work stress in the prior month [50]. Those authors explained that mental healthcare nurses may feel that WPV is an integral component of their job, and low burnout/secondary traumatic stress may be an adjusted reaction to their work environment [50,51]. Our present data showing a direct association between WPV and burnout may call this idea into question, and it may suggest that mental healthcare nurses with WPV feel a psychological overload as maladaptation to their work environment.

Interestingly, we also observed that the type of nursing license was a risk factor for WPV; the questionnaire results demonstrated that the nurses experienced more WPV than the assistant nurses. This is not consistent with a recent Japanese study investigating job-related stress [52]. In that study, assistant nurses who were working at psychiatry hospitals experienced more irritability and somatic symptoms than the nurses working there. The authors of that study speculated that stronger stress reactions of assistant nurses were observed because of their lesser education period compared to the certified nurses. In our study, we asked about the existence of WPV, which is categorized into an objective variable. The reason for the higher frequency of WPV among nurses may be because nurses tend to play a more responsible role; for example, persuading a patient to accept medication or a medical treatment or conducting forced treatment. A U.S. study investigating work-related violence based on the type of nursing license (between registered nurses and licensed practical nurses) showed that the risk of physical assault was increased for the licensed practical nurses working with neonatal/pediatric patients, whereas the registered nurses' risk was decreased; the registered nurses' risk of physical violence increased while providing patient care, whereas the licensed practical nurses' risk increased while supervising patient care [53].

Although we did not find an association in multivariate analysis, our present study revealed that psychiatric nurses working at acute wards had encountered more physical violence compared to that in other workplaces for nurses. This is consistent with a study that showed that patients with mental illness (affected by dementia, mental retardation, drug and substance abuse, or other psychiatric disorders) were the most frequent perpetrators of physical violence in a general hospital [54]. It is also of note that verbal violence was observed equally in acute wards and in other places including chronic wards in the present study.

4.2. *Recommendations for Further Research*

We raise four major challenges for further research. First, because we did not measure the severity and frequency of WPV, a study measuring them may play a role. Second, we detected an association between WPV and burnout, but we did not ask the participants about their stressors other than WPV. Moreover, our study was cross-sectional. It is thus necessary to conduct a large-scale longitudinal cohort study to assess the impacts of WPV, work-related stressors, and non-work-related stressors. It has been reported that both WPV and burnout were positively associated with turnover intention [26]. Third, not only risk factors but also factors that protect against negative psychological impacts after WPV should be examined. A study in Canada investigated the role of relational occupational coping self-efficacy against workplace incivility and burnout and revealed that self-coping is a protective factor [55]. Fourth, a program that helps reduce the psychological burden of mental healthcare nurses due to WPV should be developed. A study demonstrated that the life satisfaction of mental healthcare nurses was affected more by staff resilience, post-traumatic growth, and job stress than by WPV [56]. A program with strategies for increasing occupational coping self-efficacy, resilience, and post-traumatic growth may be effective.

4.3. *Study Limitations*

There are several limitations to be considered in this study. (1) The study's design was cross-sectional, and we cannot discuss causality. (2) We did not include a comparison group such as nurses working in an internal medicine ward. (3) We did not use validated versions of the evaluations for anger and WPV. (4) We did not obtain the sociodemographic information of the non-respondents; this may have caused selection bias.

5. Conclusions

The results of our study demonstrated that mental healthcare nurses who experienced WPV showed a poorer mental health status, and WPV was associated with burnout among mental healthcare nurses in Japan. Further research is merited, including longitudinal studies, investigations assessing risk and protective factors, and the development of an intervention program for the psychological burden experienced after WPV. An expansion of the existing call to action by the implementation of policy changes is also important to mitigate workplace violence in healthcare settings.

Author Contributions: Conceptualization, Y.K., M.O., M.M., and T.I.; methodology, M.O.; writing—original draft preparation, Y.K. and M.O.; writing—review and editing, M.M., T.I., H.C., and N.U.; project administration, M.O.; funding acquisition, H.C. and M.O. All authors have read and agreed to the published version of the manuscript.

References

1. Health and Safety Executive. Work-related Violence. Available online: http://www.hse.gov.uk/violence/index.htm. (accessed on 1 April 2020).
2. d'Ettorre, G.; Pellicani, V. Workplace Violence Toward Mental Healthcare Workers Employed in Psychiatric Wards. *Saf. Health Work* **2017**, *8*, 337–342. [CrossRef]
3. Chappell, D.; Di Martino, V. *Violence at Work*, 3rd ed.; International Labour Office: Geneva, Switzerland, 2006.
4. Schnieden, V. Violence against doctors. *Br. J. Hosp. Med.* **1993**, *50*, 9.
5. Martinez, A.J. Managing Workplace Violence with Evidence-Based Interventions: A Literature Review. *J. Psychosoc. Nurs. Ment. Health Serv.* **2016**, *54*, 31–36. [CrossRef]
6. D'Ettorre, G.; Pellicani, V.; Mazzotta, M.; Vullo, A. Preventing and managing workplace violence against healthcare workers in Emergency Departments. *Acta Biomed.* **2018**, *89*, 28–36. [CrossRef] [PubMed]
7. Edward, K.L.; Stephenson, J.; Ousey, K.; Lui, S.; Warelow, P.; Giandinoto, J.A. A systematic review and meta-analysis of factors that relate to aggression perpetrated against nurses by patients/relatives or staff. *J. Clin. Nurs.* **2016**, *25*, 289–299. [CrossRef] [PubMed]
8. Mento, C.; Silvestri, M.C.; Bruno, A.; Muscatello, M.R.A.; Cedro, C.; Pandolfo, G.; Zoccali, R.A. Workplace violence against healthcare professionals: A systematic review. *Aggress. Violence Behav.* **2020**, *51*, 101381. [CrossRef]
9. Firenze, A.; Santangelo, O.E.; Gianfredi, V.; Alagna, E.; Cedrone, F.; Provenzano, S.; La Torre, G. Violence on doctors. An observational study in Northern Italy. *Med. Lav.* **2020**, *111*, 46–53. [CrossRef] [PubMed]
10. Inoue, M.; Tsukano, K.; Muraoka, M.; Kaneko, F.; Okamura, H. Psychological impact of verbal abuse and violence by patients on nurses working in psychiatric departments. *Psychiatry Clin. Neurosci.* **2006**, *60*, 29–36. [CrossRef] [PubMed]
11. Shi, L.; Li, G.; Hao, J.; Wang, W.; Chen, W.; Liu, S.; Yu, Z.; Shi, Y.; Ma, Y.; Fan, L.; et al. Psychological depletion in physicians and nurses exposed to workplace violence: A cross-sectional study using propensity score analysis. *Int. J. Nurs. Stud.* **2020**, *103*, 103493. [CrossRef]
12. Lee, H.L.; Han, C.Y.; Redley, B.; Lin, C.C.; Lee, M.Y.; Chang, W. Workplace Violence Against Emergency Nurses in Taiwan: A Cross-Sectional Study. *J. Emerg. Nurs.* **2020**, *46*, 66–71.e64. [CrossRef]
13. Phillips, J.P. Workplace Violence against Health Care Workers in the United States. *N. Engl. J. Med.* **2016**, *375*, e14. [CrossRef] [PubMed]
14. Alshehry, A.S.; Alquwez, N.; Almazan, J.; Namis, I.M.; Cruz, J.P. Influence of workplace incivility on the quality of nursing care. *J. Clin. Nurs.* **2019**, *28*, 4582–4594. [CrossRef] [PubMed]
15. Liu, J.; Gan, Y.; Jiang, H.; Li, L.; Dwyer, R.; Lu, K.; Yan, S.; Sampson, O.; Xu, H.; Wang, C.; et al. Prevalence of workplace violence against healthcare workers: A systematic review and meta-analysis. *Occup. Environ. Med.* **2019**, *76*, 927–937. [CrossRef] [PubMed]
16. Fujita, S.; Ito, S.; Seto, K.; Kitazawa, T.; Matsumoto, K.; Hasegawa, T. Risk factors of workplace violence at hospitals in Japan. *J. Hosp. Med.* **2012**, *7*, 79–84. [CrossRef] [PubMed]
17. Fujimoto, H.; Greiner, C.; Hirota, M.; Yamaguchi, Y.; Ryuno, H.; Hashimoto, T. Experiences of Violence and Preventive Measures Among Nurses in Psychiatric and Non-Psychiatric Home Visit Nursing Services in Japan. *J. Psychosoc. Nurs. Ment. Health Serv.* **2019**, *57*, 40–48. [CrossRef]
18. Sato, K.; Wakabayashi, T.; Kiyoshi-Teo, H.; Fukahori, H. Factors associated with nurses' reporting of patients' aggressive behavior: A cross-sectional survey. *Int. J. Nurs. Stud.* **2013**, *50*, 1368–1376. [CrossRef]

19. Saeki, K.; Okamoto, N.; Tomioka, K.; Obayashi, K.; Nishioka, H.; Ohara, K.; Kurumatani, N. Work-related aggression and violence committed by patients and its psychological influence on doctors. *J. Occup. Health* **2011**, *53*, 356–364. [CrossRef]
20. Kimura, Y.; Inoue, M. Factors Associated with the Level of Psychological Impact of Patients' Offensive Language/Violence on Psychiatric Nurses Varying in Years of Experience. *Jpn. J. Occup. Med. Traumatol.* **2017**, *65*, 137–142.
21. World Health Organization. International Classification of Diseases 11th Revision. Available online: https://icd.who.int/ (accessed on 1 November 2019).
22. The World Health Organization. Burn-Out an "Occupational Phenomenon": International Classification of Diseases. Available online: https://www.who.int/mental_health/evidence/burn-out/en/ (accessed on 5 April 2020).
23. Woo, T.; Ho, R.; Tang, A.; Tam, W. Global prevalence of burnout symptoms among nurses: A systematic review and meta-analysis. *J. Psychiatr. Res.* **2020**, *123*, 9–20. [CrossRef]
24. López-López, I.M.; Gómez-Urquiza, J.L.; Cañadas, G.R.; De la Fuente, E.I.; Albendín-García, L.; Cañadas-De la Fuente, G.A. Prevalence of burnout in mental health nurses and related factors: A systematic review and meta-analysis. *Int. J. Ment. Health Nurs.* **2019**, *28*, 1032–1041. [CrossRef]
25. Gascon, S.; Leiter, M.P.; Andrés, E.; Santed, M.A.; Pereira, J.P.; Cunha, M.J.; Albesa, A.; Montero-Marín, J.; García-Campayo, J.; Martínez-Jarreta, B. The role of aggressions suffered by healthcare workers as predictors of burnout. *J. Clin. Nurs.* **2013**, *22*, 3120–3129. [CrossRef] [PubMed]
26. Liu, W.; Zhao, S.; Shi, L.; Zhang, Z.; Liu, X.; Li, L.; Duan, X.; Li, G.; Lou, F.; Jia, X.; et al. Workplace violence, job satisfaction, burnout, perceived organisational support and their effects on turnover intention among Chinese nurses in tertiary hospitals: A cross-sectional study. *BMJ Open* **2018**, *8*, e019525. [CrossRef] [PubMed]
27. Choi, S.H.; Lee, H. Workplace violence against nurses in Korea and its impact on professional quality of life and turnover intention. *J. Nurs. Manag.* **2017**, *25*, 508–518. [CrossRef] [PubMed]
28. Wu, Y.; Wang, J.; Liu, J.; Zheng, J.; Liu, K.; Baggs, J.G.; Liu, X.; You, L. The impact of work environment on workplace violence, burnout and work attitudes for hospital nurses: A structural equation modelling analysis. *J. Nurs. Manag.* **2019**. [CrossRef]
29. Figley, C.R.; Carbonell, J.L.; Boscarino, J.A.; Chang, J. A clinical demonstration model for assessing the effectiveness of therapeutic interventions: An expanded clinical trials methodology. *Int. J. Emerg. Ment. Health* **1999**, *1*, 155–164.
30. Zerach, G.; Shalev, T.B. The relations between violence exposure, posttraumatic stress symptoms, secondary traumatization, vicarious post traumatic growth and illness attribution among psychiatric nurses. *Arch. Psychiatr. Nurs.* **2015**, *29*, 135–142. [CrossRef]
31. Tirgari, B.; Azizzadeh Forouzi, M.; Ebrahimpour, M. Relationship Between Posttraumatic Stress Disorder and Compassion Satisfaction, Compassion Fatigue, and Burnout in Iranian Psychiatric Nurses. *J. Psychosoc. Nurs. Ment. Health Serv.* **2019**, *57*, 39–47. [CrossRef]
32. Topp, C.W.; Østergaard, S.D.; Søndergaard, S.; Bech, P. The WHO-5 Well-Being Index: A systematic review of the literature. *Psychother. Psychosom.* **2015**, *84*, 167–176. [CrossRef]
33. Awata, S.; Bech, P.; Yoshida, S.; Hirai, M.; Suzuki, S.; Yamashita, M.; Ohara, A.; Hinokio, Y.; Matsuoka, H.; Oka, Y. Reliability and validity of the Japanese version of the World Health Organization-Five Well-Being Index in the context of detecting depression in diabetic patients. *Psychiatry Clin. Neurosci.* **2007**, *61*, 112–119. [CrossRef]
34. Awata, S.; Bech, P.; Koizumi, Y.; Seki, T.; Kuriyama, S.; Hozawa, A.; Ohmori, K.; Nakaya, N.; Matsuoka, H.; Tsuji, I. Validity and utility of the Japanese version of the WHO-Five Well-Being Index in the context of detecting suicidal ideation in elderly community residents. *Int. Psychogeriatr.* **2007**, *19*, 77–88. [CrossRef]
35. Kessler, R.C.; Barker, P.R.; Colpe, L.J.; Epstein, J.F.; Gfroerer, J.C.; Hiripi, E.; Howes, M.J.; Normand, S.L.; Manderscheid, R.W.; Walters, E.E.; et al. Screening for serious mental illness in the general population. *Arch. Gen. Psychiatry* **2003**, *60*, 184–189. [CrossRef]
36. Furukawa, T.A.; Kawakami, N.; Saitoh, M.; Ono, Y.; Nakane, Y.; Nakamura, Y.; Tachimori, H.; Iwata, N.; Uda, H.; Nakane, H.; et al. The performance of the Japanese version of the K6 and K10 in the World Mental Health Survey Japan. *Int. J. Methods Psychiatr. Res.* **2008**, *17*, 152–158. [CrossRef] [PubMed]

37. Sakurai, K.; Nishi, A.; Kondo, K.; Yanagida, K.; Kawakami, N. Screening performance of K6/K10 and other screening instruments for mood and anxiety disorders in Japan. *Psychiatry Clin. Neurosci.* **2011**, *65*, 434–441. [CrossRef] [PubMed]
38. Reinert, D.F.; Allen, J.P. The alcohol use disorders identification test: An update of research findings. *Alcohol. Clin. Exp. Res.* **2007**, *31*, 185–199. [CrossRef] [PubMed]
39. Kawada, T.; Inagaki, H.; Kuratomi, Y. The alcohol use disorders identification test: Reliability study of the Japanese version. *Alcohol* **2011**, *45*, 205–207. [CrossRef]
40. Hiro, H.; Shima, S. Availability of the Alcohol Use Disorders Identification Test (AUDIT) for a complete health examination in Japan. *Jpn. J. Alcohol Stud. Drug Depend.* **1996**, *31*, 437–450.
41. Forbes, D.; Alkemade, N.; Hopcraft, D.; Hawthorne, G.; O'Halloran, P.; Elhai, J.D.; McHugh, T.; Bates, G.; Novaco, R.W.; Bryant, R.; et al. Evaluation of the dimensions of anger reactions-5 (DAR-5) scale in combat veterans with posttraumatic stress disorder. *J. Anxiety Disord.* **2014**, *28*, 830–835. [CrossRef]
42. Forbes, D.; Alkemade, N.; Mitchell, D.; Elhai, J.D.; McHugh, T.; Bates, G.; Novaco, R.W.; Bryant, R.; Lewis, V. Utility of the Dimensions of Anger Reactions-5 (DAR-5) scale as a brief anger measure. *Depress. Anxiety* **2014**, *31*, 166–173. [CrossRef]
43. Cheung, T.; Yip, P.S. Workplace violence towards nurses in Hong Kong: Prevalence and correlates. *BMC Public Health* **2017**, *17*, 196. [CrossRef]
44. International Labour Office; International Council of Nurses; World Health Organisation; Public Services International. Workplace Violence in the Health Sector Country Case Studies Research Instruments Survey Questionnaires. Available online: https://www.who.int/violence_injury_prevention/violence/interpersonal/en/WVfocusgroupdiscussion.pdf (accessed on 1 April 2020).
45. Stamm, B.H. *The Concise ProQOL Manual*, 2nd ed. Pocatello, ID ProQOL.org. 2010. Available online: https://proqol.org/uploads/ProQOLManual.pdf (accessed on 15 April 2020).
46. Fukumori, T.; Goto, T.; Sato, H. Development, reliability, and validity of a Japanese version of the Professional Quality of Life Scale for Nurses. *Jpn. J. Psychol.* **2018**, *89*, 150–159. [CrossRef]
47. Chen, W.C.; Hwu, H.G.; Kung, S.M.; Chiu, H.J.; Wang, J.D. Prevalence and determinants of workplace violence of health care workers in a psychiatric hospital in Taiwan. *J. Occup. Health* **2008**, *50*, 288–293. [CrossRef] [PubMed]
48. de Looff, P.; Nijman, H.; Didden, R.; Embregts, P. Burnout symptoms in forensic psychiatric nurses and their associations with personality, emotional intelligence and client aggression: A cross-sectional study. *J. Psychiatr. Ment. Health Nurs.* **2018**, *25*, 506–516. [CrossRef] [PubMed]
49. de Looff, P.; Didden, R.; Embregts, P.; Nijman, H. Burnout symptoms in forensic mental health nurses: Results from a longitudinal study. *Int. J. Ment. Health Nurs.* **2019**, *28*, 306–317. [CrossRef] [PubMed]
50. Itzhaki, M.; Bluvstein, I.; Peles Bortz, A.; Kostistky, H.; Bar Noy, D.; Filshtinsky, V.; Theilla, M. Mental Health Nurse's Exposure to Workplace Violence Leads to Job Stress, Which Leads to Reduced Professional Quality of Life. *Front. Psychiatry* **2018**, *9*, 59. [CrossRef]
51. Baby, M.; Glue, P.; Carlyle, D. 'Violence is not part of our job': A thematic analysis of psychiatric mental health nurses' experiences of patient assaults from a New Zealand perspective. *Issues Ment. Health Nurs.* **2014**, *35*, 647–655. [CrossRef]
52. Yada, H.; Abe, H.; Omori, H.; Ishida, Y.; Katoh, T. Job-related stress in psychiatric assistant nurses. *Nurs. Open* **2018**, *5*, 15–20. [CrossRef]
53. Nachreiner, N.M.; Hansen, H.E.; Okano, A.; Gerberich, S.G.; Ryan, A.D.; McGovern, P.M.; Church, T.R.; Watt, G.D. Difference in work-related violence by nurse license type. *J. Prof. Nurs.* **2007**, *23*, 290–300. [CrossRef]
54. Ferri, P.; Silvestri, M.; Artoni, C.; Di Lorenzo, R. Workplace violence in different settings and among various health professionals in an Italian general hospital: A cross-sectional study. *Psychol. Res. Behav. Manag.* **2016**, *9*, 263–275. [CrossRef]
55. Fida, R.; Laschinger, H.K.S.; Leiter, M.P. The protective role of self-efficacy against workplace incivility and burnout in nursing: A time-lagged study. *Health Care Manag. Rev.* **2018**, *43*, 21–29. [CrossRef]
56. Itzhaki, M.; Peles-Bortz, A.; Kostistky, H.; Barnoy, D.; Filshtinsky, V.; Bluvstein, I. Exposure of mental health nurses to violence associated with job stress, life satisfaction, staff resilience, and post-traumatic growth. *Int. J. Ment. Health Nurs.* **2015**, *24*, 403–412. [CrossRef]

9

Individual Circadian Preference, Shift Work and Risk of Medication Errors: A Cross-Sectional Web Survey among Italian Midwives

Rosaria Cappadona [1,2,3], Emanuele Di Simone [4,5], Alfredo De Giorgi [5], Benedetta Boari [5], Marco Di Muzio [4], Pantaleo Greco [1,2], Roberto Manfredini [1,3,5], María Aurora Rodríguez-Borrego [3,6], Fabio Fabbian [1,3,5,*] and Pablo Jesús López-Soto [3,6]

1 Department of Medical Sciences, University of Ferrara, 44121 Ferrara, Italy; rosaria.cappadona@unife.it (R.C.); pantaleo.greco@unife.it (P.G.); roberto.manfredini@unife.it (R.M.)
2 Obstetrics and Gynecology Unit, Azienda Ospedaliero-Universitaria S. Anna, 44121 Ferrara, Italy
3 Department of Nursing, Instituto Maimónides de Investigación Biomédica de Córdoba (IMIBIC), 14071 Córdoba, Spain; en1robom@uco.es (M.A.R.-B.); n82losop@uco.es (P.J.L.-S.)
4 Department of Clinical and Molecular Medicine, Sapienza University of Rome, 00185 Rome, Italy; emanuele.disimone@uniroma1.it (E.D.S.); marco.dimuzio@uniroma1.it (M.D.M.)
5 Clinica Medica Unit, Azienda Ospedaliero-Universitaria S. Anna, 44121 Ferrara, Italy; degiorgialfredo@libero.it (A.D.G.); benedetta.boari@unife.it (B.B.)
6 Department of Nursing Pharmacology and Physiotherapy, University of Córdoba, 14071 Córdoba, Spain
* Correspondence: f.fabbian@ospfe.it

Abstract: Background: In order to explore the possible association between chronotype and risk of medication errors and chronotype in Italian midwives, we conducted a web-based survey. The questionnaire comprised three main components: (1) demographic information, previous working experience, actual working schedule; (2) individual chronotype, either calculated by Morningness–Eveningness Questionnaire (MEQ); (3) self-perception of risk of medication error. Results: Midwives ($n = 401$) responded "yes, at least once" to the question dealing with self-perception of risk of medication error in 48.1% of cases. Cluster analysis showed that perception of risk of medication errors was associated with class of age 31–35 years, shift work schedule, working experience 6–10 years, and Intermediate-type MEQ score. Conclusions: Perception of the risk of medication errors is present in near one out of two midwives in Italy. In particular, younger midwives with lower working experience, engaged in shift work, and belonging to an Intermediate chronotype, seem to be at higher risk of potential medication error. Since early morning hours seem to represent highest risk frame for female healthcare workers, shift work is not always aligned with individual circadian preference. Assessment of chronotype could represent a method to identify healthcare personnel at higher risk of circadian disruption.

Keywords: circadian rhythm; chronotype; midwives; Morningness–Eveningness Questionnaire (MEQ); near misses; nurses; rhythms desynchronization; risk of medication errors; shift work; sleep

---

1. Introduction

Chronobiology is a biomedical discipline devoted to the study of biological rhythms. Biological rhythms exist at any level of living organisms and, according to their cycle length, are classified into: (a) circadian rhythms (from the Latin circa-dies, characterized by a period of ~24 h), (b) ultradian rhythms (period <24 h), and c) infradian rhythms (period >24 h) [1]. Circadian rhythms are the most commonly and widely studied biological rhythms, but they are not strictly the same in all persons, since an individual circadian preference (the so-called chronotype) closely linked to biological and psychological variables, exists. Horne & Ostberg first spoke of possible individual differences in circadian attitudes, the so-called chronotype [2]. By means of a simple a self-assessment Morningness–Eveningness Questionnaire (MEQ), they identified Morning-types (M-type, more active early in the day), Evening-types (E-type, more active later in the day), and neither type or Intermediate (I-type). As for chronotype distribution, data based on human population in the temperate region seem to show a Gaussian curve, with 10% M-type, 10% E-type, and 80% I-type [3]. Moreover, differences by sex and age exist as well, with men on average more evening-oriented than women, although these differences reduce with time [3]. In fact, young women are more morning-oriented than young men, but older women are less morning-oriented than older men [4].

Chronotype. A growing body of research indicates that evening chronotype may be associated with a series of unfavourable conditions. A review from our group analysed the available literature to evaluate the relationships between chronotype, gender, and different aspects of health, such as general health and metabolism, psychological health, and sleep and sleep-related problems (Table 1) [5,6]. As a general rule, M-types cope better with the synchrony effect than E-types and are able to adapt to unfavourable circumstances. At suboptimal times, M-types solved the analogy detection task faster, with the same accuracy and without the investment of more cognitive resources. They also showed greater alertness and wakefulness. At optimal times of day, M-types had more cognitive resources available to allocate in the case of more demanding conditions. E-types appear less able to adapt to suboptimal times, because they have to deal with social jetlag and decreased self-control [7]. In fact, a recent systematic review reported that female nurses with an evening-oriented preference suffer more problems of insomnia, sleepiness, fatigue, and anxiety [8].

Table 1. Association between chronotype and main health issues [Fabbian 2016] (Symbols: ↑ Increased; ↓ Decreased).

Main Health Issues	Chronotype	Main Findings
General and cardiovascular health	Evening-type	Unhealthy diet ↓ Physical activity ↑ Smoking Metabolic syndrome Diabetes mellitus
Psychological & psychopathological issues	Evening-type	↑ Common mental disorders ↑ Depression symptoms ↑ Anxiety symptoms Nightmares Risk-taking behaviour
	Morning-type	↑ Health-related quality of life
Sleep & sleep-related issues	Evening-type	Later bedtime and wake-up ↓ Sleep duration ↓ Sleep quality ↓ Sleep quantity ↓ Sleep efficiency

Shift work. Circadian rhythms are entrained by the light/dark alternation and a series of desynchronizing factors, such as exposure to light at night, jetlag, shift work, and daylight saving time, play a crucial role in disrupting the individual organization of circadian rhythms. Among these desynchronizing factors, shift work certainly plays crucial role, due to the wide dissemination of social request for activities warranting 24/hours/seven days a week assistance [9]. According to data from the Italian Institute of Statistics (ISTAT) survey "Working time organization: the role of atypical work schedules", shift working involves about one worker of five in Italy (20.4%). By disaggregating according to industry, social services (which includes education, health and social services, public administration) show the highest figures (26.8%), followed by manufacturing (21.9%) and trade services, including commerce, transport, and communications (21.7%). More men than women work with shifts (respectively 21.7% and 18.4%, respectively), due mainly to shift schemes which imply night work [10]. Different disorders have been associated with shift work, with stress and sleep disorders as the most frequent ones. For example, when comparing nurses and firefighters with day workers, sleep disturbances were more frequent in shift workers than day workers [11]. Moreover, different cardio-metabolic indices, including higher waist circumference, body mass index, fasting glucose, blood pressure, and cardio-metabolic risk score have been described in night workers [12], who also showed almost three times higher association with abdominal obesity independent of age and gender than day shift workers [13].

Errors. Medications errors (MEs) represent a major concern of healthcare systems worldwide, and near misses represent the most reported incidents (69.3%) [14]. According to the World Health Organization, near miss is defined as "an error that has the potential to cause an adverse event (patient harm) but fails to do so because it is intercepted" [15]. Although inadequate staffing levels, workload, and working in haste have been called the most frequent causes of increased risk for omissions and other types of error and for patient harm [16], circadian misalignment, in addition to a series of health problems in shift workers secondary to the sleep deprivation, e.g., daytime sleepiness, i.e., the difficulty maintaining wakefulness and alertness during normal waking hours [17–20], can represent a crucial favouring factor for lack of performance and any kind of errors. Attentional networks are sensitive to sleep deprivation and increased time awake, and sleep duration variability appeared to moderate the association between sleep duration with overall reaction time and alerting scores [21]. Nurses' sleep quality, immediately prior to a working 12-h shift, was shown to be more predictive of error than sleep quantity [22] and functional magnetic resonance imaging (fMRI) studies showed that task performance in nonoptimal times of the day may result in cognitive impairments leading to increased error rates and slower reaction times [23]. Moreover, sleep deprivation represents a further source of risk, not limited to the short term. In hospital shift workers, being screened positive for a sleep disorder was associated with 83% increased incidence of adverse safety outcomes in the following six months, such as motor vehicle crashes, near-miss crashes, occupational exposures, and medical errors [24].

Health professionals. Recent data from Canada, with reference to the year 2011, show that approximately 1.8 million Canadians (12% of the working population), were exposed to night shift work, and 45% were female. By occupation, professional occupations in health ranked second place (35% of workers), following occupations in protective services (37%) [25]. However, despite these numbers, and even if nurses and midwives make up almost 50% of the global healthcare shift working workforce, much of the research addressed to the shift work area used men [26]. Female nurses working in rotating night shift were found to have significantly lower mean scores in job satisfaction, sleep, and psychological well-being as compared to day shift workers [27] and even impaired sexual self-efficacy and sexual quality of life [28]. There is an extreme paucity of studies conducted on midwives, although they play an important role in medical care: a systematic review of sleep-related/fatigue-management including more than 8600 participants, 89% females, did not find studies conducted in midwives [29]. In the same year, a survey study by the American College of Nurse-Midwives Sleep and Safety Taskforce, conducted on more than 4350 certified nurse-midwives and midwives to identify sleepiness, found that midwives working shifts >12 h had higher rates of excessive daytime sleepiness compared with those who worked shifts of ≤12 h [30].

Based on these premises, the aim of this study was to evaluate the possible association between chronotype, shift work, and risk of medication errors in midwives, inviting a representative sample of these health care professionals by means of a web survey. Social media, in fact, has increased the popularity since it represents a convenient method for communicating on the Web, for recruiting participants for health research, and for conducting survey studies by questionnaires [31,32].

2. Materials and Methods

2.1. Sample

A sample of Italian midwives willing to participate in the survey were invited through the most frequently used social media, i.e., Facebook and Instagram, to complete a questionnaire. We chose this extremely smart method in order to maximize the final sample size and the willingness to fill a self-administered web survey allowed us to obtain the informed consent to take part in the survey, Thus, participation was voluntary and confidential.

Midwifes were reached through social media, and those willing to fill the questionnaire were enrolled. In this case, they were told that their personal data would not have been recorded in any way; however, we asked them to declare their job activity, and we trusted health care professionals declaring to be midwifes at the time of starting the questionnaire. We could not analyse any other data nor the reason for refusing or agreeing to participate. All cases of incomplete questionnaire were excluded from the analysis.

The survey was built on Google Forms, and sent to Italian midwifes. Data was collected starting from 14 June 2019 to 31 August 2019. The statistical power of the sample to obtain statistically significant results was determined by a freely available on-line web platform. The authors considered the appropriate sample size for an adequate study power considering a confidence level of 99% and a confidence interval of 5% on a total of about 21,000 midwifes working in Italy. The analysis computed a representative sample size of 377 midwifes. The confidence interval also called margin of error is the plus-or-minus figure usually reported in opinion poll results, whilst the confidence level suggests the level of security in excluding wrong answers.

2.2. Instruments and Procedures

The questionnaire consisted of a cover page (describing the purpose of the study, as well the methods to ensure anonymity and voluntary participation), and three special sections, including several different items each. In particular, the special sections dealt with:

A. demography, actual working schedule, and working experience information;

B. the Morningness–Eveningness Questionnaire (MEQ), consisting of 19 questions about personal daily sleep-wake habits and the times of day of preference of certain activities, with assigned points from 0 to 5, giving a possible overall score ranging from 16 to 86. Five categories can be identified: definitely E-type (16–30), moderately E-type (31–41), neither type or I-type (42–58), moderately M-type (59–69), and definitely M-type (70–86). For ease of interpretation, we considered moderately E-type as E-type (16–41 points) and moderately M-type as M-type (59–86 points). Thus, we had three final subgroups: E-types, I-types, and M-types.

C. a perception of risk of medication errors survey, based on the "seven rights" (7R) rule of medication administration (right medication, right client, right dose, right time, right route, right reason, and right documentation) [33]. As for risk evaluation, we chose "near misses", i.e., accidents that do not cause the patient harm [34], since they represent the majority of medication errors [14]. The perception of risk of medication errors was evaluated on the basis of the following questions:

    - Based on the 7R rule, during the last shift, how many times did you (or any of your colleagues) run the risk of making a medication error?
    - Why medication error was about to occur?

2.3. Statistical Analysis

For statistical analysis, first a descriptive analysis was performed, including results derived from either MEQ calculated score and personal self-perceived chronotype. The sample was classified according to the self-perception of risk of medication errors, and subgroups by age, working schedule, years of working experience, and chronotype were then compared. Second, a logistic regression analysis was done, considering the self-perception of risk of medication errors as the dependent variable and all the other parameters as the independent ones. Third, a cluster analysis was performed, to determine the phenotype of health care professionals exposed to risk of medication errors based on demography, type of work, and chronotype. IBM Statistical Package for Social Science (SPSS 13.0 for Windows, SPSS Inc., Chicago, IL, USA) was utilized.

3. Results

3.1. Participants

The final sample included 401 Italian midwives (98.8% women), and the main characteristics are summarized in Table 2.

Table 2. Characteristics of the whole population of midwifes.

Number of Participants (*n*)	401
Female (*n* (%))	396 (98.8)
Mean age (years)	38.5 ± 10.1
age 23–30 years (*n* (%))	102 (25.5)
age 31–35 years (*n* (%))	81 (20.0)
age 36–40 years (*n* (%))	79 (19.8)
age 41–45 years (*n* (%))	37 (9.2)
age 46–50 years (*n* (%))	37 (9.2)
age 51–55 years (*n* (%))	30 (7.5)
age 56–60 years (*n* (%))	35 (8.8)
University degree (*n* (%))	32 (8)
High school degree (*n* (%))	369 (92)
Shift work schedule (*n* (%))	293 (73)
Mean working experience (years)	11.7 ± 8.9

3.2. Chronotype

As for individual chronotype (MEQ score) and age, subgroups were represented as follows: age 23–30 years: 52 ± 8.3; age 31–35 years: 56 ± 8.2; age 36–40 years: 58.2 ± 7.6; age 4–45 years: 58.7 ± 9.2; age 46–50 years: 60.5 ± 8.3; age 51–55 years: 60.4 ± 8; age 56–60 years: 58.5 ± 8.2 ($p < 0.001$).

As for individual chronotype (self-perceived), subgroups were represented as follows: M-type $n = 115$ (28.7%), I-type $n = 245$ (61%), E-type: $n = 41$ (10.2%). Mean MEQ score in groups who perceived M-type, I-type, and E-type was 64.8 ± 5.1, 54.2 ± 5.1, and 44.7 ± 7.1, respectively ($p < 0.001$).

As for individual chronotype (MEQ calculated score), subgroups were represented as follows: definite M-type: $n = 25$ (6.3%); moderately M-type: $n = 156$ (39%); I-type: $n = 202$ (50.3%); moderately E-type: $n = 16$ (4%); definite E-type: $n = 2$ (0.4%).

Figure 1 reports the distribution of groups by self-perceived and calculated chronotype. For ease of comparison, the MEQ calculated score was reported considering moderately E-type plus definite E-type as E-type and moderately M-type plus definite M-type as M-type.

3.3. Perception of Risk of Medication Errors

As for perception of risk of medication errors, subjects with response "no, never" were 208 (51.9%), and subjects with response "yes, at least once" were 193 (48.1%). The MEQ score did not show significant differences between the two groups (56.7 ± 8.4 vs. 56.5 ± 8.9, p = NS). No differences between the two groups were found for subgroups by class of age, working shift, years of working experience, and chronotype either.

Logistic regression analysis did not show any independent association with perception of risk of medication errors, whereas cluster analysis showed that perception of risk of medication errors was associated with class of age 31–35 years, shift work schedule, working experience 6–10 years, and I-type MEQ score. No perception of risk of medication errors was associated with age 46–50 years, daytime working, working experience 21–25 years, or M-type MEQ score (Figure 2).

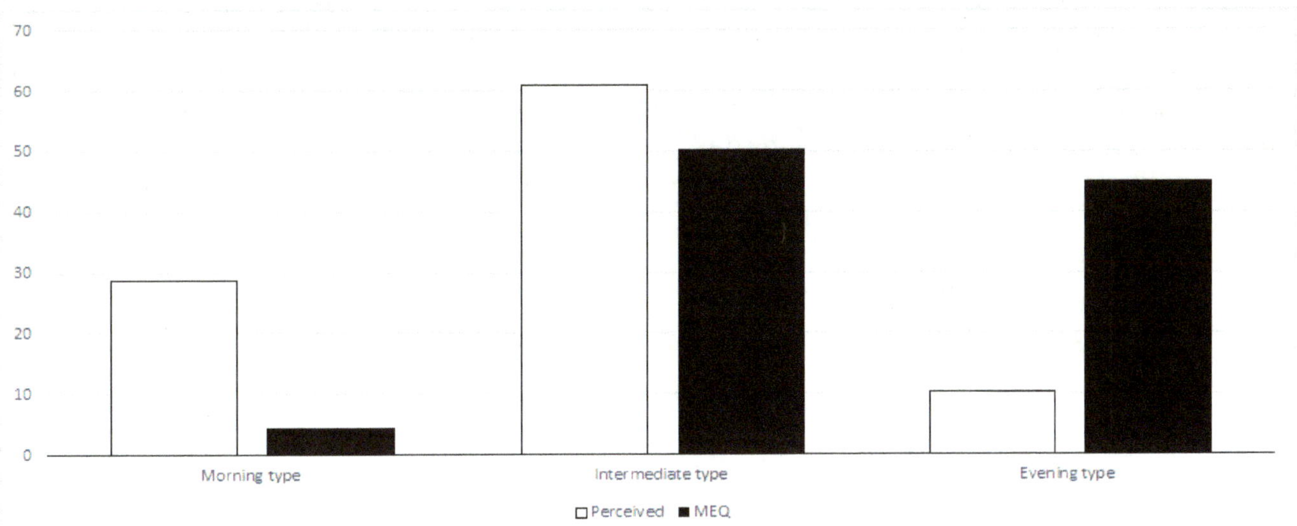

Figure 1. Self-perceived and calculated chronotype distribution of groups. For ease of comparison, the Morningness–Eveningness Questionnaire (MEQ) calculated score was reported considering moderately E-type plus definite E-type as E-type and moderately M-type plus definite M-type as M-type.

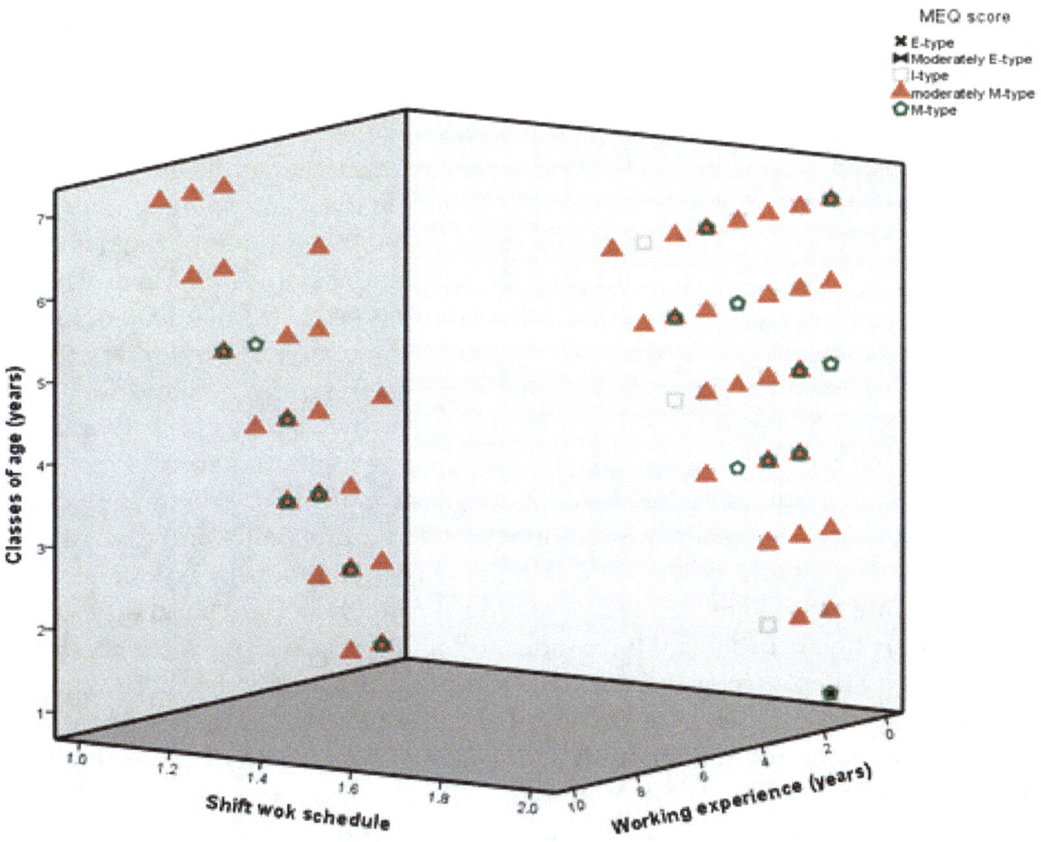

Figure 2. Cluster analysis relating age, shift work schedule, working experience, and MEQ score.

4. Discussion

The results of this study, addressed to investigate the possible relationship between chronotype and risk of medication errors in midwives, showed that the risk of medication errors was associated with younger age, shift work, relatively low working experience, and being an Intermediate chronotype. This is the first report on the association of shift work and risk medical errors in midwives. A recent multicentre Chinese study showed that sleep quality, social support, job satisfaction, occupational injuries, adverse life events, frequency of irregular meals, and employment type were statistically significant factors influencing fatigue among midwives [35]. We found that younger persons, with reduced working experiences, were more likely to report an increased risk of error. It is possible that experience may help in attenuating the decrease in performance during night shift.

Errors. Medication error incidents are more likely to be reported in the morning shift [14,36], but it is common practice that morning therapy is prearranged by the night nursing crew at the end of their shift. Rhythm desynchronization exhibits also gender-specific differences [37], and studies on the circadian and sleep-wake-dependent regulation of cognition in a forced desynchronization protocol showed that accuracy exhibited the largest sex difference in circadian modulation, with the worse performance in women in the early morning hours (at around 6 a.m.) [38]. Even risk taking, a complex form of decision-making that involves calculated assessments of potential costs and rewards, may play a role in the determination of errors. Both gender-specific and chronotype differences exist, since males report higher propensity for risk-taking, in particular E-types. However, although there is no significant difference in risk propensity or risk-taking behaviour across chronotypes in males, E-type females significantly report and take more risk than other chronotypes [39].

Chronotype. Chronotype is also strongly implicated in performance tasks, also making reference to the so-called "synchrony effects", i.e., superior performance at optimal and inferior performance at suboptimal times of day. A study aimed at evaluating the effect of individual differences in chronotype on performance task, evaluated a sample of M-type and E-type women during a driving session in morning (8 a.m.) and evening (8 p.m.). A vigilance decrement was found when E-type participants drove at their nonoptimal time of day (morning session). In contrast, driving performance in the M-type group remained stable over time on task and was not affected by time of day [40]. By contrast, studies on subjects tested for mean reaction times, error rates, and efficiency of three attentional networks (alerting, orienting, and executive control/conflict) at two time points (time 1 or baseline at 8 a.m.; time 2, after 18-h sustained wakefulness at 2 a.m.), showed that E-types participants outperformed M-types on incongruent time, i.e., deep night [21]. On one hand, negative effects of sleep impairments seem to be confirmed to affect more E-types than other chronotypes. An Australian online survey study conducted on paramedics (age 39 ± 12 years; 54% women; 85% rotating shift-workers; 57% I-types, 32% M-types, 11% E-types), showed significantly higher depression scores, anxiety, poorer sleep quality, and reduced general well-being in the E-types, compared with M-types [41]. Our study identifies Intermediate-type as the group at higher risk of error. On one hand, this result is contradictory with respect to the available literature. On the other, this result, if confirmed, is extremely interesting since Intermediate chronotype represents the most frequent circadian preference and not only in our sample. Thus, the finding that younger midwives, with relatively limited working experience, and even with chronotype extremes, are exposed to higher risk of error during their night shift, raises serious concern.

Limitations. We are aware of several limitations to this study: (a) cross-sectional design, based on data collected through a web survey, therefore the sample could be sized only by social media users only; (b) the MEQ score, even if used in the majority of studies for assessing morningness–eveningness preference, does not categorized for different ages [42]; (c) to evaluate the risk of medication error, we considered the general definition of near misses. Although it is largely the most frequent incident reported, we did not differentiate between near misses and no harm incidents [43]; (d) individual perception of the risk of medication errors is not a validated item yet; (e) logistic regression analysis did not identify independent factors; (f) we could not evaluate any gender effect, as most of the sample were women, as usually occurs for studies on nurses and midwives. However, there are also some positive aspects: (a) the web survey method warranted speed, and even in a short timeframe all different classes of age were represented; (b) we found that perception of chronotype was different from the effective profile identified by a well-validated score. This concept could help for future studies and also for practical applications since when workers (health care personnel in particular) ask for health measures, they very often make reference to personal perception.

Coping strategies. Midwifery and nursing are acknowledged as stressful occupations, and the negative impact of high stress levels often requires coping strategies. Of these, the eleven most used have been identified via interview material: drinking alcohol, smoking, using the staff social club, using social networking websites, exercising, family activities, home-based activities, outdoor activities, avoiding people, displacement, and sleep [44]. Unfortunately, it is evident that some of these coping strategies are unhealthy and extremely concerning. Moreover, due to the stress burden, absenteeism is becoming a significant global problem, and taking a "mental health day" as sickness absence is a common phenomenon, taken by more than one half of nurses and midwives, according to an online cross-sectional survey in Australia [45].

5. Conclusions

With this study, we found that younger midwives, with lower working experience, engaged in shift work and belonging to an Intermediate chronotype, seem to be at higher risk of potential medication error. At least to the best of our knowledge, this is the first web survey study addressed to the relationship between chronotype, shift work, and perceived risk of medication error in midwives. Since morning hours seem to represent highest risk frame for female healthcare workers and shift work is not always aligned with individual circadian preference, our preliminary reports could stimulate further specific research aimed to practical applications. For example, assessment of individual chronotype and sleep attitude in healthcare personnel, by means of validated questionnaires, just previously suggested in terms of prevention of metabolic diseases [46], could provide easy and inexpensive method to identify subjects at potential higher risk of circadian disruption. Again, possible countermeasures, such as time-scheduled naps during night-shifts, have been positively tested on female nurses, who showed significantly greater increments in performance between 3:00 and 7:00 a.m. on nap versus no-nap nights [47]. Last but not least, attention to shift work consequences, together with specific training programs, could help to reduce medication errors and improve patients' safety [48].

Author Contributions: Conceptualization: R.C., E.D.S., M.A.R.-B., P.J.L.-S.; Data curation: E.D.S., A.D.G., B.B.; Formal analysis: E.D.S., A.D.G., B.B., M.D.M., F.F.; Funding acquisition: P.G., M.D.M., R.M.; Investigation: R.C., E.D.S., A.D.G., B.B., M.A.R.-B., P.J.L.-S., F.F.; Methodology: R.C., E.D.S., A.D.G., P.G., M.D.M., R.M.; Project administration: R.C., E.D.S., A.D.G., B.B., F.F.; Resources: M.A.R.-B., P.G., M.D.M., R.M., P.J.L.-S.; Software: R.C., E.D.S., A.D.G., B.B., F.F.; Supervision: M.A.R.-B., P.G., M.D.M., R.M., P.J.L.-S.; Validation: R.C., E.D.S., A.D.G., B.B., M.A.R.-B., P.J.L.-S., F.F.; Visualization: R.C., A.D.G., P.G., M.D.M., R.M.; Writing—original draft: R.C., F.F.; Writing-review and editing: M.A.R.-B., P.G., M.D.M., R.M., P.J.L.-S. All authors have read and agreed to the published version of the manuscript.

Acknowledgments: We thank Isabella Bagnaresi, Clinica Medica Unit, Department of Medical Sciences, University'of Ferrara, for precious technical support. We also thank Claudia Righini and Donato Bragatto, Biblioteca Interaziendale di Scienze della Salute, Azienda Ospedaliero-Universitaria "S.Anna", Ferrara, for helpful assistance.

References

1. Manfredini, R.; Salmi, R.; Malagoni, A.M.; Manfredini, F. Circadian rhythm effects on cardiovascular and other stress-related events. In *George Fink (Editor-in-Chief) Encyclopedia of Stress*, 2nd ed.; Academic Press: Oxford, UK, 2007; Volume 1, pp. 500–505.
2. Horne, J.A.; Ostberg, O. A self-assessment questionnaire to determine morningness-eveningness in human circadian rhythms. *Int. J. Chronobiol.* **1976**, *4*, 97–110. [PubMed]
3. Ashkenazi, I.E.; Reinberg, A.E.; Motohashi, Y. Interindividual differences in the flexibility of human temporal organization: Pertinence to jetlag and shiftwork. *Chronobiol. Int.* **1997**, *14*, 99–113. [CrossRef] [PubMed]

4. Randler, C.; Engelke, J. Gender differences in chronotype diminish with age: A meta-analysis based on morningness/chronotype questionnaires. *Chronobiol. Int.* **2019**, *36*, 888–905. [CrossRef] [PubMed]
5. Fabbian, F.; Zucchi, B.; De Giorgi, A.; Tiseo, R.; Boari, B.; Salmi, R.; Cappadona, R.; Gianesini, G.; Bassi, E.; Signiani, F.; et al. Chronotype, gender and general health. *Chronobiol. Int.* **2016**, *33*, 863–882. [CrossRef] [PubMed]
6. Ki, J.; Ryu, J.; Baek, J.; Huh, I.; Choi-Kwon, S. Association between Health Problems and Turnover Intention in Shift Work Nurses: Health Problem Clustering. *Int. J. Environ. Res. Public Health* **2020**, *17*, 4532. [CrossRef]
7. Nowack, K.; Van Der Meer, E. The synchrony effect revisited: Chronotype, time of day and cognitive performance in a semantic analogy task. *Chronobiol. Int.* **2018**, *35*, 1647–1662. [CrossRef]
8. López-Soto, P.J.; Fabbian, F.; Cappadona, R.; Zucchi, B.; Manfredini, F.; Garcia-Arcos, A.; Carmona-Torres, J.M.; Manfredini, R.; Rodriguez-Borrego, M.A. Chronotype, nursing activity, and gender: A systematic review. *J. Adv. Nurs.* **2019**, *75*, 734–748. [CrossRef]
9. Sack, R.L.; Auckley, D.; Auger, R.R.; Carskadon, M.A.; Wright, K.P., Jr.; Vitiello, M.V.; Zhdanova, I.V. Circadian rhythm sleep disorders: Part II, advanced sleep phase disorder, delayed sleep phase disorder, free-running disorder, and irregular sleep-wake rhythm. An American Academy of Sleep Medicine review. *Sleep* **2007**, *30*, 1484–1501. [CrossRef]
10. European Foundation for the Improvement of Living and Working Conditions. Available online: https://www.eurofound.europa.eu/publications/report/2009/working-time-in-the-european-union-italy (accessed on 21 March 2020).
11. Choi, S.J.; Song, P.; Suh, S.; Joo, E.Y.; Lee, S.I. Insomnia symptoms and mood disturbances in shift workers with different chronotypes and working schedules. *J. Clin. Neurol.* **2020**, *16*, 108–115. [CrossRef]
12. Ritonja, J.; Tranmer, J.; Aronson, K.J. The relationship between night work, chronotype, and cardiometabolic risk in female hospital employees. *Chronobiol. Int.* **2019**, *36*, 616–628. [CrossRef]
13. Brum, M.C.B.; Dantas Filho, F.F.; Schnorr, C.C.; Bertoletti, O.A.; Bottega, G.B.; da Costa Rodrigues, T. Night shift work, short sleep and obesity. *Diabetol. Metab. Syndr.* **2020**, *12*, 13. [CrossRef] [PubMed]
14. Aseeri, M.; Banasser, G.; Baduhduh, O.; Baksh, S.; Ghalibi, N. Evaluation of medication error incident reports at a tertiary care hospital. *Pharmacy (Basel)* **2020**, *8*, 69. [CrossRef] [PubMed]
15. World Health Organization. *World Alliance for Patient Safety: WHO Draft Guidelines for Adverse Event Reporting and Learning Systems: From Information to Action*; World Health Organization: Geneva, Switzerland, 2005.
16. Härkänen, M.; Vehviläinen-Julkunen, K.; Murrells, T.; Paananen, J.; Franklin, B.D.; Rafferty, A.M. The contribution of staffing to medication administration errors: A text mining analysis of incident report data. *J. Nurs. Scholarsh.* **2020**, *52*, 113–123. [CrossRef] [PubMed]
17. Drake, C.L.; Roehrs, T.; Richardson, G.; Walsh, J.K.; Roth, T. Shift work sleep disorder: Prevalence and consequences beyond that of symptomatic day workers. *Sleep* **2004**, *27*, 1453–1462. [CrossRef] [PubMed]
18. Rosa, D.; Terzoni, S.; Dellafiore, F.; Destrebecq, A. Systematic review of shift work and nurses' health. *Occup. Med. (Lond.)* **2019**, *69*, 237–243. [CrossRef] [PubMed]
19. Di Muzio, M.; Reda, F.; Diella, G.; Di Simone, E.; Novelli, L.; D'Atri, A.; Giannini, A.; De Gennaro, L. Not only a Problem of Fatigue and Sleepiness: Changes in Psychomotor Performance in Italian Nurses across 8-h Rapidly Rotating Shifts. *J. Clin. Med.* **2019**, *8*, 47. [CrossRef]
20. Di Muzio, M.; Dionisi, S.; Di Simone, E.; Cianfrocca, C.; Di Muzio, F.; Fabbian, F.; Barbiero, G.; Tartaglini, D.; Giannetta, N. Can nurses' shift work jeopardize the patient safety? A systematic review. *Eur. Rev. Med. Pharmacol. Sci.* **2019**, *23*, 4507–4519.
21. Barclay, N.L.; Myachykov, A. Sustained wakefulness and visual attention: Moderation by chronotype. *Exp. Brain. Res.* **2017**, *235*, 57–68. [CrossRef]
22. Weaver, A.L.; Stutzman, S.E.; Supnet, C.; Olson, D.M. Sleep quality, but not quantity, is associated with self-perceived minor error rates among emergency department nurses. *Int. Emerg. Nurs.* **2016**, *25*, 48–52. [CrossRef]
23. Reske, M.; Rosenberg, J.; Plapp, S.; Kellermann, T.; Shah, N.J. fMRI identifies chronotype-specific brain activation associated with attention to motion–why we need to know when subjects go to bed. *Euroimage* **2015**, *111*, 602–610. [CrossRef]
24. Weaver, M.D.; Vetter, C.; Rajaratnam, S.M.W.; O'Brien, C.S.; Qadri, S.; Benca, R.M.; Rogers, A.E.; Leary, E.B.; Walsh, J.K.; Czeisler, C.A.; et al. Sleep disorders, depression and anxiety are associated with adverse safety outcomes in healthcare workers: A prospective cohort study. *J. Sleep. Res.* **2018** *27*, e12722. [CrossRef]

25. Rydz, E.; Hall, A.L.; Peters, C.E. Prevalence and recent trends in exposure to night shiftwork in Canada. *Ann. Work Expo. Health* **2020**, *64*, 270–281. [CrossRef]
26. Matheson, A.; O'Brien, L.; Reid, J.A. Women's experience of shiftwork in nursing whilst caring for children: A juggling act. *J. Clin. Nurs.* **2019**, *28*, 3817–3826. [CrossRef] [PubMed]
27. Verma, A.; Kishore, J.; Gusain, S. A comparative study of shift work effects and injuries among nurses working in rotating night and day shifts in a tertiary care hospital of North India. *Iran J. Nurs. Midwifery Res.* **2018**, *23*, 51–56. [CrossRef]
28. Khastar, H.; Mirrezaie, S.M.; Chashmi, N.A.; Jahanfar, S. Sleep improvement effect on sexual life quality among rotating female shift workers: A randomized controlled trial. *J. Sex. Med.* **2020**, *17*, 1467–1475. [CrossRef] [PubMed]
29. Querstret, D.; O'Brien, K.; Skene, D.J.; Maben, J. Improving fatigue risk management in healthcare: A systematic scoping review of sleep-related/fatigue-management interventions for nurses and midwives. *Int. J. Nurs. Stud.* **2019**, *106*, 103513. [CrossRef]
30. Arbour, M.; Tanner, T.; Hensley, J.; Beardsley, J.; Wika, J.; Garvan, C. Factors that contribute to excessive sleepiness in midwives practicing in the United States. *J. Midwifery Women Health* **2019**, *64*, 179–185. [CrossRef]
31. McCarthy, E.; Mazza, D. Cost and effectiveness of using Facebook advertising to recruit young women for research: PREFER (Contraceptive Preferences Study) Experience. *J. Med. Internet Res.* **2019**, *21*, e15869. [CrossRef] [PubMed]
32. Shaver, L.G.; Khawer, A.; Yi, Y.; Aubrey-Bassler, K.; Etchegary, H.; Roebothan, B.; Asghari, S.; Wang, P.P. Using Facebook advertising to recruit representative samples: Feasibility assessment of a cross-sectional survey. *J. Med. Internet. Res.* **2019**, *21*, e14021. [CrossRef]
33. Smeulers, M.; Verweij, L.; Maaskant, J.M.; de Boer, M.; Krediet, C.T.; Nieveen van Dijkum, E.J.; Vermeulen, H. Quality indicators for safe medication preparation and administration: A systematic review. *PLoS ONE* **2015**, *10*, e0122695. [CrossRef]
34. Kessels-Habraken, M.; Van der Schaaf, T.; De Jonge, J.; Rutte, C. Defining near misses: Towards a sharpened definition based on empirical data about error handling processes. *Soc. Sci. Med.* **2010**, *70*, 1301–1308. [CrossRef] [PubMed]
35. Chen, X.Q.; Jiang, X.M.; Zheng, Q.X.; Zheng, J.; He, H.G.; Pan, Y.Q.; Liu, G.H. Factors associated with workplace fatigue among midwives in southern China: A multi-centre cross-sectional study. *J. Nurs. Manag.* **2020**. [CrossRef]
36. Suclupe, S.; Martinez-Zapata, M.J.; Mancebo, J.; Font-Vaquer, A.; Castillo-Masa, A.M.; Viñolas, I.; Morán, I.; Robleda, G. Medication errors in prescription and administration in critically ill patients. *J. Adv. Nurs.* **2020**, *76*, 1192–1200. [CrossRef]
37. Cappadona, R.; Di Simone, E.; De Giorgi, A.; Zucchi, B.; Fabbian, F.; Manfredini, R. Biological rhythms, health, and gender-specific differences. *Ital. J. Gender-Specific. Med.* **2020**, in press.
38. Santhi, N.; Lazar, A.S.; McCabe, P.J.; Lo, J.C.; Groeger, J.A.; Dijk, D.J. Sex differences in the circadian regulation of sleep and waking cognition in humans. *Proc. Natl. Acad. Sci. USA* **2016**, *113*, E2730–E2739. [CrossRef] [PubMed]
39. Gowen, R.; Filipowicz, A.; Ingram, K.K. Chronotype mediates gender differences in risk propensity and risk-taking. *PLoS ONE* **2019**, *14*, e0216619. [CrossRef] [PubMed]
40. Correa, A.; Molina, E.; Sanabria, D. Effects of chronotype and time of day on the vigilance decrement during simulated driving. *Accid. Anal. Prev.* **2014**, *67*, 113–118. [CrossRef]
41. Khan, W.A.A.; Conduit, R.; Kennedy, G.A.; Jackson, M.L. The relationship between shift-work, sleep, and mental health among paramedics in Australia. *Sleep Health* **2020**, *6*, 330–337. [CrossRef]
42. Levandoski, R.; Sasso, E.; Hidalgo, M.P. Chronotype: A review of the advances, limits and applicability of the main instruments used in the literature to assess human phenotype. *Trends Psychiatry Psychother.* **2013**, *35*, 3–11. [CrossRef]
43. Sheikhtaheri, A. Near misses and their importance for improving patient safety. *Iran. J. Public. Health* **2014**, *43*, 853–854.
44. Happell, B.; Reid-Searl, K.; Dwyer, T.; Caperchione, C.M.; Gaskin, C.J.; Burke, K.J. How nurses cope with occupational stress outside their workplaces. *Collegian* **2013** *20*, 195–199. [CrossRef] [PubMed]

45. Lamont, S.; Brunero, S.; Perry, L.; Duffield, C.; Sibbritt, D.; Gallagher, R.; Nicholls, R. 'Mental health day' sickness absence amongst nurses and midwives: Workplace, workforce, psychosocial and health characteristics. *J. Adv. Nurs.* **2017**, *73*, 1172–1181. [CrossRef] [PubMed]
46. Manfredini, R.; Cappadona, R.; Fabbian, F. Nurses, shift work, and diabetes: Should late chronotype be considered as a risk factor? *BMJ* **2019**, *364*, 1178. [CrossRef] [PubMed]
47. Zion, N.; Shochat, T. Let them sleep: The effects of a scheduled nap during the night shift on sleepiness and cognition in hospital nurses. *J. Adv. Nurs.* **2019**, *75*, 2603–2615. [CrossRef] [PubMed]
48. Di Simone, E.; Giannetta, N.; Auddino, F.; Cicotto, A.; Grilli, D.; Di Muzio, M. Medication errors in the emergency department: Knowledge, attitude, behavior and training needs of nurses. *Indian J. Crit. Care Med.* **2018**, *22*, 46–352.

10

I am a Nursing Student but Hate Nursing: The East Asian Perspectives between Social Expectation and Social Context

Luis Miguel Dos Santos

Woosong Language Institute, Woosong University, Daejeon 34514, Korea; luisdossantos@woosong.org

Abstract: From the East Asian social and cultural perspectives and contexts, this study aimed to understand the relationships and behaviors between nursing students' sense of filial piety and their decision-making behind selecting nursing education as their major. Forty-two traditional-age nursing students (i.e., six men and 36 women) at their final year of a bachelor's degree program in nursing were invited. The findings indicated that many nursing students disliked their university major and the potential career pathway as a nursing professional, as none of them selected the major based on their choice and interest. The environmental context and family's recommendations were the major impacts to influence the decision-making process of the participants. The result also indicated that filial piety, parents' recommendations, and elderly people's suggestions were the key factors to influence the selections and decisions of university major and career development pathways. The study provided a blueprint for related staff and professionals to create and design career counselling and services for East Asian youths to enable life investment and development.

Keywords: career development; counselling; cultural perspective; decision-making process; East Asian perspective; filial piety; nursing education; nursing shortage; nursing student; turnover

---

1. Introduction

Nursing education and training are popular university majors for secondary school graduates, university students, and even adult returning students wishing to pursue life-long personal investment and development [1]. Every year, a large number of secondary school graduates and returning students decide to study nursing as their university major and to develop their careers. Although many individuals start their university education directly after completing secondary school, there are also a large number of adult returning students deciding to start their college and university study during mid-adulthood [2]. The selection of one's university major and career development path are decisions that impact the rest of one's life [3]. However, individuals' social, family, personal, educational, and economic patterns influence their decision-making processes, particularly for East Asian people, who have a strong sense of collectivism [4]. The expression of decision-making for career development is more likely employed when describing that process, which can happen at different stages of life [5].

Although nursing education is a very famous and popular university major, an inappropriate matching and mismatching of career development continues to happen in this profession. One study [6] collected information from 648 questionnaires at three hospitals in Taiwan about nurses' job satisfaction and intention to quit their position. The results indicated that a large number of nurses planned to leave their positions due to significant levels of stress and burnout at their workplace. Although they understand their job natures and responsibilities before entering the profession, many nurses decide to switch their career profession due to ideas of balancing work and family [7].

One study [8] employed the Ward Organizational Features Scales (WOFS) to measure the relationship between job satisfaction and work responsibilities of 834 acute ward nurses in the United Kingdom. The relationship between nurses and other medical staff was one of the most critical elements for their career decision. Additionally, many nurses indicated that the workload of their positions always negatively impacted their job satisfaction due to unbalanced responsibilities. It is worth noting that the negative measurement affected the career decisions of these nurses, who worked in a stressful environment [9].

A recent study [10] about the relationship between disappointment and nursing student retention collected data from 17 nursing students during the third year of their nursing program at university level. The report indicated that many nursing students decided to join the nursing profession because of the desire to provide a caring service, a personal background with the healthcare profession, modelling from peers, and potential career advancement. One study [11] indicated that a number of nursing students explained that negative experiences regarding their training, teaching staff, placement experience, and teammates always affected their career decisions. For example, some participants indicated that the excessive responsibilities and expectations from their supervisors could influence their career decisions due to negative placement experiences. Based on the results, it is not hard to predict that many nursing students or fresh graduate nurses may leave the nursing profession within the first few years of their career [11].

Another study indicated that nursing programs always have a high dropout rate due to the unique nature of the profession [12]. Unlike doctors who can provide individualized medical treatments to patients, nurses tend to assist other medical professionals. In other words, nurses cannot offer individual services without the supervision of other medical professionals. Therefore, once nursing students understand the nature of the profession, many decide to drop out [13].

Expectation is another element of dropout [14]. Providing a caring service is meaningful for many individuals who want to join social care and health services. However, the responsibilities of nurses are unique. Unlike social workers and counsellors who provide counselling and mental health services to individuals with problems, nurses need to provide both psychological and physical labor services from cleaning to operation room assistance. Therefore, the responsibilities are more comprehensive than for many professions in the field of social care and healthcare. As a result, after students understand the relationship between the duties and their expectations, they may drop out or leave the profession [15].

However, many individuals decide to enter the nursing profession due to stable job advancement and salary, particularly in developing countries [16]. Nursing, teaching, and social work are three demanding professions in society internationally. Many enter these fields due to financial, family, and personal considerations. Although these professions always welcome learners and second-career professionals, inappropriate matching is not uncommon. However, for various reasons, some mismatched individuals never leave their positions. In such cases, low-level performance, motivation, and morale prevail in the workplace [17].

One study [18] indicted that East Asian students are more likely to select a university major based on the interests and expectations of their parents, while most European students tend to select their major based on their own interests. Jin [19] indicated that East Asians' major selection tends to be influenced by filial piety toward parents. The researcher employed the Career-Related Filial Piety Scale (C-FPS) to investigate the relationship between parents' decisions and students' choices. The results indicated that students usually tend to study at universities their parents like and enter professional fields according to their parents' preferences. More recently, a study [20] conducted in Hong Kong reflected this as well. The study collected information from 522 undergraduate students about their reciprocal and authoritarian behaviors and senses about the relationship between students' filial piety and career decisions. The results indicated that although many students select their career pathways based on their interests, most respect their parents' wishes according to the traditional East Asian perspective [21]. Perhaps the social and cultural environment in Hong Kong influences young adults' career decisions due to the westernized nature of that society; most Chinese students and participants tend to listen to their parents in order to avoid arguments and misunderstanding [22].

Purpose of the Study

The researcher has conducted research in the fields of social care, human resource management, school administration, and organizational psychology. The personnel shortage in the areas of social caring and nursing has been an issue for decades. Although many human resource professionals, policymakers, school administrators, leaders of social care departments, and researchers always establish plans to encourage potential medical professionals to work in the field. However, the results of these plans were not always effective. Due to the social and cultural expectations, the researcher wants to understand how the East Asian perspective influenced these issues. Currently, studies with a focus on nursing education and nurses' career development tend to explore participants' elements from a westernized perspective [7,11,13,16], in which individualism is the primary social norm and practice [4]. Therefore, this study aimed to understand the relationship between East Asian nursing students' sense of filial piety and their decision-making behind selecting nursing education as their major [23–34].

There are two purposes of this study. First, every year, a significant number of students decide to enroll in nursing education programs for initial training. Based on the literature review, various reasons for this have been found among these students [7]. However, many of them drop out of the programs or leave the nursing profession within the first few years of their career development [14]. Therefore, this study sought to study a group of traditional-age nursing students enrolled in a nursing education program but who will not enter the nursing profession after graduation. Second, the study sought to understand the factors that contribute to the relationship between East Asian university students' filial piety [20,35–37] and their decision-making behind selecting their university major and career development pathway in nursing [38]. The elements studied included outcome expectations, interests, and goals [38].

As a result, little empirical evidence exists for East Asia regarding the relationships between expectations, social-economic backgrounds, social environmental factors, and personal interests of young individuals and their selection of university subjects and career paths [8–11]. It is worthwhile to note that, unlike in Western cultures, Asian young people tend to highly respect their parents' suggestions, as well as the recommendations of their elders, such as parents, grandparents, teachers, and elder siblings, due to traditions of filial piety [8]. In short, this study serves as one of the first attempts to understand the relationship between filial piety and the decision-making of East Asian university students regarding their major selection and career development [23–34]. Unlike with Westerners, the values of filial piety, collectivism, and sense of family union are essential elements for East Asian people [39]. Therefore, this study will help provide opportunities for readers, university administrators, international school staff, educators, and international student service professionals to establish effective counselling services to assist this particular group of students.

2. Materials and Methods

The employment of qualitative research methods [40] would be appropriate. Unlike quantitative research, qualitative research method allows the researcher to collect rich and in-depth data information from the participants. The researcher could access the information and lived stories which could not be answered by statistics and numbers [41]. Although the researcher had aimed to collect information from one single university counselling centre for a case study, the researcher believed the data information from one single source might not be able to express the holistic pictures of the current problem. Therefore, the researcher decided to employ the general qualitative approach [40,42–44], which may better apply to this study. Thomas [44] indicated that the general qualitative approach is an inductive approach that may meet most of the requirements for qualitative researchers. Moreover, without additional requirements, qualitative researchers could freely collect data information from the targeted groups. As the current study might not fit other qualitative methods, such as case study, the general qualitative approach would be the selection [41,44].

2.1. Participants

Fort-two traditional-age nursing students (i.e., six men and 36 women) at their final year of a bachelor's degree program in nursing were invited. All agreed to participate in this study. All the participants were local Taiwanese students. Five out of the 42 were indigenous Taiwanese. All were born and raised in Taiwanese families with the traditional East Asian conceptions. The age range was 18-22 years. The researchers invited these participants with the snowball sampling strategy [40,42,43]. In other words, the researcher invited participants based on the networking from other participants. Participants were enrolled at five different universities in Taiwan. The participants needed to meet the following criteria, which were:

1. he/she is currently enrolled at a nursing education program in Taiwan;
2. he/she is currently enrolled in the final year of the program;
3. he/she was born and raised in Taiwan;
4. he/she needed to meet the age requirement.

2.2. Data Collection

Two types of tools were employed, including individual and focus group activities [40,43,45]. The individual interviews were conducted to explore their understanding, life experience, and family issues under a private sharing environment [46–48]. The focus group activities were conducted to explore some similar background, social and family expectations, social bias, and interests. Both research tools were particularly useful in regard to listening to the voices by engaging them individually and collectively.

All participants have voluntarily participated in this study. The general inductive approach [44] was employed for qualitative data collection and analysis. The researcher was the collector of the data information. In order to seek meaningful data information, first, the semi-structured interview sessions were created. According to Seidman [49], individuals are less likely to share lived stories and personal background to others without any prior relationships. Therefore, in order to overcome this issue, the researcher decided to conduct two sessions of semi-structured, one-on-one, and private interviews in a private room at a community centre for each participant. Each interview lasted up to 40 min. One of the directions of this study was to explore the direct effect of filial piety on a career decision. Therefore, the protocol interview questions for both individual interview sessions tended to focus on the relationship between an East Asian perspective and the social context and issues. Appendix A shows the protocol interview questions for both interview sessions.

Second, after each participant completed the individual interview sections, all participants were invited into six focus group activities, each with seven participants. As the schedule of each participant was different, the focus group activity hosted seven members regardless of their university enrolments. The focus group activities were hosted at the same community centre. Appendix B shows the protocol interview questions for the focus group activities.

As it might be difficult for participants to share their understanding and experience in English language and a language other than their mother tongue, all the sections were conducted in Chinese Mandarin and translated into English. All the interview and focus group activities were audio-recorded and transcribed into written documents for data analysis. Member checking was done after the data analysis procedure. In order to protect the personal rights of each participant, all participants were given a pseudonym.

2.3. Data Analysis

After the data collection procedure, 543 pages of written transcripts were created based on the semi-structured interviews and focus group activities. Qualitative researchers [40,43,45] advocated that large-size data information should be narrowed down to meaningful themes and patterns. Therefore, the researcher followed the general inductive approach (GIA) [44] for data analysis. First, the researcher used the open-coding procedure for the initial themes. After the initial themes were formed, the axial-coding procedure was employed for the second-level themes. As a result, two themes and seven subthemes were merged.

2.4. Human Subject Protection

All the signed and unsigned agreements, personal contact, audio recording, written transcripts, computer, and related materials were locked in a password-protected cabinet. Only the researcher had the means to open it. After the study was completed, the researcher immediately destroyed and deleted all related materials for personal privacy.

Due to the agreement, the university information and place of origin was masked due to privacy. Most of the students were concerned that their university information would be disclosed. Due to the small population and closed professional networks, the researcher needed to protect the information of the participants. However, the participants allowed the researcher to show their gender for this study. Therefore, the following part will outline their gender with their discussion. It is worth noting that a small number of participants agreed to disclose their place of origin. The researcher reported this information with the discussion of the findings.

All subjects gave their informed consent for inclusion before they participated in the study. The study was conducted in accordance with the Declaration of Helsinki, and the protocol was approved by the Ethics Committee of The Youth Caring Association (2018/2019/SummerFall).

3. Findings and Discussion

During each interview and focus group activity section, the participants answered the same general semi-structured questions that asked for their opinions and feedback. Although all participants had a similar family and social background in the same country, having come from one of the Taiwanese areas, their personal sharing, lived stories, and life experiences were not the same. Unlike in other studies, which have focused on westernized cultural perspectives, all participants reported that their major selection (i.e., nursing) was influenced by their family members, parents, and social expectations. In order to help answer the research questions, the findings were categorized into two superordinate themes and seven subthemes. It is surprising to note that all 42 participants were studying a university major that was not their own selection or interest. In other words, upon graduation, they would receive a degree, initial license, and potentially develop their long-term career pathways in a direction in which they have no strong interests. More importantly, many expressed that they will leave the nursing profession after graduation. Table 1 outlines the themes and subthemes of this study.

Table 1. A list of themes and subthemes for this study.

		Themes and Subthemes
3.1.		**Influences from the Participants' Contextual Environment**
	3.1.1.	The East Asian Perspective on Occupational and Role Expectations
	3.1.2.	Academic Results
	3.1.3.	Financial Influence
3.2.		**Influences from the Participants' Family and Elders**
	3.2.1.	Parental Recommendations
	3.2.2.	Teachers' Recommendations
	3.2.3.	Pressures from Family Members
	3.2.4.	Comparison with Other Relatives

3.1. *Influences from the Participants' Contextual Environment*

Before the session began, the researcher needed to indicate that the statements about I hate nursing. I dislike the medical career had been recorded 356 times. It was very surprising that the mismatching of major and human resources (i.e., students) was significant in the current Taiwanese university environment, particularly in the faculty of nursing. Although the current study could not represent the overall situation in Taiwan and the East Asian region, the significant results from this study may explore and contribute to an understanding of how these extreme situations [14] happen in the East Asian region [31].

By listening to the stories and life experiences of the participants, the researcher identified several elements that impacted their major decisions. The findings of this study discovered that all did not follow their personal goals and interests when selecting their major (i.e., nursing). The results reflected that the participants' behaviors also tended not to follow their own interests in choosing a career, which goes against a large number of previous findings [7,15,16]. It is worth noting that in most cases in East Asia, university students are not allowed to switch their major once they have been accepted. In other words, students are required to complete the major and degree that they submitted as their choice with their application. Therefore, the contextual and environmental factors that prevailed during their secondary school period highly influenced their life-long developments and career decisions [50]. A group of participants expressed that nursing was a choice of their parents during the application period, saying, "I can apply up to six universities and majors ... But once I admitted with a school and major ... I cannot switch ... but the major application was written by my mother without my agreement ... " (P#5, Male, Interview).

The results of this study supported the idea that youth have their own ways of thinking about career developments [7,51,52]. However, because the university's constraints on their university decisions and their overall contextual factors limited their opportunities, most were unable to exercise the career pathways that they might have decided on their own [14]. A discussion of the influences on the career decisions of the participants follows.

3.1.1. The East Asian Perspective on Occupational and Role Expectations

All 42 participants expressed that the East Asian perspectives about occupational and role expectations influenced their decisions about the major they were studying, their university enrollment, and their career decisions [53]. In the traditional East Asian perspective, medical practitioners are considered to be upper-class citizens with a high level of social status [54]. Although more than half of the participants expressed their desire to become an artist, reporter, chef, journalist, or photographer, none of them selected the majors associated with those occupations. One participant expressed that almost all artists and performers in the fine arts could not become famous until their death, saying, "Although I want to be an artist, I may become a nurse and do some part-time art activities ... But I am not sure will I become a nurse become I hate this occupation now ... " (P#2, Male, Focus Group). Another participant (P#4, Female, Interview) believed her hobbies in dancing could not be a long-term occupation, sharing,

> *I chose nursing was because I think medical professionals are very smart in our society ... I really enjoy the perspective of medical professionals ... Although I want to become an artist with my wish and interests ... both athlet[e]s and dancers can only work in their occupation until the early 30s. After that, the lucky one[s] can work as [a] coach. The others are living under the poverty line ... .but now, I don't know ... should I become a nurse? I hate this career ... .* (P#4, Female, Interview)

It is worth noting that not only these two participants, but all 42 participants also expressed the ideas *I hate nursing and I dislike medical professions* in this category. Many expressed interests in other fields but had no chances and opportunities. Although the participants tried to escape from the major (i.e., nursing) they were not interested, they still needed to complete the degree and training due to the East Asian perspective and expectation from the society.

The lack of long-term career development in Taiwan always prohibited youths from joining their dream professions [55], particularly in the humanities and fine art occupations. A participant (P#24, Male, Focus Group) shared an idea:

> *I like[d] botany and plant biology from [a] young age. I wish[ed] I c[ould] become a botanist from 8 years ago . . . [but] the long-term development of [a] botanist is unclear. No one can guarantee jobs after graduation, as there are more than 3,000 graduates in this field yearly. Also, Taiwanese people don't really consider Botanist as a professional. So if I can, I [will] select nursing instead. At least the general public will consider doctors as upper professionals . . . .* (P#24, Male, Focus Group)

It was not surprising to hear that in East Asia, university subject selections were not based on the students' own interests and desires for career development [23–34]. For example, the above participants wished to join botanical biology during her secondary school period. But due to the social context and social expectation [39], she needed to select the alternative (i.e., nursing) as her sixth choice on her application. One participant (P#36, Female, Interview) shared about enrolling in a nursing school instead of an electronic engineering program based on the gender-oriented bias and social expectation of gender-oriented occupations, saying,

> *. . . my parents and the society . . . in East Asian countries believe engineers, doctors, pharmacists, and emergency medical technicians must be males. I love science and engineering . . . I want to become a medical engineer in the future . . . but I mother told me that in many Taiwanese universities, there are only a few female students in any of the engineering programmes . . . it is ugly to be the only girl . . . .* (P#36, Female, Interview)

Most described their selection of their university major as having been significantly influenced by the East Asian perspective, social context, and social expectations [23–34]. More importantly, the sense of collectivism [4] was highly represented in these groups of individuals. For example, several of the female participants refused to study one of the STEM subjects because of the social norms and social expectations of men in these areas. Female individuals, however, were expected to study and join the workforce in lesser industries, such as nursing, administration, elementary school education, and social work [56]. Due to the strong East Asian perspective, social context, and social expectation on selecting an academic major and career, it is worth noting that some young adults might give up on following their own interests merely on the basis of the enrollment of students of the opposite gender in a program for which they had prepared for more than four years [19].

3.1.2. Academic Results

Standardized exams and university admission placement tests are widely used in many countries [57]. In Taiwan, a widely used standardized exam is the General Scholastics Ability Test (GSAT). Although there are alternative pathways for enrollment, the GSAT is the most common admission exam for local Taiwanese students. Nearly 30 of the student respondents expressed that their low GSAT scores prohibited their enrollment in the university of their choice and also their selection of university subjects. Unlike in the American educational system, with the community college options, students are allowed to select an undecided major pathway. But Taiwanese students have to select their university enrollment and major during their final semester of 12th grade in secondary school. One participant (P#38, Female, Focus Group) expressed,

> *I wish I c[ould] follow my will to become a medical doctor. But my low score . . . I can only apply for the nursing program . . . However, I cannot enrol at a community college or vocational college because there are no ways to build-up to the medical doctor's programme in the future . . . If I want to study but not re-take the exam for one more year, the only selection would be nursing . . . But again, I hate nursing . . . because it is not the same . . . .* (P#38, Female, Focus Group)

It is less likely for students to switch their university major once enrolled in many East Asian contexts due to unbalanced admission requirements and university policies. Unlike universities in the United States, students started their general education requirement during the first two-year of university education. Except for in special circumstances, students can switch and re-design their university major after the first or the second year of university education. The following participant (P#10, Male, Interview) shared his negative stories about the switching issue in Taiwan, saying,

> *Once I studied nursing during my first year at university, I discovered that I don't like this subject. However, in order to change my university subject, I have to be [among] the top-rated students for the purpose of switching. Otherwise, I have to re-apply for the entire GSAT steps again . . . I hate nursing, I hate it so much . . . But I cannot switch it due to the administrative requirement . . . Also, the social expectation of my nursing career . . . What can I do . . . .* (P#10, Male, Interview)

In addition to their university enrollment and their selection of a major, the participants' academic results also limited their selection of university location. Some reported that they were forced by their parents and teachers to go to an urban university due to their high score of GSAT. One participant (P#11, Female, Interview) reported,

> *I was partially willing to study nursing actually if I could stay in my hometown . . . In the southern part of Taiwan, there is a very good university and the nursing department. The enrolment of this university is my goal. But I received a high score in my GSAT. Therefore, my mother and school principal forced me to come to the capital city with a university that I dislike. I don't like the university, the social expectation of the university, and how people believed this university should create good nurses . . . So I hate nursing because of the social expectation . . . .* (P#11, Female, Interview)

It is worth noting that this participant (P#11, Female, Interview) was willing to study nursing if she could stay in her hometown. However, the East Asian perspective, social context, and social expectation [23–34] about her testing score, university, major, and potential career development destroyed her career perspective and beliefs. Although she wanted to become a nurse, she will now suffer due to the stresses and pressures from all different directions of her life.

Almost all described their GSAT scores, regardless of the level, as being a factor in their university enrollment, the decision about their academic major, and career development. Because the GSAT score was the most significant element, the decision about university subjects, the location of the university, and even the ability to switch university subjects after enrollment were not controlled by the participants. However, more importantly, a large number of participants expressed that based on their academic results, their parents, teachers, and even school leaders [35] expected them to enroll at top-tier universities and in a specific academic major. Almost all participants were forced to study in an academic major based on the recommendations from their parents and school staff. For example, a participant (P#32, Female, Focus Group) said, "I cannot cho[ose] which school and which location [where] can I study, I have to listen to my parents and teachers".

3.1.3. Financial Influence

Everyone experienced the stress of financial factors. Due to the East Asian traditions and cultural perspectives [34], children are responsible for taking care of their parents and even grandparents after their university graduation. Although the Taiwanese government does not regulate any policies about birth control, many contemporary Taiwanese families have fewer than two children.

Nearly two-thirds of the participants expressed that they would be the one who would take care of their parents and even grandparents after graduation, so they needed to select a career pathway that would allow them to make a significant amount of money. In fact, such East Asian perspectives on family engagements and responsibilities highly influenced the decision-making processes of these participants [31]. One participant (P#33, Male, Focus Group) told the researcher that being a nurse was almost the only way to take care of his parents and four grandparents after his graduation. In the same focus-group activity section, another participant (P#35, Female, Focus Group) echoed that situation with her own, saying,

> *In many families, taking care of parents [is] expected. My parents expected me to take care of their late [years] . . . although I wanted to study music . . . I must study nursing, [in] which [I] can make money . . . But this must not be my wills . . . I really hate nursing . . . I don't want to become a nurse after university . . . I want my life back as an adult after university . . . I did not tell my mother about this yet . . . But I am sure I will not become a nurse . . . I dislike nursing not matter what . . . .* (P#35, Female, Interview)

Another Participant (P#25, Male, Focus Group) grew up in a rural community in central Taiwan. He also identified this family expectation and financial difficulties as a villager in the countryside. As mentioned above, many East Asian elderly were expected to be cared for by their children. Therefore, as a male child, the participant felt a need to send financial resources to his parents after university graduation. Consequently, this participant considered nursing as one of the occupations that could provide financial security, saying,

> *. . . my parents sent me to university due to financial stress. I wish I c[ould] work in my family-run farm. But my parents want me to work in an upper social occupation . . . I need to listen . . . Moreover, my mother is a disabled person . . . I need to take care of her after I finished my university . . . But I want to continue my study in physical therapy in the future . . . I like the medical profession, but I surely dislike nursing as my life-long career development . . . I will explore a master's degree or another qualification soon . . . .* (P#25, Male, Focus Group)

It is worth noting that this participant has a very strong sense in the field of the medical profession. Although he took nursing as his alternative during his university application period, he will continue his career development in physical therapy due to these personal goals and financial considerations.

In addition to their concerns about post-graduation financial stress, participants also experienced pre-graduation financial stress due to their lower-income status. One participant (P#9, Female, Focus Group) used to plan to study in a culinary arts and bakery programs based on her goals and interests. However, most of the culinary arts and bakery program required higher tuition fees and supplemental fees. Because her family could not afford the extra fees, she had to give up her own goals and enroll in the nursing program. Another participant (P#8, Female, Focus Group) also shared similar stories, saying,

> *I was planning to apply for the film major. But the department required [me] to have several expensive cameras and lenses, a high-quality computer, as well as the extra tuition fees for fine art lectures. I don't want to spend all the saving[s] of my family . . . I have to select a university major . . . which I hate . . . that can make money . . . .* (P#8, Female, Focus Group)

In short, the East Asian perspective, social context, and social expectation about the nursing and medical professions always limited their opportunities and career choices [6,25]. Unlike many studies conducted in the westernized societies and communities, many Taiwanese nursing students decided to enroll into one of the nursing programs based the social and cultural expectations [21]. Although university major and career development should be a selection of individuals, such preferences are not widely available in eastern societies. Furthermore, securing financial resources for their parents and elderly always forced them to enter the medical profession due to the stable salary and other financial considerations [29]. Although registered nurses may earn a reasonable salary for their family, it is unfair for both registered nurses and patients in this case in Taiwan. Although career mismatching always happens due to various reasons, this study discovered some significant findings which may gradually be detrimental to the medical and social health care system [11].

3.2. Influences from the Participants' Contextual Environment

3.2.1. Parental Recommendations

"I do this degree for my parents" (P#13, Female, Interview). It is worth noting that the perspective of "I have to do this degree for my parents" was shared 320 times based on the transcripts.

Young adults and recent secondary school graduates usually do not have significant work and life experience from which to select a major that may, in turn, be an investment in their long-term career plans. One potential way to obtain recommendations is from their parents. Due to the ideas of collectivism, many East Asian people tended to conduct activities and behaviors based on the benefits of the groups and communities. Without the permissions from family members and group members, East Asian people usually conduct nothing further because of the ideas of respectfulness.

All advocated the ideas of collectivism with the traditional East Asian perspective [4] due to their respectfulness towards family members and elders in their cohort [25]. In fact, they consulted with their parents and even grandparents about university selection, academic major, and career development before they submitted their university application. One participant (P#20, Female, Interview) recalled a story about marking her major selections, saying,

> *My mother asked me to study nursing as both of my parents are medical professionals in the national-level hospital. Perhaps I am not a good medical profession as I do not have any passion for my patients. But I have to listen to my parents as they are the one who took care of my life. I have to be respectful to them as a good child ... This is traditional of us ... Although I hate nursing ... you don't know how much I hate nursing and the career development of a registered nurse ... But I have to do this degree for my parents ....* (P#20, Female, Interview)

Another participant (P#28, Female, Interview) also shared a similar situation at the same focus group activity section, saying,

> *My father is a doctor, and my mother is a nurse ... they expected my sister and I [to] become medical practitioners ... so, my sister was asked to enrol in a nursing school and so am I ... my interest and career goal is to become a news reporter. But what can I do? Can I not listen to my parents? They spent almost half of their life for two of us ... I cannot just say no to them ... I hate nursing ... But I am doing this degree for them ... but for my own interests and goals ....* (P#28, Female, Interview)

From the above sharing, many participants selected their major and career development based on their parents' desires and recommendations instead of their own [29]. A study indicated that East Asian people tended to listen to their parents and cohort members as recommendations for their decision. Unlike people in the westernized society, East Asian people advocate the notion of respectfulness towards their parents, elders, and community members. Therefore, this study also reflected the practices of the current participants.

In addition to parental recommendations being an extension of the parents' original occupations, a large number of participants advocated that they were asked to study a major that their parents had not been able to achieve during their own youth. In fact, these expectations from parents are not uncommon in the East Asian perspective [27]. During the last century, most of the East Asian countries and regions were developing as third-world countries. Therefore, youth and students at that time did not have chances for university education. Therefore, parents of this generation and even the society have a higher-level of expectations in the current social context. One participant (P14, Female, Focus Group) was one of many with this case, saying,

> *My mother was raised in a low-income family and wished to become a nurse during her childhood ... but she couldn't ... now, she asked me to complete her dream. But she did not ask me if I want to do so. As a daughter, I hope I can complete her dream for the purpose of respectfulness ... however, I can tell you that I hate nursing ... I studied this nursing degree for my mother ... I will not join the nursing profession afterwards ... absolutely no ....* (P14, Female, Focus Group)

Similarly, another participant (P#17, Female, Focus Group) also shared a case of a comparable situation, saying,

> *My parents did not go to university during their young age ... [so they] forced me to go to university ... during my early teenage [years], they asked me to [study] medical biology. I have no interest ...*

but my mother liked this ... I [studied]. Now, my parents want me to study nursing ... I enrolled at my nursing programme now ... because I want to be a good girl ... but I am sure that I hate this nursing subject and I studies this degree for them obviously ... I will not join this nursing profession afterwards ... But I have to study this for my parents .... (P#17, Female, Focus Group)

After P#17 shared her experience in a focus-group activity section, another participant (P#18, Female, Focus Group) echoed her similar case, saying,

I am sure a lot of students selected their major based on some expectations of the East Asian perspectives ... I am sure more than half of us [classmates]' majors were selected by parents or someone at home ... at least four women in my dorm room were ... I am so surprised that four girls [roommates] in our room were forced to study nursing because of our parents' decision ... We won't join the nursing profession afterwards as we all studied that for our parents ... We all understood that we hate nursing so much .... (P#18, Female, Focus Group)

When the researcher asked questions about the interrelationships of financial responsibility, academic major, and career decision and development, one participant (P#42, Female, Interview) exclaimed that due to pressure and expectations from her parents,

I absolutely want to become an early childhood teacher ... but my mother just wanted me to study nursing in the capital city ... if I cannot complete the degree, who is going to take care of her late [in] life? I am just a machine to take care of the elderly. But I have to take care of her, due to the filial piety ... this makes me hate nursing so much .... (P#42, Female, Interview)

One participant (P#25, Female, Interview) expressed that she had to listen to her parents' suggestion to attend medical school instead of the school of agriculture, due to financial considerations. Based on her life stories, the participant showed a solid awareness of her interests and career goals in the farming industry. However, her sense of filial piety limited her arguments because her parents' suggestions were a higher consideration than her own interests and career goals [31].

In short, all participants advocated that their major selections and career developments were chosen by their parents due to the East Asian perspective, social context, and social expectation, particularly parental recommendations and respectfulness [23–34]. The finding from this section was hardly found in much of the current literature with a westernized perspective. It is worth noting that all participants always respected their parents instead of their own interests and goals. Although respectfulness is encouraged, such mismatching may damage the health and social care system.

3.2.2. Teachers' Recommendations

In addition to the recommendations from parents, teachers also controlled the participants' decisions about their university enrollment, academic major, and career development. Nearly all participants revealed that their secondary school principal and homeroom teacher[s] had forced them to go to a nursing program because their enrollment would increase the reputation of the secondary school. One participant (P#23, Female, Interview) shared,

My secondary school is located in a rural community ... I am the first graduate who receive[d] a first-rated GSAT score ... [my] school principal asked me to go to the capital city and stud[y] a bachelor's degree in nursing science, so the secondary school can promote my name and achievement in the city hall. I have asked my parents, family member[s], teachers, counsellors, and social workers about this. All of them advocated the relocation to the capital city and nursing school ... It seems like I have no choice ... but I want to study ocean studies .... (P#23, Female, Interview)

Teachers' recommendations did not influence just a single student's decision, but a large number of participants. Questions about teachers' recommendations were asked during both the individual and focus-group activity sections, and nearly two-thirds of the participants shared their opinions on how teachers' recommendation influenced their decision. Several significant opinions are listed below. For example, a participant (P#39, Female, Interview) shared negative experience, saying,

> *... my 12th grade homeroom teacher told me that the shortage of medical doctor[s] would be terminated within a decade. So I listened and obeyed her opinion and switch[ed] to nursing. This is the worst recommendation so far in my life ... I want to be a doctor ... not a nurse ... I hate nursing, I like to be a medical doctor as my career development ... It looks like I am studying for my teacher ... I am so angry and upset ....* (P#39, Female, Interview)

Another participant (P#22, Female, Interview) also told her lived stories between her teachers and herself to the focus group participants, saying,

> *... my teacher asked us to fill up the application form in front of her. She assigned us with the particular subject[s]. If we [did] not listen to her, I think that would be a little bit irresponsible? So I just listened to her. But this is certainly not my own will ... So like, I am studying this degree for my teacher or what?* (P#22, Female, Interview)

In short, nearly all participants exhibited filial piety and respectfulness to their teachers and other school professionals [23–34]. Although some of them argued that their university enrollment and academic major, and their career decisions, were not their first choice, they felt that as good students they had to show the required filial piety and respectfulness.

3.2.3. Pressures from Family Members

Besides family and teachers who had daily interactions with the participants, other family members, such as cousins, uncles, and aunts, also revealed expectations about the participants' decisions regarding their university enrollment, academic major, and career pathway. Almost all participants expressed experience in this subtheme. One participant (P#3, Female, Focus Group) shared that her decisions were forced by her uncle, saying,

> *... my uncle told my mother that he used to work in a hospital and believed the nurses can make a lot of money. So, he highly recommended [to] my mother ... [that] I select this direction. My mother and my uncle sent me the nursing brainwashing messages everyday ... respectfulness, listening, orders from the parents ... I am sure I hate nursing now ... but I am studying this degree exclusively for these two people ....* (P#3, Female, Focus Group)

Another participant (P#1, Female, Focus Group) also added to this theme and said,

> *... my uncle is [in] upper leadership in chained clinics in the capital city. He always convinced my mother, and I worked for him. So, he called my mother every day and asked me to study nursing ... nursing is a subject that I hated ... But the pressure from my uncle and mother ... I have to follow this pathway ... for them ....* (P#1, Female, Focus Group)

During the same focus group activity section, Participant (P#29, Focus Group) shared a negative experience, saying,

> *I was the only one who was forced by other family members ... in the Taiwanese society, many people believe being a doctor or medical practitioner is an excellent occupation. I agreed. But this is not something that I want to do for my whole life. I always thought I was tricked by my family as well as the society ....* (P#29, Focus Group)

In short, many participants expressed negative opinions and experiences about the influence of family [23–34]. Because East Asian people tend to respect their elders' recommendations [29], nearly all participants followed the wills of their family members instead of their own personal interests. It is worth noting that not only parents but also related family members, had the authority to order the participant to choose a particular direction for study and career choice.

3.2.4. Comparison with Other Relatives

Many participants seemed to have had common experiences about how their parents compared their (i.e., the participants') university enrollment, major, and even GSAT scores with those of other children with similar backgrounds. When one of the participants (P#19, Female) was asked how she had decided to start her undergraduate study in nursing, she said that her parents compared her GSAT score and university application form with those of other children who were living in the same neighbourhood. The following remarks made by some of the participants seem to show similar situations of negative experiences. For example, a participant (P#16, Female, Interview) shared,

> *My mother asked [about] other people's academic major selections in the community centre. Afterwards, she came back and asked me to study that nursing ... I was very surprised that my career and major are decided and selected by a group of aunts in the community centre ... I hate nursing for sure ... But as a Taiwanese girl ... I needed to listen to our cohort and members of my family ... If I don't, I cannot show the respectfulness to the community ....* (P#16, Female, Interview)

Another participant (P#1, Male, Interview) also shared that his mother brought his application form to the community centre and asked opinions from other children. Besides sending their information and report cards to the community centre, some participants told the researcher their parents had even brought all their family members and relatives to their home for discussion. One participant (P#23, Female) shared her experience, saying,

> *During the application period, my parents called everyone to my home for suggestions and discussions. My elder cousins provided more than 20 suggestions. My parents always compare[d] my scores, university enrolment, and major intentions to everyone ... they compared my scores and major ... my score was not excellent. Some of them even laughed ... after they laughed, I still had to follow my mother's decision ....* (P#1, Male, Interview)

Another participant (P#26, Female, Interview) shared a similar situation, saying,

> *My GSAT score was high enough to apply [for] most of the appropriate majors. I would like to go to a university in the southern part of Taiwan, as I wanted to escape from my family ... but my parents wanted me to study near them. So I stayed ... my parents wanted me to study medicine. Even if I want to study nursing, I have to follow their wills ... because they are my parents ....* (P#26, Female, Interview)

Last but not least, the cohort and community-based collectivism always influenced how East Asian people behave. In this case, although the participants have their own goals and interests for major and career development, they did not have many choices due to the perspective of collectivism and respectfulness from their elders, family members, and members in their community. The results of this study outlined the relationship between the East Asian perspective, social context, and social expectation. The researcher used nursing students as a sample to explore and discover how this relationship exists in contemporary society. Without a doubt, many behaviors, ideas and perspectives were influenced by this relationship [23–34].

Attention should be paid to the directives given by the parents and family members. Although filial piety is a traditional aspect of the East Asian culture that may not change in the short term in Taiwan, the opinions and expressions of youth should be respected [36]. It is important to note that individuals' academic and career interests and goals significantly influence their career pathways and career development [58,59]. Parents and family members should avoid ordering their children to base their decisions about university enrollment and university subject selections on the desires of their elders. One participant (P#41, Female, Interview) indicated that playing a musical instrument as an academic major was her desire because that hobby was developed based on the decisions of her parents. However, she had no choices due to her parents' decision and application. Therefore, parents should also learn that they need to release more authority to their children and that the children should be taught career development navigation, such as vocational skills training [60].

4. Conclusions

To the best of the knowledge, this is one of the very first nursing studies that is based on the approach of the relationship between an East Asian perspective, social context, and social expectation for East Asian university students' decision-making about their major selections and career developments. In some other countries, in which individuals do not have the significant sense of filial piety and obedience toward their parents and elders that East Asians do, individuals may follow their own interests and career goals for university enrollment and selection of their academic major, particularly in the field of nursing education [1,7,16].

In addition to the East Asian educational systems and structures that exist at the macro-level, at the micro-level filial piety and family negotiation continue to play a vital role for young adults in their decision-making about university enrollment, academic majors, and career progression, and that role could influence their long-term career investment and development [23–34]. Based on the data and experiences shared by this study's 42 participants, all students indicated that their decisions and intentions were solid but were made unwillingly. However, due to their sense of filial piety, almost all of them had tended to listen to and obey suggestions or orders from their parents, teachers, and elders [35].

Some readers may argue that parents accept opinions from the youth in contemporary society. However, because this study was conducted recently in Taiwan with several dozen young adults, it seems clear that their sense of filial piety in the decision-making process is not likely to change in the short run. In general, secondary school graduates are usually under the age of 18 years old. Therefore, their university applications and related forms must be signed by parents or guardians. Although their sense of filial piety would not change even if the students had reached the age of 18 years old, young university students in their early adulthood should have greater authority to decide their own career pathways. The study's findings indicate that some young adults choose to avoid the dictates of filial piety and instead pursue their own interests and career goals. For those interviewed here, the pursuit of their own interests and career goals combined with those directed by filial piety sometimes occurred [20,35–37]. For example, they may have pursued a double university subject major and minor study, to also satisfy their own desires.

4.1. Limitations

Every research study has its limitations. Two limitations have been found in this study. First, this study was a qualitative research study with 42 traditional-age nursing students. However, as mentioned before, nursing education and career development are famous career selections for many university students and second-career changers. Therefore, future research may expand the population to non-traditional age students, second-career changers, returning students, and adult students.

4.2. Implementations

In recent decades, some vocational higher education institutions have created vocation-oriented undergraduate degree programs for students who want to develop hands-on skills for their career pathways [61]. In addition to vocational undergraduate degree programs, some educational systems also allow individuals to take their first and second year of university education with a university subject as undecided. Both of those educational elements are significant blueprints for reforming Taiwanese and even all East Asian higher education institutions and universities, with the goal of expanding the current curriculum and policies for students with non-traditional backgrounds.

Instead of changing the sense of filial piety, the universities, departments of education, and related agencies could reform specific policies in order to avoid putting limitations on young adults. As discussed above, some participants expressed that the university policy did not allow them to switch their university subject. However, recent graduates of secondary school and young adults usually do not have enough life experience to choose appropriate career pathways during their late teenage years. Thousands of university graduates do not participate in the industry or subject area in which they received their undergraduate degree. As a result, if universities would allow enrolled students to switch their academic major after their registration and enrollment, that potentially could increase the graduation rate and interest levels of students and contribute to their learning and enjoyment. It is also worth noting that the relevant agencies should discuss creating an undecided academic major for students who encounter difficulty deciding on a specific major.

Parents also can learn skills and techniques for sharing short-term, middle-term, and long-term career goals and academic interests with their children, while providing the children with the appropriate rewards, appreciation, encouragement, support, and involvement. In addition, parents can learn the significance of helping their children explore and discover their own academic interests and career goals, by bringing them on field trips to university campuses and organizations, introducing them to various cultural backgrounds and diversities, and increasing their understanding of particular subject matters. By conducting these parenting steps, the parents can help their children to exercise filial piety by a show of respectfulness toward their parents, while at the same time making their own decisions about university enrollment, university subject selection, and career development.

Appendix A

Interview Protocol Questions: The First Interview

(1) Why do you want to study nursing as your bachelor's degree major? Please tell me more.
(2) Do you enjoy your major? Why or why not?
(3) How did you select your university major during secondary school?
(4) If you can select it again, would you select nursing as your major?
(5) How would you think filial piety for your university major selection and other related behaviors?
(6) Further questions will be asked as follow-up questions.

Appendix B

Interview Protocol Questions: The Second Interview

(1) Let's think about the biggest reasons why would you select nursing as your major?
(2) Without this reason, would you select nursing again?
(3) Who select this major (i.e., nursing)? Yourself, families, friends, peers influence, parents etc.?
(4) Would other people influence your major selection/career development/university choice etc.?
(5) Would you think filial piety take some positions in the selection process?
(6) Further questions will be asked as follow-up questions.

References

1. Foronda, C.L.; Alfes, C.M.; Dev, P.; Kleinheksel, A.J.; Nelson, D.A.; O'Donnell, J.M.; Samosky, J.T. Virtually Nursing. *Nurse Educ.* **2017**, *42*, 14–17. [CrossRef] [PubMed]
2. Dos Santos, L.M. The motivation and experience of distance learning engineering programmes students: A study of non-traditional, returning, evening, and adult students. *Int. J. Educ. Pract.* **2020**, *8*, 134–148. [CrossRef]
3. Ginzberg, E. Career development. In *Career Choice and Development: Applying Contemporary Theories to Practice*; Brown, D., Brooks, L., Eds.; Jossey-Bass: San Francisco, CA, USA, 1984; pp. 172–190.
4. Han, C.M. Individualism, collectivism, and consumer animosity in emerging Asia: Evidence from Korea. *J. Consum. Mark.* **2017**, *34*, 359–370. [CrossRef]

5. Super, D. A Life-span, life-space approach to career development. In *The Jossey-Bass Management Series and the Jossey-Bass Social and Behavioral Science Series. Career Choice and Development: Applying Contemporary Theories to Practice*; Brown, D., Brooks, L., Eds.; Jossey-Bass: San Francisco, CA, USA, 1990; pp. 197–261.
6. Tzeng, H.-M. The influence of nurses' working motivation and job satisfaction on intention to quit: An empirical investigation in Taiwan. *Int. J. Nurs. Stud.* **2002**, *39*, 867–878. [CrossRef]
7. Mohamed, L.K. First-career and second-career nurses' experiences of stress, presenteeism and burn-out during transition to practice. *Evid. Based Nurs.* **2019**, *22*, 85. [CrossRef]
8. Adams, A.; Bond, S. Hospital nurses' job satisfaction, individual and organizational characteristics. *J. Adv. Nurs.* **2000**, *32*, 536–543. [CrossRef]
9. Nantsupawat, A.; Kunaviktikul, W.; Nantsupawat, R.; Wichaikhum, O.; Thienthong, H.; Poghosyan, L. Effects of nurse work environment on job dissatisfaction, burnout, intention to leave. *Int. Nurs. Rev.* **2017**, *64*, 91–98. [CrossRef]
10. Ten Hoeve, Y.; Castelein, S.; Jansen, G.; Roodbol, P. Dreams and disappointments regarding nursing: Student nurses' reasons for attrition and retention. A qualitative study design. *Nurse Educ. Today* **2017**, *54*, 28–36. [CrossRef]
11. Connors, C.A.; Dukhanin, V.; March, A.L.; Parks, J.A.; Norvell, M.; Wu, A.W. Peer support for nurses as second victims: Resilience, burnout, and job satisfaction. *J. Patient Saf. Risk Manag.* **2020**, *25*, 22–28. [CrossRef]
12. Jones, M. Career Commitment of Nurse Faculty. *Res. Theory Nurs. Pract.* **2017**, *31*, 364–378. [CrossRef]
13. Bakker, E.J.M.; Verhaegh, K.J.; Kox, J.H.A.M.; van der Beek, A.J.; Boot, C.R.L.; Roelofs, P.D.D.M.; Francke, A.L. Late dropout from nursing education: An interview study of nursing students' experiences and reasons. *Nurse Educ. Pract.* **2019**, *39*, 17–25. [CrossRef]
14. Salmi, E.; Vehkakoski, T.; Aunola, K.; Määttä, S.; Kairaluoma, L.; Pirttimaa, R. Motivational sources of practical nursing students at risk of dropping out from vocational education and training. *Nord. J. Vocat. Educ. Train.* **2019**, *9*, 112–131. [CrossRef]
15. Jacob, E.R.; McKenna, L.; D'Amore, A. Educators' expectations of roles, employability and career pathways of registered and enrolled nurses in Australia. *Nurse Educ. Pract.* **2016**, *16*, 170–175. [CrossRef]
16. Rainbow, J.G.; Steege, L.M. Transition to practice experiences of first- and second-career nurses: A mixed-methods study. *J. Clin. Nurs.* **2019**, *28*, 1193–1204. [CrossRef] [PubMed]
17. Hama, T.; Takai, Y.; Noguchi-Watanabe, M.; Yamahana, R.; Igarashi, A.; Yamamoto-Mitani, N. Clinical practice and work-related burden among second career nurses: A cross-sectional survey. *J. Clin. Nurs.* **2019**, *28*, 1–11. [CrossRef] [PubMed]
18. Tang, M.A. Comparison of Asian American, Caucasian American, and Chinese College Students: An Initial Report. *J. Multicult. Couns. Devel.* **2002**, *30*, 124–134. [CrossRef]
19. Jin, L. *The Role of Personality and Filial Piety in the Career Commitment Process among Chinese University Students*; The University of Hong Kong: Hong Kong, China, 2009.
20. Hui, T.; Yuen, M.; Chen, G. Career-related filial piety and career adaptability in Hong Kong university students. *Career Dev. Q.* **2018**, *66*, 358–370. [CrossRef]
21. Vuong, Q.-H.; Bui, Q.-K.; La, V.-P.; Vuong, T.-T.; Nguyen, V.-H.T.; Ho, M.-T.; Nguyen, H.-K.T.; Ho, M.-T. Cultural additivity: Behavioural insights from the interaction of Confucianism, Buddhism and Taoism in folktales. *Palgrave Commun.* **2018**, *4*, 143. [CrossRef]
22. Cubillo, M.; Sanchez, J.; Cervino, J. International students' decision-making process. *Int. J. Educ. Manag.* **2006**, *20*, 101–115. [CrossRef]
23. Cooper, C.E.; McLanahan, S.S.; Meadows, S.O.; Brooks-Gunn, J. Family structure transitions and maternal parenting stress. *J. Marriage Fam.* **2009**, *71*, 558–574. [CrossRef]
24. Sung, K. Filial Piety in Modern Times: Timely Adaptation and Practice Patterns. *Australas. J. Ageing* **1998**, *17*, 88–92. [CrossRef]
25. Li, H.; Lin, Y.; Lee, I. The impact of traditional filial piety between older people and their children in Taiwan. *J. Compr. Nurs. Res. Care* **2016**, *1*, 103.
26. Hwang, K.K. Filial piety and loyalty: Two types of social identification in Confucianism. *Asian J. Soc. Psychol.* **1999**, *2*, 163–183. [CrossRef]
27. Cheung, C.K.; Kwan, A. The erosion of filial piety by modernisation in Chinese cities. *Ageing Soc.* **2009**, *29*, 179–198. [CrossRef]

28. Sung, K.-T. A New Look at Filial Piety: Ideals and Practices of Family-Centered Parent Care in Korea. *Gerontologist* **1990**, *30*, 610–617. [CrossRef]
29. Canda, E.R. Filial Piety and Care for Elders: A Contested Confucian Virtue Reexamined. *J. Ethn. Cult. Divers. Soc. Work* **2013**, *22*, 213–234. [CrossRef]
30. Sung, K. Elder respect: Exploration of ideals and forms in East Asia. *J. Aging Stud.* **2001**, *15*, 13–26. [CrossRef]
31. Croll, E. The Intergenerational Contract in the Changing Asian Family. *Oxford Dev. Stud.* **2006**, *34*, 473–491. [CrossRef]
32. Chong, A.M.L.; Liu, S. Receive or give? Contemporary views among middle-aged and older Chinese adults on filial piety and well-being in Hong Kong. *Asia Pac. J. Soc. Work Dev.* **2016**, *26*, 2–14. [CrossRef]
33. Sun, Y. Among a Hundred Good Virtues, Filial Piety is the First: Contemporary Moral Discourses on Filial Piety in Urban China. *Anthropol. Q.* **2017**, *90*, 771–799. [CrossRef]
34. Zhang, M.; Lin, T.; Wang, D.; Jiao, W. Filial piety dilemma solutions in Chinese adult children: The role of contextual theme, filial piety beliefs, and generation. *Asian J. Soc. Psychol.* **2019**. [CrossRef]
35. Kwan, K. Counseling Chinese peoples: Perspectives of filial piety. *Asian J. Couns.* **2000**, *7*, 23–41.
36. Chen, W.-W. The relations between filial piety, goal orientations and academic achievement in Hong Kong. *Educ. Psychol.* **2016**, *36*, 898–915. [CrossRef]
37. Sun, P.; Liu, B.; Jiang, H.; Qian, F. Filial piety and life satisfaction among Chinese students: Relationship harmony as mediator. *Soc. Behav. Personal. Int. J.* **2016**, *44*, 1927–1936. [CrossRef]
38. Lent, R.W.; Brown, S.D.; Hackett, G. Toward a unifying social cognitive theory of career and academic interest, choice, and performance. *J. Vocat. Behav.* **1994**, *45*, 79–122. [CrossRef]
39. Nguyen, V.; Nguyen, N.; Khuat, T.; Nguyen, P.; Do, T.; Vu, X.; Tran, K.; Ho, M.; Nguyen, H.; Vuong, T.; et al. Righting the Misperceptions of Men Having Sex with Men: A Pre-Requisite for Protecting and Understanding Gender Incongruence in Vietnam. *J. Clin. Med.* **2019**, *8*, 105. [CrossRef]
40. Merriam, S.B. *Qualitative Research: A Guide to Design and Implementation*; Jossey Bass: San Francisco, CA, USA, 2009.
41. Sharan, B.; Merriam, E.J.T. *Qualitative Research: A Guide to Design and Implementation*, 4th ed.; Jossey-Bass: San Francisco, CA, USA, 2015.
42. Creswell, J. *Qualitative Inquiry and Research Design: Choosing Among Five Approaches*; SAGE Publications: Thousand Oaks, CA, USA, 2007.
43. Creswell, J. *Qualitative Inquiry and Research Design: Choosing Among Five Approaches*; Sage: Thousand Oaks, CA, USA, 2012.
44. Thomas, D.R. A general inductive approach for analyzing qualitative evaluation data. *Am. J. Eval.* **2006**, *27*, 237–246. [CrossRef]
45. Tang, K.H.; Dos Santos, L.M. A brief discussion and application of interpretative phenomenological analysis in the field of health science and public health. *Int. J. Learn. Dev.* **2017**, *7*, 123–132. [CrossRef]
46. Dos Santos, L.M. Experiences and expectations of international students at historically black colleges and universities: An interpretative phenomenological analysis. *Educ. Sci.* **2019**, *9*, 189. [CrossRef]
47. Dos Santos, L.M. Rural Public Health Workforce Training and Development: The Performance of an Undergraduate Internship Programme in a Rural Hospital and Healthcare Centre. *Int. J. Environ. Res. Public Health* **2019**, *16*, 1259. [CrossRef]
48. Dos Santos, L.M. Promoting safer sexual behaviours by employing social cognitive theory among gay university students: A pilot study of a peer modelling programme. *Int. J. Environ. Res. Public Health* **2020**, *17*, 1804. [CrossRef] [PubMed]
49. Seidman, I. *Interviewing as Qualitative Research: A Guide for Researchers in Education and the Social Sciences*, 4th ed.; Teachers College Press: New York, NY, USA, 2013.
50. Dos Santos, L.M. Mid-life career changing to teaching profession: A study of secondary school teachers in a rural community. *J. Educ. Teach.* **2019**, *45*, 225–227. [CrossRef]
51. Kim, M.S.; Seo, Y.S. Social cognitive predictors of academic interests and goals in South Korean engineering students. *J. Career Dev.* **2014**, *41*, 526–546. [CrossRef]
52. Evans, V.; Salcido, K. *Career Paths: Nursing*; Express Publishing: Newbury, UK, 2019.
53. Yu, M.; Lee, M. Managers' career development recognition in Taiwanese companies. *Asia Pac. Manag. Rev.* **2015**, *20*, 11–17. [CrossRef]

54. Chen, L.; Reich, M. *Medical Education in East Asia: Past and Future*; Indiana University Press: Bloomington, IN, USA, 2017.
55. Remmert, D. *Young Adults in Urban China and Taiwan: Aspirations, Expectations, and Life Choices*; Routledge: London, UK, 2016.
56. Milliken, E. Feminist theory and social work practice. In *Social Work Treatment: Interlocking Theoretical Approaches*; Turner, F.J., Ed.; Oxford University Press: Oxford, UK, 2017; pp. 191–208.
57. Gökdağ Baltaoğlu, M.; Güven, M. Relationship between self-efficacy, learning strategies, and learning styles of teacher candidates (Anadolu University example). *S. Afr. J. Educ.* **2019**, *39*, 1–11. [CrossRef]
58. Dickinson, J.; Abrams, M.D.; Tokar, D.M. An examination of the applicability of social cognitive career theory for African American college students. *J. Career Assess.* **2017**, *25*, 75–92. [CrossRef]
59. Carrico, C.; Matusovich, H.M.; Paretti, M.C. A qualitative analysis of career choice pathways of college-oriented rural central appalachian high school students. *J. Career Dev.* **2019**, *46*, 94–111. [CrossRef]
60. Bodycott, P.; Lai, A. The role of Chinese parents in decisions about overseas study. In *Understanding Higher Education Internationalization. Global Perspectives on Higher Education*; Mihut, G., Altbach, P., Wit, H., Eds.; Sense Publishers: Rotterdam, The Netherlands, 2017; pp. 197–201.
61. Lapan, R.; Shaughnessy, P.; Boggs, K. Efficacy expectations and vocational interests as mediators between sex and choice of math/science college majors: A longitudinal study. *J. Vocat. Behav.* **1996**, *49*, 277–291. [CrossRef]

11

Living with the Memories—Parents' Experiences of their Newborn Child Undergoing Heart Surgery Abroad

Ólöf Kristjánsdóttir [1,*], Annica Sjöström-Strand [2] and Gudrún Kristjánsdóttir [1]

1 Faculty of Nursing, University of Iceland, Eirberg, Eiriksgata 34, 101 Reykjavík, Iceland; gkrist@hi.is
2 Department of Health Sciences, Faculty of Medicine, Lund University, Box 157, 22100 Lund, Sweden; annica.sjostrom-strand@med.lu.se
* Correspondence: olofk@hi.is

Abstract: Parents of children with a congenital heart defect needing complex heart surgery are at high risk of developing health problems. One can assume that parents whose child undergoes heart surgery abroad will undoubtably face added and unique stressors and health vulnerabilities. The aim of this qualitative study was to explore the transition experiences of parents of children who underwent a complex heart surgery abroad as newborns 1–5 years ago. The qualitative content analysis methodology by Graneheim and Lundman was used. A purposive sample of twelve parents, whose child had undergone a heart surgery abroad, participated in face-to-face, semi-structured interviews. Interviews were transcribed and analyzed using inductive qualitative content analysis. The overarching theme of "living with the memories" emerged from parents' experiences, emphasizing the long-lasting impact this stressful event had on their lives. These experiences were characterized by four main categories: (1) being in an unknown situation; (2) feeling connected; (3) wishing to be accepted; and (4) finding closure. The findings show that the transition of having a newborn child undergo heart surgery abroad superimposed on the expected parenthood. That parents need to feel connected and included as legitimate clients was highlighted in their stories of experienced vulnerabilities. The results highlight the need for interdisciplinary teams to support these vulnerable families, particularly with follow-up care.

Keywords: child; parent; congenital heart disease; heart surgery; qualitative research; content analysis; cross-border care; transitions

---

1. Background

Having a child with a critical congenital heart defect (CCHD) is recognized as an extremely distressing experience for parents [1], inevitably leading to vast supportive care needs that begin at the child's congenital heart defect (CHD) diagnosis and continue through surgery and childhood [2,3]. CHDs are the most common congenital abnormality among infants, with the global yearly prevalence estimated at about 1% [4]. Of these, 25% are predicted to have CCHD, which is a life-threatening condition requiring urgent heart surgery and intensive care at birth, followed by life-long medical follow-ups and often further surgery [5]. It is estimated that up to 30% of parents of children with CCHD develop post-traumatic stress disorder and 25–50% develop depression or anxiety [6]. This is problematic because a parent's ability to care for their child diminishes if their own needs are not met [2,7]. Unfortunately, these parents continue to be at a higher risk of developing mental health problems due to a lack of social support, information, and mental support [2,3].

Transitions in hospital environments (e.g., from the pediatric intensive care unit (PICU) to a clinical ward) are known as challenging experiences for parents of critically ill children [8], including those with CCHD [9,10]. Under these circumstances, insecurity, fear, stress, and anxiety are reported to be experienced by parents due to, for example, the unfamiliarity and uncertainty of the new environments. Subsequently, these may result in various changes, impacting parental and child health and well-being [8–10].

Due to the highly specialized hospital treatments complex pediatric heart surgeries require, this medical service is not always available "at home". In these instances, children may be referred overseas, where they receive state-funded cross-border care [11,12]. These unprecedented circumstances inevitably introduce heightened stress, and unique challenges to already vulnerable families. Currently, our understanding of state-funded cross-border care for children with CCHD and their families is limited. Given this dearth of knowledge, using a qualitative approach to the parental transition experience, is seen as a prerequisite for understanding the supportive care needs of these families. State-funded cross-border, or the transfer of patients between two health care systems where funding agreements are in place, is different from medical tourism, which implies patients traveling abroad to receive "out-of-pocket and third-party payments medical treatments" [13]. Both cross-border care and medical tourism involve the movement of patients and families between countries, cultures, and health care systems. This inevitably creates added stress, challenges, and burden. Even so, the contexts are very different, for example, the severity and acuity of newborn's CCHD needing cross-border care is inevitably different from medical tourism.

Scarce literature exists regarding child medical tourism [14,15]. Only three studies were found looking at parents' experiences [16–18], all focusing on older children (not newborns) receiving cancer or blood-related treatments in the United States. Two include Spanish-speaking parents from low-income countries [16,17] and one English-speaking parents from a high-income country [18]. Overall, these studies showed that transitions into new cultural environments create stress and extra burdens on families [16–18].

According to Meleis's transitions theory [19], transition is the movement from one life condition to another and involves an adaption to change. Transitions can be triggered by events that require geographical changes (e.g., relocation), where sudden and rapid adjustments to different environments are needed. This inadvertently increases individuals' stress and depletes and disrupts their usual sources of support. Therefore, creating an imbalance which can affect individual's vulnerability risk, health, and wellbeing [19]. The transitions experienced by parents of newborn children with CCHD needing heart surgery abroad, surely create an imbalance. Understanding these experiences is thus an important first step in developing quality health care for these families. Therefore, the aim of this study was to elucidate and describe parents' transition experiences of having a newborn suffering from a heart defect and having to undergo heart surgery abroad.

2. Methods

2.1. Design and Sample

A qualitative exploratory design, based on Graneheim and Lundman's content analysis methodology, was chosen to describe parents' experiences of their child undergoing heart surgery abroad [20,21]. This approach is well suited to capture a deeper understanding of a topic and to obtain a sense of individuals' experiences from their own perspective. Here, the meaning of an experience is described in terms of what and how it is experienced, and surfaces from the actual text using manifest (categories) and latent (themes) content analysis. This type of analysis is preferable when populations or topics have limited research because it helps create new knowledge that can be woven into a new or existing theory [20,21]. To ensure quality, the consolidated criteria for reporting qualitative research (COREQ) guidelines were followed in preparing this manuscript, and are provided in Supplementary Table S1.

A purposive sampling method was used to select the participants based on whether parents identified as having a child (0–18 years old) with CHD who underwent heart surgery at a university hospital in the southern part of Sweden between 2014 to 2019. Participants were included if they were over 18 years, able to speak and understand Icelandic, and if no more than 5 years had passed since their child underwent heart surgery in Sweden.

2.2. Setting and Recruitment of Participants

Participants were initially recruited from a patient database at the largest hospital in Reykjavik, Iceland. After participating in a survey, parents were asked if the researchers could contact them again in the future for an interview study. Those who provided consent were contacted by the first author (Ó.K.) via email, during which they were informed about the current study's goal and invited to participate. In total, 25 parents were invited to participate, and of these, 11 declined to participate. The final study sample consisted of 12 parents because two parents dropped out due to unforeseen events conflicting with the study.

Table 1 shows the sociodemographic and specific characteristics of the parents with regards to the travel and their child. Of the 12 participants, 7 were mothers and 5 fathers. Of these, three traveled abroad more than once, two had a child that underwent more than one surgery, one had a child that experienced severe complications and disability after surgery, and one parent had a child that died. All children were newborns when they traveled abroad for the first time for surgery. The time from child's heart surgery abroad and parents interview ranged from 1-to-5 years.

Table 1. Family demographics and background (n = 12).

Parent Information	*n* (%)
Role	
Mother	7 (58)
Father	5 (42)
Age [a]	
20–29 years	5 (45)
30–39 years	5 (45)
40–49 years	1 (10)
Marital status [a]	
Married/common law	7 (63)
Living separately	3 (27)
Divorced	1 (10)
Education	
Highschool diploma or vocational education	5 (42)
Tertiary (collage/university)	5 (42)
Advanced college/university	2 (16)
Total monthly family income [a]	
≤789,000 ISK	4 (37)
790,000–1.29 million ISK	5 (45)
≥1.3 million ISK	2 (18)
Other children at the time (no)	8 (67)
Both parents traveled abroad (yes)	12 (100)
Relatives traveled abroad with parents (yes)	8 (67)
Length of stay abroad [a]	
≤14 days	4 (36)
15–21 days	5 (46)
>22 days	2 (18)
Multiple travels abroad (no)	9 (75)
Time from travel abroad to study [a]	
1–2 years	5 (45)
3–5 years	6 (55)

Table 1. *Cont.*

Child Information	*n* (%)
Gender (boy)	10 (83)
Age of child at first travel abroad	
1–10 days old	7 (58)
11–30 days old	3 (25)
>31 days old	2 (17)
Delivery type (vaginal)	7 (58)
Time of diagnosis (postnatal)	9 (75)
Diagnosed heart defect (ICD-10) [b]	
Congenital malformations of great arteries (Q25)	6 (50)
Congenital malformations of pulmonary and tricuspid valves (Q22)	2 (17)
Congenital malformations of cardiac septa (Q21)	3 (25)
Discordant ventriculoarterial connection (Q20.3)	1 (8)

[a] Demographic data missing for one participant. [b] Category based on the International Classification of Diseases, Tenth Revision.

2.3. Data Collection

Data were collected between November 2019 and February 2020 via 12 individual face-to-face semi-structured interviews. The interview guide used was developed by the authors, informed by their previous work [22], confirmed in the authors group, and pilot tested both with one mother and during the first three interviews, which resulted in minor revisions. Each interview started with the broad question: "Can you please describe how you experienced having to travel to Sweden for your infant's heart surgery?" Probing questions were asked to encourage participants to describe their experience as much as possible (e.g., "Could you please explain what you mean by that?"). Selected interview questions are listed in Table 2.

Table 2. Selected interview questions.

- Could you tell me what it was like learning that your child needed heart surgery abroad?
- Could you please tell me what it was like while you were waiting to travel abroad for your child in surgery?
- Could you please tell me what it was like traveling abroad for your child surgery abroad?
- Could you tell me what it was like while you were waiting for your child in surgery?
- Could you tell me how you experienced the hospital stay abroad?
- Could you tell me how you experienced the support provided by the health care staff?
- Could you tell me what it was like being away from your family (e.g., other children)?
- Could you tell me about the things that made this experience stressful for you?
- Could you tell me about what helped you during stressful time periods?
- Could you tell me your experiences with the discharge process?
- Could you tell me how this experience has affected your health? Relationships?
- Could you tell me your experience of flying with your child back home?
- Could you tell me how it was like coming back home after the surgery?
- Could you please describe your life after you were discharged from the hospital abroad and back home?

Before the interviews started, a written informed consent form was provided and signed by the participants, and the interviewer explained her role in the research. No prior personal relationship existed between any of the researchers and the participants. All authors are female, registered pediatric nurses, with clinical experience and a research background (Masters and Doctorate degrees).

All of the interviews were carried out by the first author (Ó.K.) and took place in accordance with the parents' wishes. That is to say, 11 were conducted in a separate interview room at a university in Iceland, and one was conducted in a private room at the participant's workplace. The interviews lasted between 45 and 136 min, during which time only the interviewer and interviewee were present in the room. At the end of the interview, parents were thanked for their time and willingness to share their stories. Parents did not receive any financial reward for participating in the study.

2.4. Data Analysis

The data were analyzed using Graneheim and Lundman's [20,21] content analysis approach. The codebook was developed from the initial analysis of the data (a posterior) using an inductive method. All interviews were audio recorded, transcribed verbatim by a professional transcriber, checked for accuracy, and translated from Icelandic to English to make them available to all of the authors. The data analysis process started with the three authors reading and rereading the transcribed text individually to familiarize themselves with the material. Next, the three authors created meaning units from the text that comprised of several words or sentences that helped answer the research question. The meaning units were then condensed and labeled with codes that were understood in relation to the context (i.e., an open coding process). Initial codes were created by the three authors, who also referred to the literature when creating the final coding list. These codes facilitated the identification of concepts. Next, the authors used a categorization process to identify categories and subcategories, followed by the identification of a theme. The authors used a process of reflection and discussion to agree on the codes, categories, and themes. This resulted in the creation of a coding tree; provided as a Supplementary Table S2. This process was well documented throughout.

2.5. Ethical Considerations

Each potential participant was provided with verbal and written information stating that: (a) participation was voluntary; (b) withdrawal from the study could be made at any time without reason; and (c) all data were confidential. Each participant was provided with a written informed consent form. All parents were informed that a registered psychologist would be available to them following the interview. Permission for the study was obtained from the National Bioethics Committee of Iceland (no. 18/204) and the Icelandic Data Protection Authority.

3. Results

The overarching theme of "living with the memories" emerged from parents' closeness with their experiences, and its lasting presence in their lives. Although up to five years had passed since parents had traveled abroad for their child's heart surgery, their memories and emotions were still vivid. In all instances, parents became emotional at some point during their interview. Table 3 illustrates the overarching theme, and the four categories and eight subcategories from which this theme emerged.

Table 3. Overarching theme, main categories, and subcategories.

Overarching Theme: Living with the Memories	
Categories	**Subcategories**
1. Being in an unknown situation	a. Disrupted life b. Life on hold
2. Feeling connected	a. Supportive environment b. Handling the experience
3. Wishing being accepted	a. Parenting roles and needs b. Feeling overlooked: Culture and system
4. Finding closure	a. Surviving b. Showing compassion

3.1. Being in an Unknown Situation

Parents memories of their child's CHD diagnosis and heart surgery abroad revealed the superimposition of unanticipated and unwanted transitions on an expected transition of parenting a healthy and normal newborn. One father described this unexpected transition of the news vividly: *"just a complete shock to hear this just like that ... [you thought] your child was going for a 15-minute routine test [at the hospital], but comes home 16 days later somehow ... this is like [being on] a rollercoaster, you have no control. You just have to sit."* (Father 5). In these unknown situations, parents' lives were disrupted and somehow placed on hold.

3.1.1. Disrupted Life

All parents were shocked upon receiving the news of their child's CHD diagnosis and stunned when told that their child needed to travel overseas for complex heart surgery. Parents previous envision and expectations of a normal parenthood were superimposed by previously unknown reality, or as one mother described, *"it was surreal when he [doctor] said: He must go to Sweden. We just stared at him: What are you talking about? ... Go to Sweden? He was just born."* (Mother 7). In this situation, parents' lives changed instantaneously and often without any warning, leaving them feeling powerless. The chain of unanticipated changes and disruption was described as overwhelming and leaving parents at a loss for what to do, *"there was this overwhelming overflow of anxiety of all the tasks that lay ahead. You just asked yourself: What am I supposed to do now."* (Father 2).

In such strange and unknown situations, parents' habitats were constantly changing, which forced them to adjust to new environments, with new rules and regulations. Hospital rules, such as only allowing one parent to stay overnight at the cardiac ward, having to share a room with other families, were felt to restrict parents' ability to share habitats freely. Access to healthy food was also described as problematic, and sometimes it seemed that parents lived in a suitcase and sleep was a luxury: *"We got a room to stay in ... Of course, she [the mother] just wanted to be next to him ... I checked on them several times during the night. So, I did not sleep much, but it was still good to get a room and a shower, and we were there with the suitcases."* (Father 5). Within these changing circumstances parents had to learn how to care for their child and themselves, in addition to maintaining a healthy relationship with their support systems in Iceland and Sweden. Creating an equilibrium within these situations was difficult.

Following the surgery and throughout childhood, the child's illness continued to create disruptions in parents' lives. This was exemplified by parents' descriptions of their child's continuous follow-up medical appointments, long-term therapies, and multiple surgeries abroad. The daily stress was evident in parents' interviews, described by one mother as feeling like *"a balloon about to burst"* (Mother 3) following the aftermath, but today, three years post-surgery, her daughter goes *"weekly to physiotherapy and occupational therapy, then there are regular team meetings at the kindergarten ... and then she naturally has regular follow-ups with her cardiologist and an orthopedic surgeon, an ophthalmologist, and the neurologist."* (Mother 3).

3.1.2. Life on Hold

Amidst this turmoil of changes, parents simultaneously experienced the feeling that their lives were on hold. This feeling was mostly described as waiting for event to happen or milestones to be hit. The events and milestones identified as important, varied by parents.

However, all parents talked about the day of the surgery as particularly hard. The anxiety and uncertainty before were followed by either joy and thankfulness when the outcome was positive, but grief, sadness, and anger when it was negative. The stress of waiting was perhaps most palpable in parents' stories as 'phone-call': *"we just wandered around and kill time. And then he [surgeon] phoned when the surgery was over ... Everybody jumped up when the phone rang and just Oh My God!"* (Mother 12).

Following the surgery, parents then began waiting for the child's recovery. In this regard, the PICU discharge was a significant milestone for parents. Although this time-point created anxiety, parents also understood how significant this milestone was for the child and the family as a whole. As described by one mother, *"it was a big step for him to get there [cardiac ward], it was just amazing, just for all the three of us to be together."* (Mother 7).

Parents with other children at home expressed the stress of being separated from them. Some parents had never been away from their children before, and for the smaller children, explaining their absence was hard. Waiting to return home and reunite with their children, but not knowing at what date, was very distressing for the whole family: "*What was hardest was not knowing when we would go back home ... every night she [the daughter at home] asked: Mama when are you coming home?*" (Mother 1).

This feeling of waiting continued for parents. Parents described anxiety as they waited for the child to hit developmental milestones and their worries as they waited for child's next follow-up appointment with the cardiologist: "*But before the follow-up appointments, I become nervous. I always got a headache afterwards, sort of like de-stressing.*" (Mother 7). This waiting placed a strain on parents and put their lives on hold.

3.2. Feeling Connected

As parents moved through their unexpected and unwanted transitions of their child's illness, supportive environment that provided comfort, familiarity, and connection, appeared in parents' interviews as a situational condition that facilitated a healthy transition. In particular, the importance of feeling connected—to the child, the siblings, the spouse, the grandparents, the health professionals, and other families of peers—was evident.

3.2.1. Supportive Environment

As parents prepared for the travel to Sweden, they asked questions and sought support from various sources. The pediatric cardiologist was described by all parents as their key person within the health care system that provided them support, being referred to as the "*rock*" (Father 4) and "*the main man*" (Father 5). Following parents return home, the cardiologist continued to be that key person and almost the only professional support.

Spark, a nonprofit CHD parent organization, was mentioned by all parents as instrumental in preparing and supporting them throughout the journey. Their peer-to-peer program, parental Facebook groups, website, and staff was described as immaculate for seeking knowledge and information, as well as being a safe space in which parents were understood and able to envision the future. One father described Spark as a "*rescue squad*" (Father 10); a metaphor exemplified in mother's rumination of her struggles leading up to the travel on of how to explain the situation, and say goodbye to her other daughters: "*we disagreed [she and her husband] ... so I sought advice from other mothers [via Spark's website] about how to best explain this to my daughters ... I didn't want to lie to them about where we were going.*" (Mother 3).

Parents always sheltered themselves by seeking closeness and support from the grandparents, who traveled abroad with the parents, except if they needed to care for the siblings at home. Both parents traveled with their child to Sweden in all instances, but siblings always stayed at home. But a supportive spouse was likely the most important source of support for all parents: "*We [he and his wife] were just going to solve this together and just hope for the best.*" (Father 2).

As parents transitioned between countries, hospitals, and wards, it was important for them to build a safe and comforting habitat for the family. Here, the Ronald McDonald House was described as having the welcoming "home away from home" environment they needed. Furthermore, Icelandic countrymen in Sweden (i.e., grandparents, other families, and health professionals) were instrumental in creating familiarity and security: "*And our moms were also there with us. They often prepared food for us which was home-like and very helpful ... as was having other three Icelandic families staying at the same time, also with children undergoing heart surgery.*" (Mother 11).

All parents felt that their child received quality health care both by health professionals in Sweden and Iceland, and were remembered for their competence and skills: "*The staff ... was wonderful ... I experienced so much professionalism and security while I was there and if I'd need to do this again, I'd insist on it being in Lund.*" (Mother 9). However, in seeking support for themselves, Icelandic health professionals working at the hospital in Sweden were frequently described as a significant source of support and help. Parents portrayed them as selfless and voluntary; these professionals provided the parents with what seemed like a crucial yet unofficial support network. They stepped in and touched many parents' lives: *"And during that time ... an Icelandic anesthesiologist, he ... just stepped into a role, he had not needed to do this. I don't know how we would have coped without having him there."* (Father 6). The Icelandic health professional provided important security in their cultural familiarity, both in the care setting or as a support during medical meetings. It was clear that parents welcomed and preferred support from Icelandic health professionals because it helped them to better understand their situation: *"Because you knew nothing [prior to transferring to a cardiac ward] ... we got some brochures and stuff ... but there was an Icelandic nurse working on that ward, which was very nice. And she spoke to us in Icelandic about exactly everything."* (Mother 12).

3.2.2. Handling the Experience

Parents' ability to cope following the news of their child's CHD diagnosis and surgery abroad varied. Some parents seemed more resilient and quickly found their new normal. The unknown situation and challenges were seen as an assignment and personal qualities a facilitator: *"I was incredibly strong ... I was so convinced that this would work out well."* (Mother 1). Furthermore, parents took charge and became engaged in their healing. They created *"photo album"* (Father 2) of the journey, intentionally accepted help offered to them by the community, *"My boss said: Just go and as see a psychologist, just pick one you like ... So we [him and his wife] went together to see a psychologist."* (Father 10), as well as seeking out and asking for the help they felt they needed, *"I asked if it would not be a good idea if I talked to a psychologist or something ... "* (Mother 1).

Parents' ability to face their fears, however varied. They struggled with the unexpected path their life had taken. Parents were worried about their child's future and how their own future would be influenced by the illness, as illustrated by one father: *"If all goes wrong ... then you'll naturally go to a dark place ... even if you decide not to hang yourself, you're going to live with it, then life is still useless, so you're just such a passenger."* (Father 10).

Knowledge and skills helped parents face the fear and handle their experiences. The act of knowing symbolized a need for control and hope. Parents' need for knowledge varied, however. Some sought a deeper understanding of their situation, while others felt that too much information created fear and anxiety. Parents described how their own education enabled them to seek and gain resources. However, a lack of knowledge (e.g., of the Swedish language) created vulnerability and a feeling of disconnect. One father explained this when he said: *"Some of the Swedish nurses, just didn't want to speak English ... they just avoided talking [to us]."* (Father 4). Further, knowledge and information were often described in opposition. For example, information was provided or not received, or was helpful or paradoxical. When information contradicted parents' hopes for a normal future for their child, it was described as threatening, even when signs of their child's permanent disability were evident.

Talking about their experiences was a coping mechanism used by all parents. However, their readiness to share this experience varied, and some needed a long time before they were ready, *"Yes, at that time there were no tears ... I really do not remember much from this time. And it was not until after a year had passed [since the heart surgery abroad] that I could talk about it."* (Mother 11). Memories also emerged, that parents did not want to talk about. One father described how he wanted to forget some memories: *"[There are] unspeakable things I've ... forgotten and blocked out, this is somehow such a tribulation."* (Father 6).

After returning home, some parents sought help from professionals to handle their experiences and help them to recover. No parent, however shared memories of faith or religion in their coping. Furthermore, with the exception of walking, physical or spiritual activities were seldom mentioned by parents as a way of coping, although one father found it helpful: *"I started to meditate ... sometimes I did yoga ... I started to run long distance."* (Father 10).

3.3. Wishing Being Accepted

Parents situational conditions could also inhibit a healthy transitional experience. In the interviews, not being seen as a legitimate client, emerged as an important inhibitor. Overall parents did not feel accepted, neither by the Icelandic or Swedish health care systems. They expressed a need to be accepted as a legitimate client, meaning both as a parent—with continuous and multiple parenting roles, and as a client—with complex health care needs. When overlooked, parents' vulnerabilities emerged, and their risk of developing traumatic experiences seemed to increase.

3.3.1. Parenting Roles and Needs

Parents felt it was important for them to fulfill their parenting roles of presence and caretaking as best they could throughout the child's traveling and hospitalization. If overlooked by health professionals, parents described feeling distressed and dismissed: *"I found it very difficult that someone [at the PICU] could just drive me away from my child ... that all of a sudden [somebody could] just [say]: You can't be with your daughter, now you just have to leave."* (Mother 3).

At the same time, the extremely stressful situations, and environments that parents found themselves in made parenting a challenge. Understanding how best to care for their child was not only difficult but also frightening: *"We just sat with him [in the PICU], which was extremely strange and surrealist to be sitting there and he was attached to 300 lines and all kinds of drugs and everything is beeping, and you do not know what is actually happening. That was a strange life experience. And you are like, should I be here or not? You just do not know how to behave."* (Mother 1).

Parenting also involved creating relationships with health professionals. Here transparency and honesty about the child's condition was a fundamental component of trust building. When parents were not included in the decision making concerning their child, as described by one father regarding his son's critical condition, they felt as if their parental rights were being violated: *"You'd never keep such information [CHD condition severity] from a patient, you'd tell him exactly what the situation was. And I think it should be exactly the same for parents."* (Father 6).

Furthermore, the disruption of the illness put a strain on spousal relationships. Parents described disagreements in their understanding of the illness and its ramifications. It seemed that if an underlying relationship problem existed previously, it was magnified by this stressful situation. In some cases, it triggered the disintegration of the family: *"I got sick [in Sweden] ... and my ex's reaction was so upsetting, that like, I got this kind of confirmation that we couldn't be married anymore."* (Mother 1). Of the 12 parents interviewed, four separated following their arrival back home.

As parents transitioned between health care systems, they often felt their needs were overlooked by health professionals both in Iceland and Sweden. The needs parents were overlooked varied, but mothers more than fathers talked about their psychological issues during and following their child's hospitalization. Parents described how they felt alone in dealing with their health problems and their need for support: *"There is nobody thinking about the parents ... I realized that there was no mental support provided abroad. And not here at home either."* (Mother 8).

Parents' vulnerabilities were expressed in their memories of distress. All mothers were recovering from childbirth when they traveled the first time with their infant to Sweden. Nevertheless, mother's postpartum problems such as *"lactation mastitis"* (Mother 1), *"lactation suppression"* (Father 6), *"post-partum depression"* (Mother 3), and *"postpartum pain"* (Mother 12) were always secondary. Mothers described how they experienced physical pain and became sick following childbirth. Memories of this physical suffering were frequently associated with the traveling: *"I remember this extreme pain; I was walking down some long [airport] terminals."* (Mother 1). This left first-time mothers feeling particularly vulnerable. Overall, parents were sleep deprived and tired during the child's hospitalization period. However, the fatigue and emotional aftershock usually appeared after they arrived back home, following which, some mothers described they developed psychological problems: *"When she was eight months old, then I began experiencing traumatic stress and anxiety ... It had been escalating since she came home."* (Mother 3). For some, these health problems were only short-term, whereas in others they became long-term health issues.

3.3.2. Feeling Overlooked: Culture and System

On their arrival in Sweden, parents had to adjust to a foreign environment, language, costumes, and regulations. In this situation, parents inevitably experienced cultural barriers. However, the parents' ability to speak or understand English or Swedish was not assessed before they traveled to Sweden. These abilities were simply assumed.

Language barriers were the most common issues raised by parents. While most parents were able to communicate in English or Swedish, some were not. Those that were unable to speak English did not seek help from a translator. Indeed, the mere idea of a translator seemed awkward and even shameful; rather, parents described how they did their best or relied on other family members to help them: *"I'm very poor in English ... but my mom and her boyfriend ... helped me understand."* (Mother 12).

Most parents felt welcomed during their stay in Sweden, although some mentioned cultural insensitivities from health professionals. In a few cases, parents noted that health professionals' proficiency in English was lacking. This was surprising to parents and in retrospect they regretted not asking for better service.

Parents talked about how they felt that unrealistic expectations and responsibilities were being placed on them. Sometimes parents felt as if they were being taken for granted, even treated as employees: *"We were just in a part-time job, actually we were providing intensive care by watching over her the whole night."* (Mother 3). Parents described how health professionals expected them to cope, under what they felt were unrealistic and extreme circumstances for them, that left them traumatized. These traumatic events were mostly related to their child's suffering during medical procedures: *"My only memory is when a line was being removed, this was a long line, all the way into the heart. I just remember how much he screamed."* (Mother 11).

When in Iceland, parents did not receive any follow-up support and there was no interdisciplinary team assigned to help the families. Parents were mostly left to navigate the systems and bureaucracy on their own to find help and support. They expressed surprise at the scarcity of resources available to them and described a gap in the system: *"Perhaps the biggest problem with the process is what happened afterwards. Because he died ... We just came home and there was nobody that contacted us ... We had to seek everything ourselves like psychological help and all that."* (Father 6). Some parents were so concerned with these systemic flaws that they sought ways to help repair the system. These parents advocated for a multidisciplinary health care team to assist the whole family.

3.4. Finding Closure

The time span of parent's situational transitions varied, but *"[getting] off the rollercoaster"* (Father 5) and finding closure was desired by all parents. Parents did not always describe a specific endpoint, but when they did it seemed fluid and sometimes attached to 'ritual(s)'. The process of finding closure was expressed in surviving and compassion, with personal growth indicating a healthy transition.

3.4.1. Surviving

All parents interviewed were survivors, they had been through tremendous challenges, stress, and even trauma, and were able to share this. The meaning parents placed on survival varied, however. For some, the stressful life event itself was their focus: *"It is a huge undertaking to go abroad. When I think back to this time, I just get shivers down my spine and if I had to do this again, I would have a nervous breakdown."* (Mother 9). This was also exemplified in one father's recollection of this time: *"we as parents, so often think back to this time with a sense of horror, it was a really dreadful time."* (Father 4). In other cases, parents described this stressful experience as something they needed to endure in order to survive: *"I just wanted this to be over. Just to get through this and have it over with."* (Mother 7).

Parents also described survival as a process of moving on and finding a new normal. This was illustrated by for example in growing their families or ending a spousal relationship. However, this process was perhaps most clearly illustrated by one father: *"Then you go off the rollercoaster and you just know: Wow! ... but then you just keep going, just forward, and finally you start picking up the threads of a healthy life."* (Father 5). In addition, recovering was also found in parents interviews as an indicator of closure: *"This is such a huge shock ... recovering could've been much harder for us ... but I think we're just lucky."* (Mother 7).

Parents who struggled the most were grieving some type of loss. To be able to move on, they had to reevaluate their experience and even reshape their memories. This was illustrated by one mother, whose daughter developed long term complications, in her statement that, *"my existence now is trying to make peace with my life ... you know her difficult life. The life she will lead ... trying to find meaning ... "* (Mother 3).

3.4.2. Showing Compassion

Parents expressed their compassion for parents in the same situation as them, especially those who were more vulnerable. They questioned whether the current system was tailored for these specific groups and had concerns: *"[It] is absolutely necessary to ask people before they travel abroad [about English skills], because individuals with intellectual disabilities are having children for example, or parents who didn't even finish elementary school and or aren't good in languages. Then it is necessary ... to have someone to translate for them."* (Mother 9).

Following their experiences of traveling abroad, some parents joined peer-to-peer groups to support other parents and others even started lobbying within the Icelandic hospital system, for health care reforms: *"we have criticized the process, asked for changes ... we are told a new protocol is in place ... I just hope that if something like this happens again [child dies abroad], it goes better for those people."* (Father 6).

Empathy-based survival guilt towards the suffering of other parents was also expressed by many parents. This empathy was directed towards other parents who either lost their child or had a much sicker child: *"After the funeral ... the guilt I felt towards my sister- and brother-in-law. We'd just got through this and it went so well and then ... their son just dies."* (Mother 9).

4. Discussion

This study elicited parents' experiences of their child's CHD diagnosis, heart surgery abroad, and journey beyond. The overarching theme, living with the memories, highlighted the superimposition of this stressful live event on the expected transition to parenthood, where parents' vivid memories still impacted their lives up to five years later. The most concerning finding was parents' negative memories of the transition back home and their descriptions of roadblocks to recovery that followed.

According to Meleis's transitions theory [19], the constructs that define transitions are its nature (e.g., critical event), conditions (i.e., facilitators and inhibitors), and patterns of response (e.g., indicators of a healthy transition). Furthermore, all transitions are believed to build on universal commonalities, where disconnectedness is seen as the most pervasive one [19].

A parental transition triggered by child's CCHD and need for heart surgery abroad has not been previously documented. However, other types of parental transitions focusing on child medical tourism [16–18] and hospitalizations of critically ill children [8–10] have been studied. Concurrently, our findings support the diverse and universal nature of transition experiences [19], although all parents experienced situational transitions, its nature—complexity, suddenness, degree of stress, and social support required —was particularly different. Thus, the uniqueness of our findings relates to the transitional conditions experienced by our parents.

Our findings showed both facilitators and inhibitors in parents' environmental conditions. Connectivity represented itself both as a facilitator (e.g., in networks of health professionals and peer-groups) and an inhibitor (e.g., separation from child's siblings). Separation or feeling separated is associated with personal, familial, socio-cultural, and geographical factors. However, separation from family and home life is hard on individuals in hospital settings and can lead to vulnerability, loneliness, and dependency [23].

The distance between home and hospital created a feeling of disconnection in parents in our study. Concurrently, others have shown that separation caused by geographical distance can negatively impact family relationships during child's hospitalization. Specifically, parents' likelihood of relationship difficulties with other family members tend to grow as the distance between hospital and home increases [24]. In our study, several parents described relationship tensions during their stay in Sweden, with some attributing this tension to the distance from home. Further, the separation from the child's siblings at home was also hard on parents, and aligns with the findings of others [16]. Parents used modern technology (e.g., Facebook, Skype, Facetime) to connect with the left-behind siblings. This seemed however disjointed to their feeling of disconnectedness due to the physical distance. Another contributing factor may be siblings age, as all were relatively young, which might have made the utilization of technology perplexing.

In hospital settings, separation from home triggers a need for comfort and support that can be found through cultural connection. This includes seeking familiarity in terms of language and food, in addition to developing a sense of belonging in terms of social support networks [23]. Consistent with a meta-analysis and systematic reviews of parental coping with their child's CHD [3], our participants used various coping strategies from surgery to childhood. However, their means of becoming culturally connected while abroad—particularly in the security, safety, and trust they placed in countrymen—is unique to our findings. Here, child's grandparents and the health professionals working at the hospital abroad were of significance in creating this cultural connection.

Similar to that in other studies [3,25], grandparents were a significant source of support to parents in our study. Grandparents were a cornerstone in their habitat building, either caring for the child's siblings at home or traveling with them abroad, thus creating familiarity through food and language. In hospital settings, such comfort can counterbalance negative emotions associated with being away from home and home life [23]. Importantly, the findings showed that the support provided by countrymen working as health professionals at the hospital abroad, created unique networks and relationships essential to the parents. These professionals provided parents with services ranging from direct medical care to assistance with practical matters, all seemingly done voluntarily. The shared culture and language appear to have created a feeling of safety, understanding, and familiarity, and a sense of belonging. Cultural competence in health care involves streamlining care and facilitating communication [26]. This could be done by matching patients and providers based on their cultural similarities [27,28]. Our results suggest that cultural competence in health care can be achieved by providing families traveling abroad with access to the medical care of health professionals who are fellow countrymen.

A key element facilitating healthy parental transitions from the PICU to a clinical ward is effective communication and information flow [8]. Furthermore, clarity in patient-provider communication is needed for facilitating and managing transitions, also imperative to securing quality care [29]. Our findings show that parents' experienced communication challenges with health professionals while abroad, which amplified the imbalance of social capitals inherent in the client-providers encounters. The clearest communicational challenges reported related to language and other cultural barriers. Similar findings are reported in child medical tourism [16,17]. Although no participant asked for medical translator, they sought assistance from their fellow countrymen (i.e., family and health professionals) when needed.

Language discrepancies between clients and health clinicians contribute to communication errors, especially if both speak a second language [30,31]. Furthermore, within these language-discrepant medical communication settings, individuals' distress and vulnerabilities are likely to increase [30,32]. This is problematic and implies that assessing and anticipating families' need for support prior to traveling (e.g., a medical translator) is necessary, as has been suggested by others [14]. It is therefore surprising that our participants and apparent health professionals did not anticipate this, even though both parties had to communicate in a second language (i.e., English).

The transitions experienced by our parents following their child's CHD diagnosis and cardiac surgery were extremely stressful. In a brief period, parents transitioned from expecting to go home with a healthy baby to having a critically ill newborn needing cardiac surgery abroad. Some even had to make this journey abroad three times. Parents' descriptions of their aftershock, unmet needs, and short- and long-term health problems following their arrival back home, concur with the pediatric cardiac literature [6]. Similar findings are however not reported in the child medical tourism literature [16–18].

Personal growth and empowerment are a positive outcome of transitions [19], described by few parents in our study. This growth was best exemplified in the compassion and empathy parents showed toward their peers in similar situations, and in parents' efforts to reform the current health care system. Concurrently, in a qualitative study, looking at parents mostly from low-income countries, majority of parents experienced personal growth (e.g., greater compassion for others) as a result of coming to the United States to seek medical treatment for their child [16]. In addition, a quantitative study [33] reported nearly 40% of parents experienced posttraumatic growth after their child's admission to PICU. The different contexts and samples used in these studies compared to ours, may explain the inconsistency of experienced personal growth by our parents. Even so, all parents in our study described a path to recovery as they tried to fit the transition into their life story in a meaningful way.

Our findings suggest an urgent need for follow-up care and support for this population, but currently, no such support is provided by health professionals in either Iceland or Sweden. A significant feature of transitional care is comprehensive and continued follow-up care for patients and families [19]. This is in line with pediatric cardiology guidelines [34] which recommend that a multidisciplinary health team supports children with CHD and their parents throughout their whole journey, including with follow-up care. Systematic reviews examining parents after their child's PICU admission [35] and meta-analyses examining adult ICU survivors and their relatives [36] have indicated that follow-up appointments can improve mental health for these groups. These findings stress the urgency of offering the same follow-up service for families of children with CHD, particularly for at-risk groups such as those traveling abroad.

eHealth is considered a promising aid to lower psychiatric morbidity in families of children with CHD [34,37] and is particularly relevant for the population of the current study. This mode of health care creates opportunities for interactive communication between all stakeholders, allowing health care teams at home and abroad to collaborate more easily with parents as they transition between systems. Furthermore, via website apps, psychological follow-up care could, for example, permit parents to make virtual revisits to the hospital abroad.

This study has both limitations and strengths for consideration. Of the seven mothers and five fathers who participated, only eight children with CHD were represented. The range of possible experiences might thus have been restricted because both parents could participate. However, parent couples' experience of a stressful event often varies greatly [38]. A written request was sent to 25 parents via e-mail. Fifteen parents replied to the e-mail, but only 12 parents participated in the study. It is unclear whether the 13 parents who did not participate are in some way demographically different from those who did. The nearly equal number of mothers and fathers, and the wide range of sociodemographic characteristics in the participant sample, however, strengthened the study findings. Additionally, the primary categories reappeared in all of the interviews, thus creating a saturation that strengthened the results. The study findings may not be generalized to other populations, but may be transferable to other parents of children with CHD traveling abroad for cardiac surgery. The sample size was relatively small. However, the fact that similar sample sizes have been used in other studies [39,40] and the emphasis on richness rather than sample size in content analysis [41] provides strength to our findings. The trustworthiness of the study findings lies in the methods used and the experience of the three authors. All authors are registered nurses with pediatric clinical experience. The second author (A.S.S.) has extensive experience with pediatric acritical care cardiology and working with parents of children with CCHD. Although all authors are experienced researchers, the second author also has extensive experience in qualitative content analysis methods.

5. Conclusions

The lived experiences of parents when their child underwent complex heart surgery abroad are filled with difficult memories and emotions. Parents' readiness and need for support was heightened after arriving home from abroad. However, these needs were not met by either of the health care systems involved. Culturally competent care for the families must be designed and implemented, starting with an assessment of language skills prior to the travel. Assigning families to multidisciplinary health care teams and providing them with follow-up support are necessary. Here, the use of eHealth interventions to improve interactive communication between all stakeholders is promising.

Author Contributions: Conceptualization, Ó.K., G.K. and A.S.-S.; methodology, Ó.K., G.K. and A.S.S.; validation, Ó.K., G.K. and A.S.-S.; formal analysis, Ó.K., G.K. and A.S.-S.; investigation, Ó.K.; resources, G.K.; data curation, G.K.; writing—original draft preparation, Ó.K.; writing—review and editing, Ó.K., G.K. and A.S.-S.; visualization, Ó.K.; supervision, G.K. and A.S.-S.; project administration, Ó.K.; funding acquisition, Ó.K. and G.K. All authors have read and agreed to the published version of the manuscript.

Acknowledgments: The researchers are most grateful to the parents who shared their experiences, and all those who supported this project.

References

1. McMahon, E.; Chang, Y.-S. From surviving to thriving—Parental experiences of hospitalised infants with congenital heart disease undergoing cardiac surgery: A qualitative synthesis. *J. Pediatr. Nurs.* **2020**, *51*, 32–41. [CrossRef] [PubMed]
2. Biber, S.; Andonian, C.; Beckmann, J.; Ewert, P.; Freilinger, S.; Nagdyman, N.; Kaemmerer, H.; Oberhoffer, R.; Pieper, L.; Neidenbach, R.C. Current research status on the psychological situation of parents of children with congenital heart disease. *Cardiovasc. Diagn.* **2019**, *9*, S369–S376. [CrossRef] [PubMed]
3. Lumsden, M.R.; Smith, D.M.; Wittkowski, A. Coping in parents of children with congenital heart disease: A systematic review and meta-synthesis. *J. Child. Fam. Stud.* **2019**, *28*, 1736–1753. [CrossRef]
4. Liu, Y.; Chen, S.; Zühlke, L.; Black, G.C.; Choy, M.-K.; Li, N.; Keavney, B.D. Global birth prevalence of congenital heart defects 1970–2017: Updated systematic review and meta-analysis of 260 studies. *Int. J. Epidemiol.* **2019**, *48*, 455–463. [CrossRef] [PubMed]
5. Bakker, M.K.; Bergman, J.E.; Krikov, S.; Amar, E.; Cocchi, G.; Cragan, J.; De Walle, H.E.; Gatt, M.; Groisman, B.; Liu, S. Prenatal diagnosis and prevalence of critical congenital heart defects: An international retrospective cohort study. *BMJ Open* **2019**, *9*, e028139. [CrossRef] [PubMed]
6. Woolf-King, S.E.; Anger, A.; Arnold, E.A.; Weiss, S.J.; Teitel, D. Mental health among parents of children with critical congenital heart defects: A systematic review. *J. Am. Heart Assoc.* **2017**, *6*, e004862. [CrossRef]
7. Bruce, E.; Lilja, C.; Sundin, K. Mothers' lived experiences of support when living with young children with congenital heart defects. *J. Spec. Pediatr. Nurs.* **2014**, *19*, 54–67. [CrossRef]
8. Suleman, Z.; Evans, C.; Manning, J.C. Parents' and carers' experiences of transition and aftercare following a child's discharge from a paediatric intensive care unit to an in-patient ward setting: A qualitative systematic review. *Intensive Crit. Care Nurs.* **2019**, *51*, 35–44. [CrossRef]
9. Obas, K.A.; Leal, J.M.; Zegray, M.; Rennick, J.E. Parental perceptions of transition from intensive care following a child's cardiac surgery. *Nurs. Crit. Care* **2016**, *21*, e1–e9. [CrossRef]
10. Gaskin, K.L. Patterns of transition experience for parents going home from hospital with their infant after first stage surgery for complex congenital heart disease. *J. Pediatr. Nurs.* **2018**, *41*, e23–e32. [CrossRef] [PubMed]

11. Neistinn. Hjartagáttin, Meðfæddur Hjartagalli. Available online: http://neistinn.is/hjartagattin/ (accessed on 30 January 2020).
12. Gunnarsdóttir, B. Greining alvarlegra meðfæddra hjartagalla á Íslandi 2014–2017. Bachelor's Thesis, University of Iceland, Reykjavik, Iceland, 14 May 2018.
13. World Health Organization. *Cross-Border Health Care in the European Union: Mapping and Analysing Practices and Policies*; World Health Organization. Regional Office for Europe: Geneva, Switzerland, 2011.
14. Hamlyn-Williams, C.; Lakhanpaul, M.; Manikam, L. Child medical tourism: A new phenomenon. In *Handbook on Medical Tourism and Patient Mobility*; Lunt, N., Horsfall, D., Hanefeld, J., Eds.; Edward Elgar: Cheltenham, UK, 2015; pp. 360–369. [CrossRef]
15. Lorraine Culley, N.H.; Baldwin, K.; Lakhanpaul, M. Children travelling for treatment: What we don't know. *Arch. Dis. Child.* **2013**, *98*, 442–444. [CrossRef]
16. Margolis, R.; Ludi, E.; Pao, M.; Wiener, L. International adaptation: Psychosocial and parenting experiences of caregivers who travel to the United States to obtain acute medical care for their seriously ill child. *Soc. Work Health Care* **2013**, *52*, 669–683. [CrossRef] [PubMed]
17. Crom, D.B. The experience of South American mothers who have a child being treated for malignancy in the United States. *J. Pediatric Oncol. Nurs.* **1995**, *12*, 104–112. [CrossRef]
18. Cockle, S.G.; Ogden, J. The 'radiation vacation': Parents' experiences of travelling to have their children's brain tumours treated with proton beam therapy. *Health Psychol. Open* **2016**, *3*, 2055102916649767. [CrossRef] [PubMed]
19. Meleis, A.I. *Transitions Theory: Middle Range and Situation Specific Theories in Nursing Research and Practice*; Springer Publishing Company: New York, NY, USA, 2010.
20. Graneheim, U.H.; Lundman, B. Qualitative content analysis in nursing research: Concepts, procedures and measures to achieve trustworthiness. *Nurse Educ. Today* **2004**, *24*, 105–112. [CrossRef] [PubMed]
21. Graneheim, U.H.; Lindgren, B.M.; Lundman, B. Methodological challenges in qualitative content analysis: A discussion paper. *Nurse Educ. Today* **2017**, *56*, 29–34. [CrossRef] [PubMed]
22. Terp, K.; Sjostrom-Strand, A. Parents' experiences and the effect on the family two years after their child was admitted to a PICU—An interview study. *Intensive Crit. Care Nurs.* **2017**, *43*, 143–148. [CrossRef] [PubMed]
23. Wensley, C.; Botti, M.; McKillop, A.; Merry, A.F. A framework of comfort for practice: An integrative review identifying the multiple influences on patients' experience of comfort in healthcare settings. *Int. J. Qual. Health Care* **2017**, *29*, 151–162. [CrossRef]
24. Yantzi, N.; Rosenberg, M.W.; Burke, S.O.; Harrison, M.B. The impacts of distance to hospital on families with a child with a chronic condition. *Soc. Sci. Med.* **2001**, *52*, 1777–1791. [CrossRef]
25. Rempel, G.R.; Ravindran, V.; Rogers, L.G.; Magill-Evans, J. Parenting under pressure: A grounded theory of parenting young children with life-threatening congenital heart disease. *J. Adv. Nurs.* **2013**, *69*, 619–630. [CrossRef]
26. White, J.; Plompen, T.; Tao, L.; Micallef, E.; Haines, T. What is needed in culturally competent healthcare systems? A qualitative exploration of culturally diverse patients and professional interpreters in an Australian healthcare setting. *BMC Public Health* **2019**, *19*, 1096. [CrossRef] [PubMed]
27. Hsueh, L.; Hirsh, A.T.; Maupomé, G.; Stewart, J.C. Patient–provider language concordance and health outcomes: A systematic review, evidence map, and research agenda. *Med. Care Res. Rev.* **2019**. [CrossRef] [PubMed]
28. Flores, G. The impact of medical interpreter services on the quality of health care: A systematic review. *Med. Care Res. Rev.* **2005**, *62*, 255–299. [CrossRef] [PubMed]
29. Meleis, A. Facilitating and Managing Transitions: An Imperative for Quality Care. *Investig. En Enfermería: Imagen Y Desarro.* **2018**, *21*. [CrossRef]
30. de Moissac, D.; Bowen, S. Impact of language barriers on quality of care and patient safety for official language minority francophones in Canada. *J. Patient Exp.* **2019**, *6*, 24–32. [CrossRef]
31. Gudykunst, W.B. *Theorizing about Intercultural Communication*; Sage: Thousand Oaks, CA, USA, 2005.
32. Bowen, S. *Language Barriers in Access to Health Care*; Health Canada: Ottawa, ON, Canada, 2001.
33. Rodríguez-Rey, R.; Palacios, A.; Alonso-Tapia, J.; Pérez, E.; Álvarez, E.; Coca, A.; Mencía, S.; Marcos, A.M.; Mayordomo-Colunga, J.; Fernández, F.; et al. Posttraumatic growth in pediatric intensive care personnel: Dependence on resilience and coping strategies. *Psychol. Trauma Theory Res. Pract. Policy* **2017**, *9*, 407–415. [CrossRef]

34. Utens, E.; Callus, E.; Levert, E.M.; Groote, K.; Casey, F. Multidisciplinary family-centred psychosocial care for patients with CHD: Consensus recommendations from the AEPC psychosocial working group. *Cardiol. Young* **2018**, *28*, 192–198. [CrossRef]
35. Baker, S.C.; Gledhill, J.A. Systematic review of interventions to reduce psychiatric morbidity in parents and children after PICU admissions. *Pediatr. Crit. Care Med.* **2017**, *18*, 343–348. [CrossRef]
36. Rosa, R.G.; Ferreira, G.E.; Viola, T.W.; Robinson, C.C.; Kochhann, R.; Berto, P.P.; Biason, L.; Cardoso, P.R.; Falavigna, M.; Teixeira, C. Effects of post-ICU follow-up on subject outcomes: A systematic review and meta-analysis. *J. Crit. Care* **2019**, *52*, 115–125. [CrossRef]
37. Williams, T.S.; McDonald, K.P.; Roberts, S.D.; Chau, V.; Seed, M.; Miller, S.P.; Sananes, R. From Diagnoses to Ongoing Journey: Parent Experiences Following Congenital Heart Disease Diagnoses. *J. Pediatr. Psychol.* **2019**, *44*, 924–936. [CrossRef]
38. Feinberg, M.E.; Jones, D.E.; McDaniel, B.T.; Liu, S.; Almeida, D. Chapter II: New fathers' and mothers' daily stressors and resources influence parent adjustment and family relationships. *Monogr. Soc. Res. Child. Dev.* **2019**, *84*, 18–34. [PubMed]
39. Sjostrom-Strand, A.; Terp, K. Parents' experiences of having a baby with a congenital heart defect and the child's heart surgery. *Compr. Child. Adolesc. Nurs.* **2017**, *42*, 10–23. [CrossRef] [PubMed]
40. David Vainberg, L.; Vardi, A.; Jacoby, R. The experiences of parents of children undergoing surgery for congenital heart defects: A holistic model of care. *Front. Psychol.* **2019**, *10*, 2666. [CrossRef] [PubMed]
41. Bengtsson, M. How to plan and perform a qualitative study using content analysis. *Nurs. Open* **2016**, *2*, 8–14. [CrossRef]

12

Relief Alternatives during Resuscitation: Instructions to Teach Bystanders

María José Pujalte-Jesús [1], César Leal-Costa [2,*], María Ruzafa-Martínez [2,*], Antonio Jesús Ramos-Morcillo [2,*] and José Luis Díaz Agea [3]

1 Faculty of Nursing, Universidad Católica de Murcia UCAM, 30107 Murcia, Spain; mjpujalte@ucam.edu
2 Faculty of Nursing, University of Murcia, 30107 Murcia, Spain
3 Faculty of Nursing, Catholic University of Murcia, 30107 Murcia, Spain; jluis@ucam.edu
* Correspondence: cleal@um.es (C.L.-C.); maruzafa@um.es (M.R.-M.); ajramos@um.es (A.J.R.-M.)

Abstract: To analyze the quality of resuscitation (CPR) performed by individuals without training after receiving a set of instructions (structured and unstructured/intuitive) from an expert in a simulated context, the specific objective was to design a simple and structured CPR learning method on-site. An experimental study was designed, consisting of two random groups with a post-intervention measurement in which the experimental group (EG) received standardized instructions, and the control group (CG) received intuitive or non-standardized instructions, in a public area simulated scenario. Statistically significant differences were found ($p < 0.0001$) between the EG and the CG for variables: time needed to give orders, pauses between chest compressions and ventilations, depth, overall score, chest compression score, and chest recoil. The average depth of the EG was 51.1 mm (SD 7.94) and 42.2 mm (SD 12.04) for the CG. The chest recoil median was 86.32% (IQR 62.36, 98.87) for the EG, and 58.3% (IQR 27.46, 84.33) in the CG. The use of a sequence of simple, short and specific orders, together with observation-based learning makes possible the execution of chest compression maneuvers that are very similar to those performed by rescuers, and allows the teaching of the basic notions of ventilation. The structured order method was shown to be an on-site learning opportunity when faced with the need to maintain high-quality CPR in the presence of an expert resuscitator until the arrival of emergency services.

Keywords: cardiopulmonary resuscitation; chest compression; method; experiential learning; observation; CPR

---

1. Introduction

The out-of-hospital cardiorespiratory arrest (OHCA) is a frequent health problem in developed countries, and only a small percentage of the victims receive cardiopulmonary resuscitation (CPR) by the bystanders [1]. Early and high-quality resuscitation maneuvers can double, or even quadruple, survival [2], however, CPR training of the general population is scarce. The current protocols differ depending if they are directed towards professionals or laypersons, and the health services continue exploring alternatives to improve bystander CPR rates when witnessing out-of-hospital cardiorespiratory arrests. Among these alternatives, we find mass training and telephone-based CPR, to such an extent that in 2015, the European resuscitation guidelines [3] recognized the important role of dispatcher-assisted CPR in the diagnosis and providing of telephone-assisted, early cardiopulmonary resuscitation.

From that point on, the attempts to combine standardized communication in CPR have increased [4,5], with supporters [6] and critics [7] until 2019, when the International Liaison Committee on Resuscitation (ILCOR) [8] recommended that the dispatchers provide instructions to the bystanders.

From that point on, many research studies provided information about the increased survival rate [9,10], and affirmed that the provision of dispatch cardiopulmonary resuscitation instructions, instead of no instructions at all, improved the results from cardiopulmonary arrest [11].

However, all of these studies suggest that the clinical results after out-of-hospital cardiac arrest have a greater possibility of improving when dispatcher assistance is available; the scientific societies identify, in their knowledge gap, the preferred CPR instruction sequence for Dispatcher-Assisted Cardiopulmonary Resuscitation (DA-CPR) [8], because an optimal sequence of orders is not yet available for those who are limited to receiving instructions from emergency services personnel. At present, the ILCOR is still seeking the best evidence through the Consensus on Science with Treatment Recommendations (CoSTR) [12].

Between the CPR observed by an expert and telephone-based CPR, we find real-life situations where only one expert/healthcare worker performs resuscitation maneuvers surrounded by people without training, but who could play an important role in maintaining high-quality CPR if they could learn how to do so on-site. These possible scenarios would need to have certain essential elements, described by Bandura [13,14], when learning a skill through observation: attention and motivation. If motivated people were available who are willing to relieve the expert resuscitator, then this expert could provide the necessary instructions to teach CPR to the bystanders for the benefit of the patient. The exhaustion of a single resuscitator could reduce the possibilities of maintaining high-quality CPR until the arrival of the emergency services.

Recent studies back the use of standardized communication in resuscitation maneuvers to improve the communication and care of the patient during life-support maneuvers [15], and other research studies have associated the use of "action-linked phrases" such as "shock delivered, start compressions" with a decreased start time of the chest compressions [16].

The general objective of our study was to analyze the quality of the CPR, performed by individuals who had no prior knowledge on resuscitation, after receiving a set of instructions (structured and unstructured/intuitive) from an expert within a context of simulated CPR. The specific objective was to design a simple and structured method for the fast learning of CPR on-site.

2. Materials and Methods

2.1. Study Design and Settings

A post-intervention two-group post-test-only randomized experiment [17–20] was designed, in which the experimental group (EG) received standardized instructions, and the control group (CG) received intuitive, unstructured instructions. This is one of the simplest experimental designs [21]. The groups (experimental and control) were randomly assigned. One group received the training; the other group did not receive the training, and was used for comparison. A previous trial was not required for this design, as participants were randomly assigned to the groups, and thus it was assumed that both groups were statistically equivalent. In this design, the objective was to determine whether differences existed between the two groups after the training program. Therefore, a prior trial was not considered for this study design. Although this test could have been used to determine whether the groups were comparable before the experiment, this was not done, to avoid the possible negative effects entailed by the trail to the internal validity, which could be detrimental for the participants' learning. On the other hand, the participants were randomly assigned to the groups and the experimental conditions, ensuring that the groups were equivalent (they had the same socio-demographic characteristics, particularly not having any previous training or prior knowledge about resuscitation).

2.2. Selection of Participants

The target population was the university population from the Region of Murcia (Spain); volunteers were solicited through announcements in the virtual campus among the students from the Catholic

University of Murcia. The collection of data was performed between the months of November 2019 and February 2020.

The study included all the volunteer participants older than 18 who had signed the informed consent form and who did not comply with the exclusion criteria. These exclusion criteria were: physical limitation that could impede them from performing chest compressions and ventilation for 2 min, intellectual limitation that could impede them from following and performing the orders, refusing to participate in the study, being a healthcare worker or a healthcare student, and having received CPR training at least 5 years prior. The participants were informed about the purpose of the study to evaluate the efficacy of a method to teach CPR on-site in the least amount of time. The participants were not informed about the results of their intervention until the end of the study. The expert resuscitators were selected from clinical simulation teaching staff volunteers at the university. The inclusion criteria were: being an instructor in basic life support (BLS) and automated external defibrillation (AED) accredited by the European Resuscitation Council (ERC), and/or being a CPR professor for more than 2 years. Ultimately, this group was comprised of eight experts, of which six were women and two were men.

2.3. Intervention

After complying with the eligibility criteria to participate in the study, the participants were randomly assigned to the experimental group "structured orders" or to the control group "unstructured orders". This assignment was performed using a random assignment tool (sealedenvelope.com, London, UK). Likewise, once assigned to a group, the roles of ventilation (VR) or chest compression (CR) were randomly assigned. Participants were blinded to the allocation until randomization. For performing the mouth-to-mouth ventilations, face protection devices (Laerdal® Face Shield, Laerdal Medical Corporation, Stavanger, Norway) were made available to the participants. When the research was conducted, knowledge about the COVID-19 pandemic was unknown in Spain.

A total of 138 individuals comprised the final sample. Of these, 12 were excluded because they had received CPR training in the last 5 years. Of the remaining 126 participants, 64 were randomly assigned to the structured orders group (experimental group, EG) and 62 to the unstructured orders group (control group, CG). Of the 64 EG participants, 32 were assigned the ventilation role (VR) and 32 to the chest compression role (CR); after the randomization, two VR participants were excluded when they refused to perform mouth-to-mouth ventilation, one CR participant was excluded for fatigue which impeded concluding the trial, and one participant was excluded due to loss of data. From the 62 participants in the GC group, 30 were assigned to the VR group and 32 to the CR group; after the randomization, two CR participants were excluded due to fatigue that impeded them from finishing the trial. Lastly, the 120 remaining participants received the training planned, and the results were analyzed. A CONSORT study flow diagram is shown in Figure 1.

2.4. Experimental Group: Structured Orders

Before starting, the participants were told that they were dealing with a simulated scenario on the street, and that they were witnessing how an expert performed CPR on a person in OHCA. They were told that the expert would ask for their help after two cycles of 30 compressions/2 ventilations (30:2) after their arrival. After this period, they would receive a series of orders that they had to follow to provide CPR for the next 2 min.

Only compressions were performed during the time the expert gave orders. The orders provided (adapted from the main guides in CPR terminology) [16,22–25] to the participants with the chest compressions role (CR) were:

1. "Kneel in front of me".
2. "Interlock your hands, one over the other, and straighten your arms".

3. "When I count to three, you have to place your hand in the middle of the chest and compress "hard and fast" [25] 30 times".
4. "Have you understood?" (If the participant answered "NO" to this question, the order would be repeated again without any changes).
5. "1, 2, 3, now!"

The orders provided to the participants with the ventilation role (VR) were given, while the CR participants performed the first chest compressions. These orders were:

1. "Put your hand on the forehead".
2. "Put the other hand on the chin and lift".
3. "Cover the nose and blow two times when your partner reaches 30".

In this sequence of instructions, to warn the rest of the participants and the resuscitators that the end of the compressions was near and to minimize the interruptions, the expert had the added requisite of counting the last five compressions aloud.

The expert who participated in the experimental group was trained in the structured learning method, and had previously practiced in simulation. The expert was the same for the completely experimental group.

2.5. Control Group: Structured Orders

To conduct the trial with the unstructured orders group (CG), the expert and the participants were informed about the same simulation scenario. The experts were told that they could ask for help after two cycles of 30:2, and they were asked to give the sequence of orders they thought to be faster and more opportune, following their intuition and previous knowledge, in order for the participants to relieve them in the following 2 min.

To eliminate the learning effect [13], meaning the familiarization of the experts with the procedure, and therefore improving the results in later trials, the pretest trials were dispensed with [26], and eight different experts were selected to interact with the CG participants, so that they were not allowed to repeat the trial more than four times. The experts were not study participants, and they did not have prior knowledge of the structured orders utilized with the EG or the hypothesis of the study.

Comments, corrections, or explanations were not allowed in any of the two groups once the orders were given and the CPR started by the participants.

2.6. Analysis Parameters

The main result of the study was the time needed for giving orders (seconds). The secondary result variables were: pauses between compression and ventilation (seconds), depth (mm), rate (compressions/minute), effective rate of ventilation (% between 500–600 mL), rate of chest recoil (%), positioning of the hands (% of success with respect to the center of the chest), scores reached in the mannequin (compression score (0–100), of ventilation (0–100), total/final (0–100)), age (years), sex (male/female), weight (kg), height (meters), and body mass index (BMI) (kg/m2).

2.7. Measurements

The demographic data were collected in questionnaires after the informed consent. For collecting the data relative to the quality of the CPR, the Resusci Anne QCPR® manikin (Laerdal Medical Corporation, Stavanger, Norway) was utilized, which was calibrated and checked before conducting the experiment, and periodically during the experimental phase.

2.8. Analysis

The continuous variables with a normal distribution were expressed as mean and standard deviation (SD); the data without a normal distribution were described as median and interquartile range (IQR). A difference in means analysis was performed for independent samples with the Student's *t* test or the Mann–Whitney U test, according to the distribution of the data. The categorical variables were described as frequencies and percentages (%). The results were considered statistically significant at $p < 0.05$. The data were reported according to the CONSORT guidelines [27]. The processing and analysis of the data were conducted with the statistical package IBM SPSS® for Windows version 22.0 (IBM Corporation, Armonk, DA, USA).

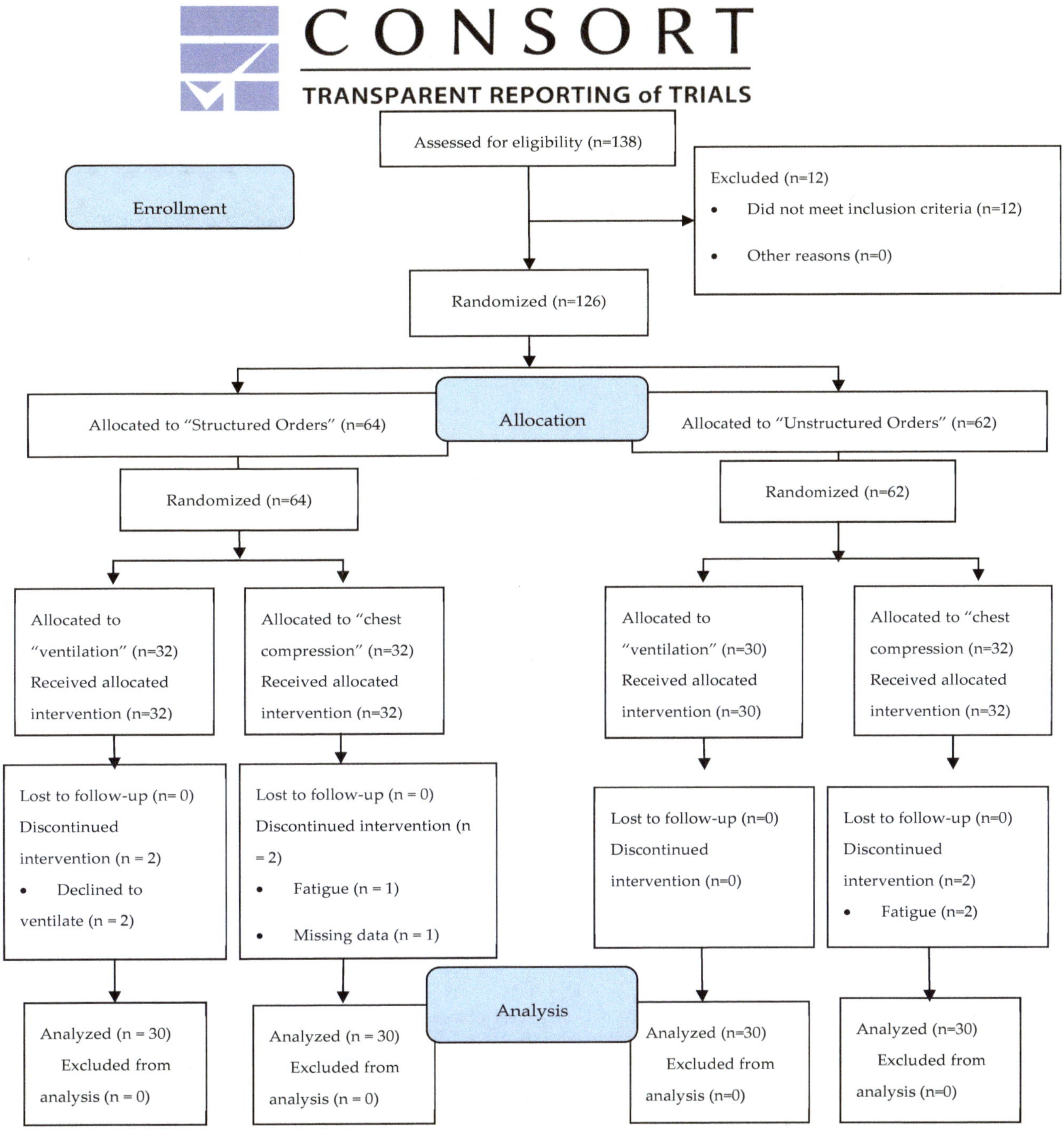

Figure 1. Study CONSORT flow diagram.

2.9. Ethical Considerations

All the participants gave their informed consent for inclusion before participating in the study. The study was conducted in accordance with the Declaration of Helsinki, and the protocol was approved by the Ethics Committee of Catholic University of Murcia (CE031901).

3. Results

The mean age of the participants was 21 years old (SD 4.75), the mean height was 1.71 m (SD 0.08), the mean weight was 66.1 kg (SD 12.14), and the mean BMI was 22.5 kg/m^2 (SD 2.92). Of these, 60% (n = 72/120) of the participants were women. Table 1 shows the demographic data according to groups (CG and EG).

Table 1. Baseline demographics (n = 120).

Demographic Variables	Unstructured Orders Group (n = 60)	Structured Orders Group (n = 60)	*p*-Value
Age (years)—mean (SD)	21 (5.07)	21 (3.78)	0.669
Sex (% female)	36 (60)	36 (60)	0.574
Height (m)—mean (SD)	1.72 (0.09)	1.70 (0.09)	0.31
Weight (kg)—mean (SD)	67.3 (13.46)	64.3 (11.68)	0.209
BMI (kg/m^2)—mean (SD)	22.7 (3.20)	22.1 (2.77)	0.236

Statistically significant differences were obtained ($p < 0.0001$) between the EG and CG for the variables: time needed to give orders (Figure 2A), pauses between chest compressions and ventilations (Figure 2B), depth, overall score, chest compression score, and chest recoil.

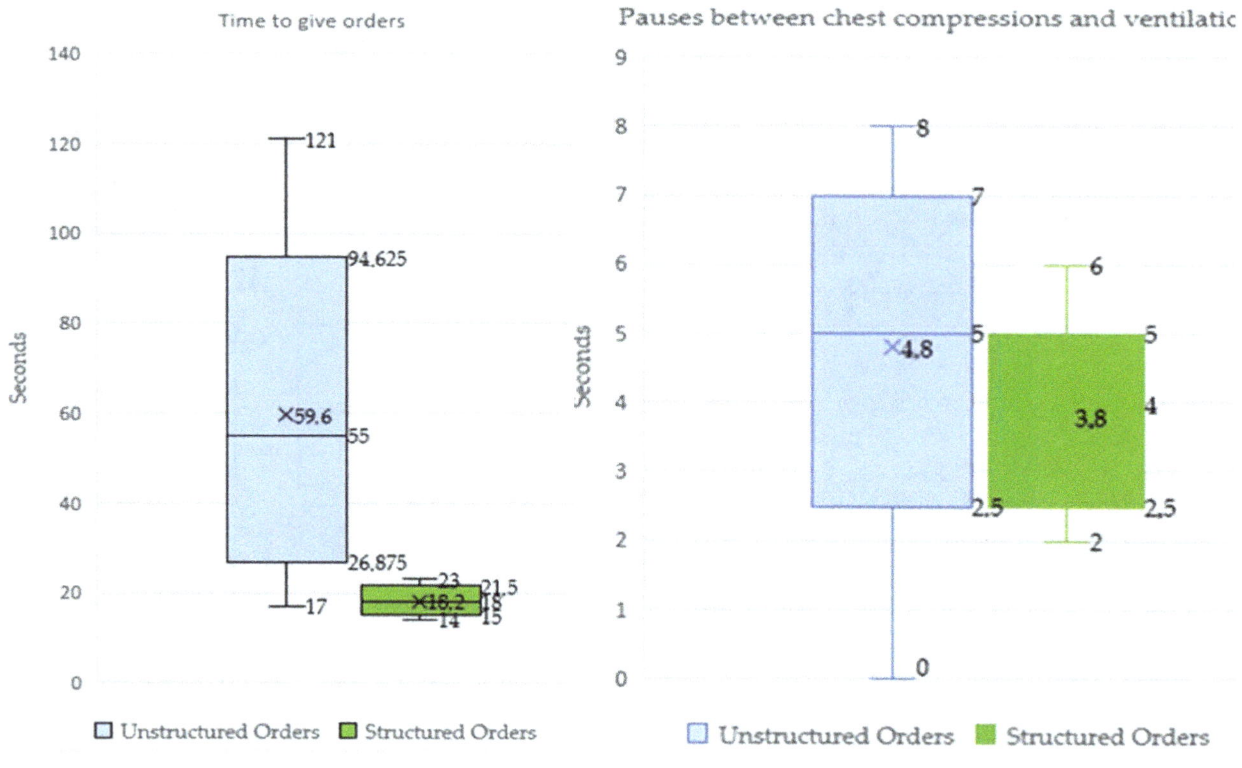

(A) (B)

Figure 2. (**A**) Time needed to give orders. (**B**) Pauses between chest compressions and ventilations.

The mean depth was 51.1 mm (SD 7.94) for EG, and 42.2 mm (SD 12.04) for the CG (Table 2).

The median of the variable rate for the EG was 121 compressions per minute (IQR 110, 130), and 121 compressions per minute (IQR 113, 132) for the CG. The median of effective ventilation (% between 500–600 mL) was 20% (IQR 5, 50) for the EG, and 40% (IQR 0, 60.42) for the CG. The median for chest recoil was 86.32% (IQR 62.36, 98.87) for the EG, and 58.3% (IQR 27.46, 84.33) for the CG. From the participants, 83.3% (25/30) correctly positioned their hands in the EG, and 80% (24/30) in the CG (Table 2).

No statistically significant differences were found according to sex, age, height, weight, or BMI between the CG and the EG, or the VR or CR groups.

As for the scores achieved (Figure 3), the means/medians obtained were: 67 points (IQR 49, 83) for the EG, and 65 points (IQR 34, 81.5) for the CG in ventilation; 78.5 points (IQR 61.5, 87.25) for the EG, and 53 points (IQR 37.25, 61) for the CG in compression; 73 points (SD 14.5) for the EG, and 45 points (SD 22.47) for the CG in the overall CPR score.

Table 2. Study outcome data.

Variables of Study	Unstructured Orders	Structured Orders	t-Test/Mann–Whitney U	p-Value
Time needed to give orders (seconds)—mean (SD)	55.3 (26.09)	17.9 (2.34)	t = 7.813	<0.001
Pauses between chest compressions and ventilations (seconds)—median (IQR)	5 (5, 6)	4 (3, 4)	U = 152	<0.001
Depth (mm)—mean (SD)	42.2 (12.04)	51.1 (7.94)	t = 3.38	0.001
Rate (comp/min)—median (IQR)	121 (113, 132)	121 (110, 130)	U = 443.5	0.923
Overall score (0–100)—mean (SD)	45.03 (22.5)	73 (14.5)	t = 5.73	<0.001
Ventilation score (0–100) [a]—median (IQR)	65 (34, 81.5)	67 (49, 83)	U = 370.5	0.437
Chest compression score (0–100)—median (IQR)	53 (37.25, 61)	78.5 (61.5, 87.25)	U = 171	<0.001
Hands position—median (IQR)	100 (100, 100)	100 (100, 100)	U = 437.5	0.784
% Effective ventilation (500–600 mL) [a]—median (IQR)	40 (0, 60.42)	20 (5, 50)	U = 394.5	0.682
% Chest recoil—median (IQR)	58.3 (27.46, 84.33)	86.32 (62.36, 98.87)	U = 263.5	0.006

[a] Two cases with missing data.

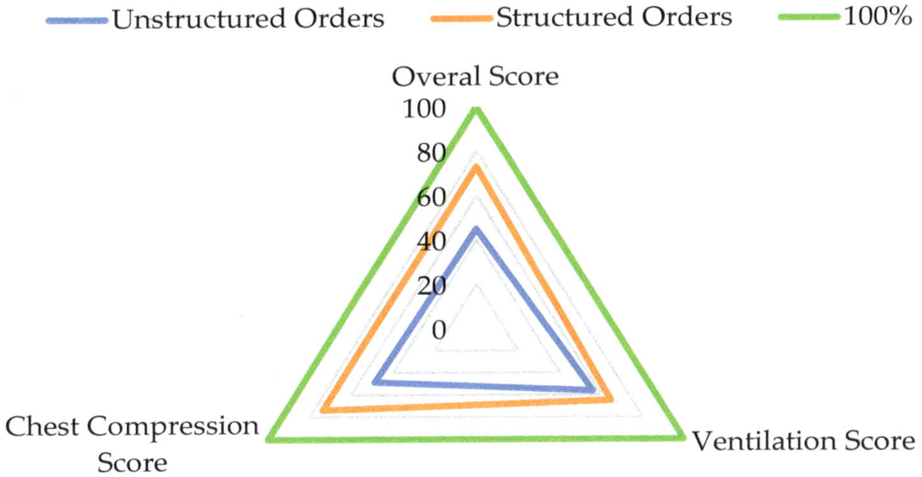

Figure 3. Comparison of the scores reached by each group, with respect to the maximum score.

As for ventilation, 40% (12/30) of the CG participants correctly performed the head-tilt/chin-lift maneuver to ventilate. In the EG, this maneuver was performed by 66.67% (20/30) of the participants. Statistically significant differences were found in effective ventilation after performing the head-tilt/chin-lift maneuver ($p < 0.0001$).

4. Discussion

Increasing the rates of resuscitation when witnessing cardiorespiratory arrests is still a challenge in Spain [28]. This study intended to demonstrate the efficiency of a fast and structured method of communication on-site for situations in which an expert is performing CPR in the presence of bystanders who are willing to provide relief, either in the compression, or in ventilation maneuvers.

Observation-based, vicarious, or through-demonstration learning [13] are some one of the most-commonly utilized methods for learning motor skills [29]. Diverse studies have suggested that visual orientation can accelerate the acquisition of complex motor skills [30]. In our case, we believe that this visual guide offered advantages over instructions that were not provided in person (such as through the phone, for example). We also believe that observational learning had effects (in both the experimental groups as well as the control group) on the quality of resuscitation; this is the reason why the co-variation of the results attributed to the independent variable (structure method) is even more powerful, as this observational learning was found in both groups (experimental and control). Therefore, it is thought that there could be a causal attribution of the structured method towards the improvement of CPR. Thus, it can be concluded that the use of structured orders results in the better performance of CPR, compared to intuitive or unstructured orders of individuals without prior knowledge of CPR.

The main finding of our study consisted of the statistically significant decrease in the time needed to provide the orders that allowed relieving the expert and performing high-quality CPR. The time invested by the expert in the experimental group was significantly less compared to the unstructured orders group. The pauses between compressions and ventilations also decreased. In addition, an improvement was registered in the mean depth and the chest recoil, compared to the set of unstructured orders.

From our point of view, the decrease in these times could be related to the simplicity of the orders, in agreement with the results from Hunt et al. [16], insofar as it was suggested that there was a greater chance that the appropriate action could occur when short, easy, and specific phrases were utilized. The pauses between compression and ventilation were significantly reduced in the experimental group, with this result possibly due to the implementation of improvements proposed by Lauridsen et al. [15], such as the use of backwards counting before the relief, or counting out loud of the last five compressions.

The simplification of the orders can also improve the quality of the chest compressions [31]. This could help in the understanding and discussion of the results from other studies [32] that suggest that non-trained bystanders are not useful during CPR.

As for ventilation, achieving the volunteer's relief of the compression expert relies on a margin of 30 compressions (between 15–17 s) for the ventilation volunteer to receive the indications correctly. The participants who performed the head-tilt/chin-lift maneuver performed effective ventilations (500–600 mL) that were significantly better than those who did not. However, for the ventilation skills, no significant differences were found between the groups; in fact, the scores reached by the unstructured orders group were higher. Thus, it seems possible that although a layperson resuscitator performs the head-tilt/chin-lift maneuver correctly, this does not ensure proper ventilation, but could result in mistakes in the volume ventilated (hyperventilation or hypoventilation).

This makes us believe that on the one hand, ventilation is a skill that requires more training time compared to compression, and on the other hand, that compression-only CPR in the presence of an expert is also a valid alternative; not only for those people who are reticent about performing mouth-to-mouth ventilation [33], but also for the notable public interest in learning CPR [34]. All of these improvements resulted in higher scores, provided by the simulator, of the experimental group than the control group.

The variables rate and hand positioning did not show significant differences between both groups, and were within the range accepted by scientific societies [35].

Our study was conducted with the aim of assessing the effectiveness of providing orders. However, this method has an added benefit, in that in a real-life situation in which the expert has to be relieved, a layperson could be properly corrected fast. Thus, during the resuscitation procedure, the strong points could be emphasized, and the weak points improved, in order to provide high quality CPR until the arrival of the emergency services. This advantage is shown in studies, such as those from González-Salvado et al. [36], which affirms that practical learning guided by an instructor provides better results.

In conclusion, the learning of technical skills seems to be greatly simplified when the layperson or beginner is allowed to observe an expert, as pointed out in other studies [37,38], which associate a greater ability of response and performance of the layperson after viewing ultra-brief videos.

Limitations

Among the main limitations of the study, we find the extrapolation of the results due to the characteristics of the sample and the type of experiment. The external validity could be improved with a representative sample of a real population, not only with a healthy university population. In the second place, we believe that the validity of the experiments with simulation is limited, as it does not occur in a real-life context, and other variables, such as stress or the interference from other spectators, could not be taken into account. Another limitation that should be mentioned is the lack of a pre-test to assess the resuscitation skills of the participants, beyond their statement of being a layperson. In this case, the design of the study would have been more complex. Thus, this was not done, to avoid the threat to the internal validity known as learning. However, if properly managed, it could have provided a greater internal validity of the study, which could have helped establish, with greater precision, if the groups were homogeneous for their comparison.

5. Conclusions

The use of a sequence of simple, short and specific orders, together with observation-based learning, makes possible the execution of chest compression maneuvers that are very similar to those performed by rescuers, and allows the teaching of the basic notions of ventilation.

Improvements were identified in the variables "time needed to give orders", "pauses between chest compressions and ventilations", and "chest recoil" when CPR was performed by laypersons in the experimental group.

The method of structured orders was shown to provide an on-site learning opportunity when faced with the need to maintain high-quality CPR in the presence of an expert resuscitator before the arrival of emergency services, and after their arrival, in case further help is needed.

More research studies are needed to assess these findings in a non-university population, and to measure other variables that could have an influence on the results, such as the role of the layperson's stress when facing this situation in a non-simulation context.

Author Contributions: Conceptualization: M.J.P.-J. and C.L.-C.; formal analysis: M.J.P.-J., C.L.-C., M.R.-M., A.J.R.-M., and J.L.D.A.; investigation: C.L.-C. and J.L.D.A.; methodology: C.L.-C., M.R.-M., A.J.R.-M., and J.L.D.-A.; project administration: C.L.-C. and J.L.D.-A.; resources: M.J.P.-J.; supervision: J.L.D.A.; validation: C.L.-C., M.R.-M., and J.L.D.A.; writing—original draft: M.J.P.-J.; writing—review and editing: M.J.P.-J., C.L.-C., M.R.-M., A.J.R.-M., and J.L.D.A. All authors have read and agreed to the published version of the manuscript.

Acknowledgments: Our most sincere thanks to the people who agreed to participate in this research.

References

1. Hawkes, C.; Booth, S.; Ji, C.; Brace-McDonnell, S.J.; Whittington, A.; Mapstone, J.; Cooke, M.W.; Deakin, C.D.; Gale, C.P.; Fothergill, R.; et al. Epidemiology and outcomes from out-of-hospital cardiac arrests in England. *Resuscitation* **2017**, *110*, 133–140. [CrossRef] [PubMed]
2. Hasselqvist-Ax, I.; Riva, G.; Herlitz, J.; Rosenqvist, M.; Hollenberg, J.; Nordberg, P.; Ringh, M.; Jonsson, M.; Axelsson, C.; Lindqvist, J.; et al. Early Cardiopulmonary Resuscitation in Out-of-Hospital Cardiac Arrest. *N. Engl. J. Med.* **2015**, *372*, 2307–2315. [CrossRef]
3. Zideman, D.A.; De Buck, E.D.J.; Singletary, E.M.; Cassan, P.; Chalkias, A.F.; Evans, T.R.; Hafner, C.M.; Handley, A.J.; Meyran, D.; Schunder-Tatzber, S.; et al. European Resuscitation Council Guidelines for Resuscitation 2015 First aid. *Resuscitation* **2015**, *95*, 278–287. [CrossRef] [PubMed]
4. Pek, J.H.; de Korne, D.F.; Hannawa, A.F.; Leong, B.S.H.; Ng, Y.Y.; Arulanandam, S.; Tham, L.P.; Ong, M.E.H.; Ong, G.Y.-K. Dispatcher-assisted cardiopulmonary resuscitation for paediatric out-of-hospital cardiac arrest: A structured evaluation of communication issues using the SACCIA® safe communication typology. *Resuscitation* **2019**, *139*, 144–151. [CrossRef] [PubMed]

5. Yamada, N.; Fuerch, J.; Halamek, L. Impact of Standardized Communication Techniques on Errors during Simulated Neonatal Resuscitation. *Am. J. Perinatol.* **2015**, *33*, 385–392. [PubMed]
6. Yamada, N.K.; Halamek, L.P. On the Need for Precise, Concise Communication during Resuscitation: A Proposed Solution. *J. Pediatrics* **2015**, *166*, 184–187. [CrossRef]
7. Wu, Z.; Panczyk, M.; Spaite, D.W.; Hu, C.; Fukushima, H.; Langlais, B.; Sutter, J.; Bobrow, B.J. Telephone cardiopulmonary resuscitation is independently associated with improved survival and improved functional outcome after out-of-hospital cardiac arrest. *Resuscitation* **2018**, *122*, 135–140. [CrossRef]
8. Soar, J.; Maconochie, I.; Wyckoff, M.H.; Olasveengen, T.M.; Singletary, E.M.; Greif, R.; Aickin, R.; Bhanji, F.; Donnino, M.W.; Mancini, M.E.; et al. 2019 International Consensus on Cardiopulmonary Resuscitation and Emergency Cardiovascular Care Science with Treatment Recommendations: Summary From the Basic Life Support; Advanced Life Support; Pediatric Life Support; Neonatal Life Support; Education, Implementation, and Teams; and First Aid Task Forces. *Circulation* **2019**, *140*. [CrossRef]
9. Ro, Y.S.; Shin, S.D.; Song, K.J.; Hong, K.J.; Ahn, K.O.; Kim, D.K.; Kwak, Y.H. Effects of Dispatcher-assisted Cardiopulmonary Resuscitation on Survival Outcomes in Infants, Children, and Adolescents with Out-of-hospital Cardiac Arrests. *Resuscitation* **2016**, *108*, 20–26. [CrossRef]
10. Goto, Y.; Maeda, T.; Goto, Y. Impact of Dispatcher-Assisted Bystander Cardiopulmonary Resuscitation on Neurological Outcomes in Children with Out-of-Hospital Cardiac Arrests: A Prospective, Nationwide, Population-Based Cohort Study. *J. Am. Heart Assoc.* **2014**, *3*, e000499. [CrossRef]
11. Bohm, K.; Vaillancourt, C.; Charette, M.L.; Dunford, J.; Castrén, M. In patients with out-of-hospital cardiac arrest, does the provision of dispatch cardiopulmonary resuscitation instructions as opposed to no instructions improve outcome: A systematic review of the literature. *Resuscitation* **2011**, *82*, 1490–1495. [CrossRef] [PubMed]
12. Olasveengen, T.M.; Mancini, M.E.; Vaillancourt, C.; Brooks, S.C.; Castren, M.; Chung, S.P.; Couper, K.; Dainty, K.N.; Escalante, R.; Gazmuri, R.J.; et al. Emergency Care: Dispatcher Instruction in CPR: Systematic Review. Available online: https://costr.ilcor.org/document/emergency-care-dispatcherinstruction-in-cpr (accessed on 25 February 2019).
13. Lyons, P.; Bandura, R.P. Case-based modeling for learning: Socially constructed skill development. *Educ.+ Train.* **2018**, *60*, 139–154. [CrossRef]
14. Domjan, M. *Principios de Aprendizaje y Conducta*; Paraninfo: Madrid, Spain, 2007; ISBN 9788497325844.
15. Lauridsen, K.G.; Watanabe, I.; Løfgren, B.; Cheng, A.; Duval-Arnould, J.; Hunt, E.A.; Good, G.L.; Niles, D.; Berg, R.A.; Nishisaki, A.; et al. Standardising communication to improve in-hospital cardiopulmonary resuscitation. *Resuscitation* **2020**, *147*, 73–80. [CrossRef] [PubMed]
16. Hunt, E.A.; Cruz-Eng, H.; Bradshaw, J.H.; Hodge, M.; Bortner, T.; Mulvey, C.L.; McMillan, K.N.; Galvan, H.; Duval-Arnould, J.M.; Jones, K.; et al. A novel approach to life support training using "action-linked phrases". *Resuscitation* **2015**, *86*, 1–5. [CrossRef]
17. Research Methods Knowledge Base. Available online: http://anatomyfacts.com/Research/ResearchMethodsKnowledgeBase.pdf (accessed on 25 February 2019).
18. Salazar, L.F.; Crosby, R.A.; DiClemente, R.J. *Research Methods in Health Promotion*; John Wiley & Sons: Hoboken, NJ, USA, 2015.
19. Experimental Research Designs. Available online: https://psycnet.apa.org/record/2015-10205-005 (accessed on 25 February 2019).
20. Allen, M. *The SAGE Encyclopedia of Communication Research Methods*; Sage Publications: Southend Oaks, CA, USA, 2017.
21. Trochim, W.M.K.; Donnelly, J.P. *Research Methods Knowledge Base*, 3rd ed.; Atomic Dog: New York, NY, USA, 2020.
22. Painter, I.; Chavez, D.E.; Ike, B.R.; Yip, M.P.; Tu, S.P.; Bradley, S.M.; Rea, T.D.; Meischke, H. Changes to DA-CPR instructions: Can we reduce time to first compression and improve quality of bystander CPR? *Resuscitation* **2014**, *85*, 1169–1173. [CrossRef]
23. Chen, K.-Y.; Ko, Y.-C.; Hsieh, M.-J.; Chiang, W.-C.; Ma, M.H.-M. Interventions to improve the quality of bystander cardiopulmonary resuscitation: A systematic review. *PLoS ONE* **2019**, *14*, e0211792. [CrossRef]
24. García del Águila, J.; López-Messa, J.; Rosell-Ortiz, F.; de Elías Hernández, R.; Martínez del Valle, M.; Sánchez-Santos, L.; López-Herce, J.; Cerdà-Vila, M.; Roza-Alonso, C.L.; Bernardez-Otero, M.

Recomendaciones para el soporte telefónico a la reanimación por testigos desde los centros de coordinación de urgencias y emergencias. *Med. Intensiva* **2015**, *39*, 298–302. [CrossRef]

25. Trethewey, S.P.; Vyas, H.; Evans, S.; Hall, M.; Melody, T.; Perkins, G.D.; Couper, K. The impact of resuscitation guideline terminology on quality of dispatcher-assisted cardiopulmonary resuscitation: A randomised controlled manikin study. *Resuscitation* **2019**, *142*, 91–96. [CrossRef]
26. Fontes, S.; García-Gallego, C.; Quintanilla, L.; Rodríguez, R.; Rubio, P.; Sarriá, E. Fundamentos de investigación en psicología. In *Diseños y Estrategias*; UNED: Madrid, Spain, 2010.
27. Schulz, K.F.; Altman, D.G.; Moher, D. CONSORT 2010 Statement: Updated guidelines for reporting parallel group randomised trials. *BMJ* **2010**, *340*. [CrossRef]
28. Ortiz, F.R.; Roig, F.E.; Navalpotro Pascual, J.M.; Iglesias Vázquez, J.A.; Sucunza, A.E.; Cordero Torres, J.A.; Cobos, E.; del Valle, M.M.; Rozalen, I.C.; martín Sánchez, E.; et al. Out-of-Hospital Spanish Cardiac Arrest Registry (OHSCAR). Results of the first year. *Resuscitation* **2015**, *96*, 100. [CrossRef]
29. Williams, A.M.; Hodges, N.J. Practice, instruction and skill acquisition in soccer: Challenging tradition. *J. Sports Sci.* **2005**, *23*, 637–650. [CrossRef] [PubMed]
30. D'Innocenzo, G.; Gonzalez, C.C.; Williams, A.M.; Bishop, D.T. Looking to Learn: The Effects of Visual Guidance on Observational Learning of the Golf Swing. *PLoS ONE* **2016**, *11*, e0155442. [CrossRef] [PubMed]
31. Rodriguez, S.A.; Sutton, R.M.; Berg, M.D.; Nishisaki, A.; Maltese, M.; Meaney, P.A.; Niles, D.E.; Leffelman, J.; Berg, R.A.; Nadkarni, V.M. Simplified dispatcher instructions improve bystander chest compression quality during simulated pediatric resuscitation. *Resuscitation* **2014**, *85*, 119–123. [CrossRef] [PubMed]
32. Li, S.; Kan, T.; Guo, Z.; Chen, C.; Gui, L. Assessing the quality of CPR performed by a single lifeguard, two lifeguards and a lifeguard with a bystander after water rescue: A quasi-experimental trial. *Emerg. Med. J.* **2020**. [CrossRef] [PubMed]
33. Taniguchi, T.; Sato, K.; Fujita, T.; Okajima, M.; Takamura, M. Attitudes to Bystander Cardiopulmonary Resuscitation in Japan in 2010. *Circ. J.* **2012**, *76*, 1130–1135. [CrossRef]
34. Chang, M.P.; Gent, L.M.; Sweet, M.; Potts, J.; Ahtone, J.; Idris, A.H. A novel educational outreach approach to teach Hands-Only Cardiopulmonary Resuscitation to the public. *Resuscitation* **2017**, *116*, 22–26. [CrossRef]
35. Olasveengen, T.M.; de Caen, A.R.; Mancini, M.E.; Maconochie, I.K.; Aickin, R.; Atkins, D.L.; Berg, R.A.; Bingham, R.M.; Brooks, S.C.; Castrén, M.; et al. 2017 International Consensus on Cardiopulmonary Resuscitation and Emergency Cardiovascular Care Science with Treatment Recommendations Summary. *Circulation* **2017**, *136*, e424–e440. [CrossRef]
36. González-Salvado, V.; Rodríguez-Ruiz, E.; Abelairas-Gómez, C.; Ruano-Raviña, A.; Peña-Gil, C.; González-Juanatey, J.R.; Rodríguez-Núñez, A. Training adult laypeople in basic life support. A systematic review. *Revista Española de Cardiología (Engl. Ed.)* **2020**, *73*, 53–68. [CrossRef]
37. Beskind, D.L.; Stolz, U.; Thiede, R.; Hoyer, R.; Robertson, W.; Brown, J.; Ludgate, M.; Tiutan, T.; Shane, R.; McMorrow, D.; et al. Viewing an ultra-brief chest compression only video improves some measures of bystander CPR performance and responsiveness at a mass gathering event. *Resuscitation* **2017**, *118*, 96–100. [CrossRef]
38. Benoit, J.L.; Vogele, J.; Hart, K.W.; Lindsell, C.J.; McMullan, J.T. Passive ultra-brief video training improves performance of compression-only cardiopulmonary resuscitation. *Resuscitation* **2017**, *115*, 116–119. [CrossRef]

13

Analyzing the Job Demands-Control-Support Model in Work-Life Balance

Virginia Navajas-Romero [1,*], Antonio Ariza-Montes [2] and Felipe Hernández-Perlines [3]

1 Department of Statistics, Management and Applied Economy. Universidad de Córdoba, 14014 Córdoba, Spain
2 Management Departament, Universidad Loyola Andalucía, 14014 Córdoba, Spain; ariza@uloyola.es
3 Departament of Business Administration; Universidad de Castilla La Mancha, 13071 Ciudad Real, Spain; felipe.HPerlines@uclm.es
* Correspondence: vnavajas@uco.es

Abstract: The balance of personal life with professional life is a topical issue that is increasingly worrisome due to globalization, the rapid introduction of new technologies into all areas of human life, the overlap between time between work and family, new organizational systems, and changes in the nature of work. This problem is accentuated by professions subjected to intense labor demands, as is the case of nurses. Adopting the Job Demand–Control–Support model, the main purpose of this research is to analyze how these factors lead to a greater or lesser degree of work–life balance. The research proposes a logistic regression model, which was constructed with a sample of 991 nursing professionals from the V European Working Conditions Survey. The results obtained confirm, on the one hand, that there is a significant effect of physical demands (but not psychological demands) on work–life balance. On the other hand, the moderating effects of job control are partially confirmed for psychological demands, and those of supervisor support (but not co-worker support) are partially confirmed for physical demands. In conclusion, the present research shows that effective management of nurses' work context can decisively contribute to finding the difficult balance between personal and professional time.

Keywords: job demands; job control; social support; work–life balance; nurses

---

1. Introduction

The balance of personal life with professional life is a topical issue that is increasingly worrisome due to globalization, the intrusion of new technologies into personal life, the overlap between work time and family time, new organizational systems, and changes in the nature of work [1]. This problem is accentuated in professions with intense working hours or schedules [2]. Nursing professionals are without a doubt in this situation. The role of a nurse is very demanding, as quick and effective responses are required to deal with the health needs of the community. Furthermore, it is an industry with an intensive work environment, which operates 24 h a day, 365 days a year, and sometimes requires exceeding the standard 40 h week of full-time employment for the production of services [3].

Work–life balance (WLB) is understood as several individual and structural constraints of their way of harmonizing work time and personal time according to an individual system of values, goals, and aspirations [4]. Although much research on the WLB has focused its analysis on the challenge of caring for children and the elderly [5–7], this is a topic of great importance in current academic research [8] because achieving an optimal WLB is critical to personal well-being [9,10]. Despite this, given the intense interconnectedness of work and personal time, many workers have serious difficulties defining the boundaries between them and often cross those boundaries, which has harmful consequences to their health and well-being [11]. Due to the changing nature of the current workforce, the WLB has a broader and higher perspective on the EU political agenda, encompassing aspects such as business organizational culture in terms of gender equality and social protection. In fact, at the Social Summit for Fair Employment and Growth held in Gothenburg in November 2017, the WLB was proclaimed as a European pillar of social rights [12]. Despite this, the peculiarities of the work environment that surrounds the nursing profession makes it difficult to reconcile work and family life, preventing a high level of work satisfaction from being achieved [13,14].

The job demand–control–support model (JDCS) [15–18] constitutes a very useful theoretical approach for understanding the characteristics of work and its consequences for the occupational health of employees [19]. In fact, this model has been used in many professions with the aim of studying a wide range of reactions that provoke tension in workers [20–27]. In particular, the JDC model establishes that factors such as the level of labor demands and the control the workers have over their work will affect the development of WLB. In subsequent model improvements, the level of perceived support at work was included as another relevant factor (the JDCS model).

Following this idea, the present study analyzes the effects caused by certain factors related to the context of work in nursing personnel (demands, control, and social support) and how they influence the WLB of these professionals. According to the JDCS model approach, the worst situation of WLB for workers would be manifested in those occupations characterized by high job demands, low control, and little social support. Previous studies with this model support the association between poor work results (for example, exhaustion, stress, poor well-being, etc.) with high levels of demands or work load (for example, [28–30]), low control over work, or the degree of autonomy in the application of labor decisions (for example, [31–33]). In addition, the low level of support perceived by colleagues or supervisors also influences (for example, [27,34]). The literature in general terms suggests that a low family–work balance is related to lower job satisfaction, higher turnover intentions, exhaustion, and deterioration of health [35,36], and a high family–work balance is related to higher levels of professional commitment and lower intentions to leave the profession [28,37,38]. However, although there are some studies that have tested the JDCS model with nursing personnel [28,39,40], the investigations that have related the model with the WLB are practically nonexistent.

Undoubtedly, nursing professionals carry out work of special interest to society, given the leading role of the health system in the welfare of any nation. Despite this, the work of nurses is characterized by high job demands: direct contact with patients, exhausting workdays, night shifts [41], and limited job control over the tasks they perform. This last circumstance is a result of the numerous regulations and operating protocols that regulate and limit the activity of these professionals, regulations that tend to be more rigorous when written by personnel outside the health care profession [42]. The other pillar on which the JDCS model is built is social support. Nursing requires much collaboration and teamwork. In this context, perceived social support is of great importance because, as Schwarzer and Knoll (2007) note, conflicts in work teams multiply when employees perceive little support from their supervisors and/or co-workers [43–45].

The consequences of the scenario described above are multifaceted: stress, alienation, low organizational commitment, and burnout. One of the least researched outcomes in academia from the perspective of the JDCS model is the problem that nurses have with balancing work time with personal time. Studies in other occupations suggest that the combination of high job demands and a great deal of autonomy can help reduce work–life conflict [46]. In contrast, individuals in professions that face many job demands within a context of low autonomy will have more difficulty achieving an adequate WLB [44]. Additionally, various studies suggest that supervisor and/or co-worker support contributes decisively to improving WLB [47].

Unlike other professionals, nurses offer an intangible service that is inextricably linked with the professional who performs it. Good management of work–family conflicts will improve the WLB of these professionals, which will translate into positive effects for the worker and the organization [48].

The purpose of this study is to contribute on the idiosyncrasies of the profession and the value the profession provides for citizens and the welfare state. The majority of studies on WLB adopt an approach based on worker health [49]. However, in the European context, there is little empirical research that analyzes both the main effects of the JDCS model and the multiplicative model in their relationship with WLB, which means that the impacts of job demands, job control, and social support have not received the attention they deserve in a profession so relevant in the European context [50]. Taking into account everything raised so far, this research seeks to (i) analyze job demands, job control, and social support in nursing staff, as well as assess whether these factors lead to a greater or lesser degree of WLB in European hospitals; and (ii) explore whether these models differ from those identified in the previous literature. The following research question is derived from these objectives: Does this organizational model allow its workers to have a high WLB according to the JDCS model that relates labor demands, labor control, and social support?

2. Managing Demands, Control and Support in an Organizational Context in Nursing

Health is one of the fundamental pillars of a welfare society. The World Health Organization estimates that the health care sector workforce in 2013 included 20.7 million nurses out of a total of 43.5 million health workers worldwide [51,52]. The well-being of workers is essential for the health of society [49]. Balancing work and family life in the nursing sector to achieve a high degree of well-being is crucial for the development of the service [53], since well-being impacts the quality of patient care [54], with poor well-being increasing the risk of negligence and/or abuse [55].

The sector is characterized by high job demands, both physical and psychological. The situation with respect the physical demands of nurse workers reflects the need to work with limited resources, both in terms of personnel and equipment [56], which causes a level of emotional strain that approaches exhaustion [52,53]. The nursing sector is the sector with the highest rate of nonfatal occupational diseases and injuries, which causes an increase in sick leave [57]. Factors such as stress, poor health, and depression negatively affect WLB [58,59]. Regarding the psychological demands, nurses must make urgent and critical decisions that involve a vital risk for the patient [60]; thus, nursing professionals are continuously exposed to traumatic events [61]. Health care services are needed 24 h a day, seven days a week. This need may contribute to greater job stability in health care than in other sectors [62], but it also implies an internal organization based on exhausting workloads and 12 h continuous work shifts, which hinder the conciliation of work with personal and family life [63].

From the perspective of job control, it deepens knowledge of the skill discretion and the decision authority of this sector, and nursing work requires multiple skills [64]. According to Ulrich, Barden, Cassidy, and Varn-Davis, there are different skills that workers in this sector have to have, such as communication, collaboration, and resource management and leadership skills [65]. At the same time, nursing professionals usually have little autonomy in carrying out their work activities [66], which greatly limits their decision-making capacity [67]. However, nurses who have higher levels of work autonomy tend to be high-performing, satisfied, and committed workers [68]. With respect to social support in health, Olmedo (2009) reports the presence of a complex web of interpersonal relationships with conflicting power dynamics between physicians (who are mostly male) and nurses, whose profession is still highly feminized [69,70]. Work pressures, limited control, and the complex social system trigger deterioration of the work environment [71], resulting in absenteeism, high turnover, depression, and even suicide [72]. Nurses who consider these conditions unsustainable eventually abandon the profession in search of jobs with fewer demands and better working conditions that will improve their personal quality of life, including the balance between work and family time [73].

Although some previous studies have applied the JDCS model in the nursing sector, they have generally done so from analytical approaches and perspectives that differ from those presented in this article. From the perspective of job demands, Heijden et al. (2018) confirm that job demands are positively correlated with job turnover, while the availability of resources and the experience of nurses are inversely related to turnover [74]. At the end of the last century, De Jonge et al. (1999) claimed that the combination of job demands and job control can predict the health of employees [75,76]. From the perspective of job control, the work of Yamaguchi et al. (2016) confirms that the absence of job control increases the likelihood that nursing personnel will abandon nursing as a career [77]. More recently, Mark and Smith (2012) have added that rewards, decision-making skills, and skill discretion decrease depression and anxiety among these professionals, which is often motivated by a lack of resources and a lack of time to attend to patients [78,79]. Finally, from social support perspective, Sigurdardottir et al. (2015) show that training programs improve nursing professionals' perceptions of social support (from both supervisors and co-workers) [80,81]. Stress is another topic of interest analyzed with this model. Thus, Nabirye et al. (2011) note that the role conflict and ambiguity that characterize the work of more experienced nurses lead to increased stress [82,83].

The effects that such a demanding profession exerts on health and well-being have also been the subject of analysis in academia [84]. The study of Xanthopoulou et al. (2009) provides key evidence of pathways leading to the well-being of nursing personnel in general hospitals [85]. Another study using the JDCS model in Uganda concluded that younger nurses are more satisfied than older nurses [82]. These authors suggest that with age, family responsibilities increase, and consequently, the likelihood of conflicts between personal and professional life increases. Other authors focus on analyzing the most important antecedents of the psychosocial well-being of nurses, highlighting the importance of social support to improve job satisfaction and stress [86]. Following this idea, two studies carried out in Sweden show the positive effect that empowerment [87] and social support [88] exert against burnout in nursing personnel.

3. Research Hypotheses

The three previously described job strain variables should have an interactive effect on the WLB of nurses. Additionally, the interaction among these variables can reduce the relationship between job demands and employees' WLB. Against the reference framework described in the previous paragraphs and based on the literature review, the following research hypotheses are proposed:

Hypothesis 1. *The high job demands faced by nursing professionals will be negatively associated with work–life balance.*

Hypothesis 2. *Job control will reduce the effects of job demands on work–life balance.*

Hypothesis 3. *Supervisors/co-workers will reduce the effects of job demands on work–life balance.*

The following Figure 1 summarizes the theoretical model and research hypotheses.

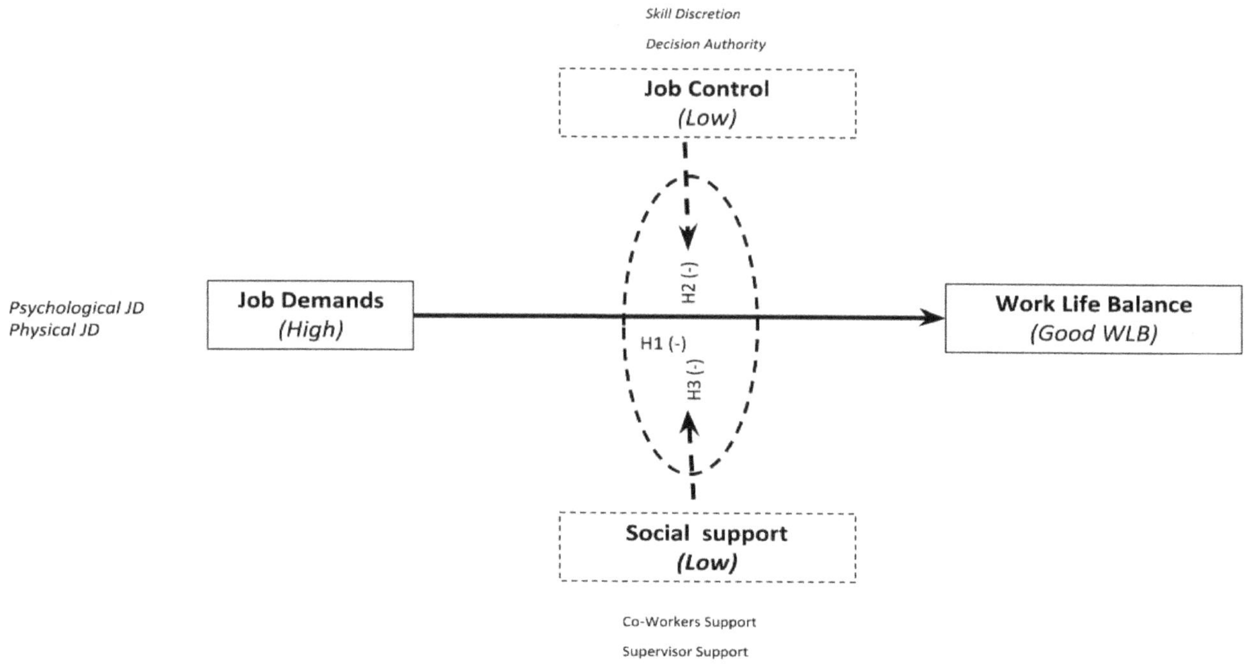

Figure 1. Research model. Source: Prepared by the authors.

4. Methodology

4.1. Data Collection and Sampling

For the development of this research, information collected by the European Foundation for the Improvement of Living and Working Conditions regarding the work environment and working conditions in 35 European countries was used (EU28, Norway, Switzerland, Albania, the former Yugoslav Republic of Macedonia, Montenegro, Serbia, and Turkey during the period from February to September 2015. The European Working Conditions Survey (EWCS) (The complete questionnaire can be found in the European Foundation for the Improvement of Living and Working Conditions (2019). See the following link: https://www.eurofound.europa.eu/sites/default/files/page/field_ef_documents/6th_ewcs_2015_final_source_master_questionnaire.pdf) is conducted every five years based on a questionnaire-based interview. A subsample of 991 nursing professionals (ISCO Code 222) (Classification structure of the International Labor Organization (ILO) that organizes jobs according to tasks and functions. Specifically, group 222 includes "Nursing and midwifery professionals") was extracted to achieve the objectives of this study. The majority of the respondents were women (89.1% of the total), with an average age of 42.8 years (SD = 11.0).

4.2. Measures and Methodology: The Binary Logistic Regression Model

The dependent variable of this study was WLB, measured by an indicator composed of four items that ask the following: (a) How are your working time arrangements set? (b) How do your working hours fit in with your family or social commitments outside work? (c) How often have you worked during your free time to meet work demands? (d) Would you say that arranging to take an hour or two off during working hours to take care of personal or family matters is easy or not? The Cronbach's α of the four-item scale was 0.898. Subjects with good WLB were coded as 1, while those with a lower level of WLB were coded as 0.

As indicated by Rugulies et al. (2010), the Copenhagen Psychosocial Questionnaire is considered a very effective tool for assessing the psychosocial work environment [89]. Different authors, such as Widerszal-Bazyl (2017), have demonstrated the psychometric properties of this questionnaire [90]. The extensive information provided by the European Working Conditions Survey permits the rigorous reproduction of the different scales included in the Copenhagen Psychosocial Questionnaire [9]. To meet the objectives of the present study, five indexes related to job demands, work organization, relationships, leadership, etc. were calculated. Twenty-three items from the EWCS were used to generate five indexes: (1) Psychological Job Demands (Cronbach's $\alpha = 0.736$); (2) Skill Discretion (Cronbach's $\alpha = 0.695$); (3) Decision Authority (Cronbach's $\alpha = 0.770$); (4) Co-worker Support (only one item); and (5) Supervisor Support (Cronbach's $\alpha = 0.905$).

Finally, physical job demands were measured with the Job Content Questionnaire (JCQ). This scale evaluates the social and psychological characteristics of a particular job. Some examples of the 13 items used to measure the risk of physical job demands are the following: "Are you exposed at work to high temperatures that make you perspire even when you are not working?", "Do you handle or have skin contact with chemical products or substances?" or "Does your main job involve lifting or moving people?" Cronbach's Alpha for this scale was 0.772.

The statistical analysis applied in this study was the binary logistic regression model. This method is one of the most frequently applied statistical approaches for developing social prediction models with binary results [91,92]. Logistic regression has been used with the Karasek model for example [93–95] and specifically in the field of nursing (for example, [96–98]). This method allows the determination of the probability that a certain event—good balance between personal and professional life—will occur compared with the probability that the opposite event will occur. In this study, the Hosmer–Lemeshow goodness of fit test was used as a measure of overall validity, and the Wald test was used for the analysis of individual variables.

5. Results

In the initial estimate of the central variable of this study, the general sample of the nursing professionals appears to present some problems balancing their personal time and work time, with an average score of only 0.5071 on a scale of 0 (poor WLB) to 1 (good WLB). In addition, this problem seems slightly more pressing among women (0.5067) than among men (0.5102).

In relation to the demands to which nursing professionals are subjected, it must be emphasized that the weight of psychological demands (0.3513) is, in all cases, greater than that of physical demands (0.2384). Additionally, women perceive more demands than men, both physical (0.2387 vs. 0.2364) and psychological (0.3524 vs. 0.3421).

Nursing professionals have greater skill discretion (0.6607) than decision authority (0.5698). This general trend does not differ by gender, although male nurses have greater skill discretion than female nurses (0.6667 vs. 0.6600), while female nurses have greater decision authority than male nurses (0.5714 vs. 0.5563).

Finally, the perceived supervisor support (0.2564) is much higher than the perceived support from co-workers (0.1893), a circumstance that should be the subject of analysis and deep debate within the profession. In addition, male nurses have more social support mechanisms than female nurses in regard to support from both supervisors (0.2617 vs. 0.2558) and co-workers (0.1952 vs. 0.1886).

5.1. Job Demand–Control–Support Factors and Work-Life Balance

The individual relationships between the different factors of the JDCS model and WLB are presented in Table 1. First, it should be noted that the fundamental principles of the JDCS model are confirmed. The high job demands, the low job control, and the low social support are negatively correlated with the outcome variable, i.e., the WLB indicator. However, these results must be taken with caution because the only variables that are statistically significant are those related to the physical ($\beta = -0.613$, $p = 0.000$) and psychological demands ($\beta = -0.520$, $p = 0.001$) on the nursing professionals. In fact, these two scales have the strongest relationship with the outcomes variable, followed by the two scales of social support and, finally, the measures of job control.

An examination of each of the individual components shows that physical demands are more important than psychological demands for predicting WLB among nursing and professionals.

In addition, the association between "low decision authority" (β = −0.188, $p = 0.250$) and WLB is more intense than the association between "low skill discretion" (β = −0.087, $p = 0.555$) and WLB. Likewise, the influence of supervisor support on WLB balance (β = −0.412, $p = 0.178$) is greater than the association between support from co-workers and WLB (β = −0.257, $p = 0.260$).

Table 1. Logistic regression: factors that determine work–life balance (high/low score).

Variables in the Model					Odds Ratios		
						95% C.I. for OR	
Variables	**B**	**Standard**	**Wald**	***p***	**OR**	**Lower**	**Upper**
Job Demands							
Psychological JD (high)	−0.520	0.151	11.863	0.001	0.594	0.442	0.799
Physical JD (high)	−0.613	0.15	16.711	0.000	0.542	0.404	0.727
Job Control							
Skill discretion (low)	−0.087	0.148	0.348	0.555	0.917	0.686	1.224
Decision authority (low)	−0.188	0.163	1.324	0.250	0.829	0.602	1.141
Social Support							
Co-worker support (low)	−0.257	0.228	1.271	0.260	0.773	0.494	1.209
Supervisor support (low)	0.412	0.306	1.811	0.178	0.662	0.364	1.207

5.2. *Strain Model*

The original proposal of the Karasek model (1979) is presented in Table 2, which shows the analysis of the association between WLB and job demands (physical and psychological) and job control (skill discretion and decision authority) and the interaction between both dimensions [16].

Table 2. Adjusted association between job demands, decision latitude, their interaction, and work–life balance index (Strain Model).

Variables in the Model					Odds Ratios		
						95% C.I. for OR	
Variables	**B**	**Standard**	**Wald**	***p***	**OR**	**Lower**	**Upper**
Job Demands							
Psychological JD (high)	0.025	0.321	0.006	0.937	1.026	0.546	1.926
Physical JD (high)	−0.397	0.193	4.223	0.040	0.672	0.460	0.982
Job Control							
Skill discretion (low)	0.320	0.248	1.673	0.196	1.377	0.848	2.237
Decision authority (low)	−0.095	0.216	0.192	0.661	0.917	0.596	1.389
Moderator effect of JC							
PhyJD x JC (Skill)	−0.257	0.329	0.541	0.462	0.785	0.412	1.495
PhyJD x JC (Dauth)	0.007	0.320	0.000	0.983	1.007	0.538	1.886
PsyJD x JC (Skill)	−0.533	0.195	7.467	0.006	0.587	0.400	0.860
PsyJD x JC (Skill)	−0.302	0.313	0.929	0.335	0.739	0.400	1.366

The results show a direct negative relationship between physical job demands and WLB (β = −0.397, $p < 0.05$). These results partially confirm Hypothesis 1.

Additionally, to test for interaction effects, interaction terms were introduced in the logistic regression model. Table 2 shows that the effect of psychological job demands on WLB is moderated when skill discretion is involved (β = −0.533, $p < 0.01$). This means that control over work (discretion to solve problems on your own and performing varied activities for which it is necessary to learn new skills) enriches nurses' work and possibly their personal life, cushioning the negative effect that the psychological demands of the profession exert on WLB. In other words, in the presence of low job control, the negative effect of psychological demands on WLB is more intense (β = −0.533, Sig. 0.006) than when greater job control is present (β = −0.520, Sig. 0.001). These results partially support Hypothesis 2 because the moderating effect of decision authority in the job demands–WLB relationship does not obtain statistically significant results for physical demands (β = 0.007, Sig. 0.983) or for psychological demands (β = −0.302, Sig. 0.335).

5.3. *Iso-Strain Model*

Subsequently, variables related to social support were incorporated into the model to contrast the hypotheses of the iso-strain model. Table 3 shows the adjusted association between WLB and job demands (physical and psychological), job control (skill discretion and decision authority), and social support (co-workers and supervisors) and their respective interactions.

Table 3. Adjusted association between job demands, decision latitude, social support, and their interaction and work–life balance index (iso-strain model).

Variables in the Model					Odds Ratios		
						95% C.I. for OR	
Variables	**B**	**Standard**	**Wald**	***p***	**OR**	**Lower**	**Upper**
Job Demands							
Psychological JD (high)	−0.122	0.466	0.069	0.793	0.885	0.355	2.206
Physical JD (high)	−0.397	0.193	4.223	0.040	0.672	0.460	0.982
Job Control							
Skill discretion (low)	−0.041	0.351	0.014	0.906	0.960	0.483	1.908
Decision authority (low)	−0.175	0.301	0.337	0.562	0.840	0.466	1.515
Moderator effect of JC							
PhyJD x JC (Skill)	0.259	0.485	0.285	0.594	1.295	0.500	3.354
PhyJD x JC (Dauth)	−0.341	0.461	0.548	0.459	0.711	0.288	1.754
PsyJD x JC (Skill)	−0.348	0.487	0.511	0.475	0.706	0.272	1.834
PsyJD x JC (Skill)	−0.621	0.264	5.543	0.019	0.538	0.321	0.901
Social Support							
Co-worker support (low)	0.029	0.466	0.004	0.950	1.03	0.413	2.566
Supervisor support (low)	−0.215	0.485	0.196	0.658	0.807	0.312	2.087
Moderator effect of Social Support							
PhyJD x JC (Skill)	0.769	0.521	2.178	0.140	2.157	0.777	5.989
PhyJD x JC (Dauth)	−0.749	0.267	7.848	0.005	0.473	0.280	0.799
PsyJD x JC (Skill)	−0.814	0.519	2.457	1.117	0.443	0.160	1.226
PsyJD x JC (Skill)	0.522	0.492	1.126	0.289	1.686	0.642	4.423

The new model presents some novelties regarding the formulated hypotheses. The most notable results are as follows. First, the direct relationship of job demands with WLB disappears from the overall model. The association of physical and psychological demands with WLB occurs in interaction with variables related to job control and social support. Thus, Table 3 shows that the strain-by-control interaction term at the 0.05 level only manifests when decision authority is present. This variable exerts a moderating effect on the psychological job demands–WLB relationship (β = −0.621, $p < 0.05$). This result partially confirms research hypothesis 2 as it indicates that decision authority, but not skill discretion, has a modulating effect.

Finally, the strain-by-support interaction term at the 0.05 level was analyzed. Table 3 shows that supervisor support moderates the effect of physical demands on WLB (β = −0.749, $p < 0.01$). This result partially confirms research hypothesis 3 as it indicates that supervisor support, but not co-worker support, has a moderating effect.

6. Discussion

The main objective of the present study was to test the efficacy of the JDCS model for predicting WLB among nursing professionals. Nursing presents its own particularities and is critical for maintaining the welfare state in Europe; however, nursing care takes place in one of the most stressful work environments that exists [96]. As noted by Karatepe and Uludag (2007), the health care sector is unique due to its high level of stress and its intense physical, psychological, and emotional demands [99].

Some studies, such as that of Ghislieri et al. (2017) performed with a sample of 500 nurses working in an Italian hospital, confirm that nurses have difficulties balancing work time and personal time [100]. To examine this issue among nursing professionals, the current study adopts the JDCS model as a reference framework, developing several logistic regression models that attempt to explain the direct and interactive effects of three fundamental variables: job demands, job control, and social support. The results obtained from a large sample of 991 European nursing professionals partially confirm both the strain hypothesis and the iso-strain hypothesis of the Johnson and Hall (1988) and Karasek (1979) models [16,17].

First, with respect to Hypothesis 1, a significant effect of physical (but not psychological) demands on WLB is confirmed. The physical demands that most affect nurses are, in the following order, handling or being in direct contact with materials that can be infectious, such as waste, bodily fluids, laboratory materials, etc.; lifting or moving people; having to maintain tiring or painful positions; performing repetitive hand or arm movement; handling or being in skin contact with chemical products or substances; and carrying or moving heavy loads. Being subjected to such physical demands causes nurses to feel that their work does not fit well with family or social commitments. The high physical demands cause a decrease in the well-being of workers linked to the work–family conflict because it includes aspects of physical fatigue, pain, and insecurity in the work environment [101], reducing the physical resources that a worker has to their WLB [47]. According to the World Health Organization, poor well-being in the workplace is one of the most important causes of absenteeism, turnover, and poor performance in the workplace [51]. This result is consistent with the study by Hussain et al. (2012), who highlight the high job demands that nurses face as well as the very poor working conditions, which translate into serious difficulties reconciling work and family time [102]. These authors warn of the risk that nurses will abandon the profession in search of less demanding and stressful options. The physical and psychological demands that nursing professionals face are well known and are overwhelmingly related to their close interactions with patients [103,104]. The results of our study indicate that nurses experience greater strain from physical demands than from psychological demands, perhaps because, as Qureshi (2018) warns, direct contact with patients requires high physical effort to lift or move people or heavy objects, maintain tiring or uncomfortable positions, and perform repetitive tasks or movements with one's hands or arms [105]. Similarly, Greenglass et al. (2001) and Garrett and McDaniel (2001) suggest that high physical demands may originate from the excessive workload and atypical schedules that include shift work, weekends, and nights [106–109]. These factors cause an imbalance between professional and personal demands, which manifests as lower organizational commitment, exhaustion, work stress, dissatisfaction, and, directly related to the object of this research, a worse personal–professional life balance [110].

Hypothesis 2 of this research was examined in a second phase intended to demonstrate the modulating effect of job control on WLB. The results of this study confirm this moderating effect in the case of psychological demands, which suggests that increasing the decision-making capacity of nursing professionals will improve their mood, vitality, and general interest, thus cushioning the direct effect that the demanding work exerts on stress, overwork, and personal life–professional life conflict [111]. Therefore, this research empirically confirms that being able choose the order in which one will perform tasks, being able to work at one's own pace and using one's own methods, being consulted about objectives that affect one's work, being able to influence the decisions that are important, or having the opportunity to apply one's own ideas at work, among other discretionary acts, cushions the negative effect that the psychological pressure of nursing work exerts on WLB. These results are in line with the study by Pisarski et al. (2006), who show that increased control in the workplace generates better WLB, especially when the individual is able to control his or her work hours and/or experiences an increase in schedule flexibility [112–115]. For many health professionals, their commitment to their work and professional career is a priority that takes them away from family and social relationships and causes them to dedicate less time than they would like to family responsibilities [116]. This extreme and rigid dedication causes a high level of exhaustion and a sensation of lethargy and depersonalization [117]. The debate on the effects of this professional dedication on WLB as one's health care career advances has a long history, but the issue seems far from a closed topic [118]. Decades ago, Hirschman (1970) reported the need to introduce changes in hospital work practices to correct this problem [119]. More recently, Mushfiqur et al. (2018) emphasize the moral obligation to change matters related to the management of health institutions, including work hours and locations, the relationship with the environment, and, of course, better balance between personal life and professional life [120]. Increasing the flexibility of work schedules is one of the most common strategies to mitigate this problem. Thus, the Medical Women's Federation (MWF) (2018) and Adisa et al. (2017) promote part-time work as a way to effectively improve WLB and create a positive impact on both Social Security and the lives of workers [118–121].

Finally, Hypothesis 3 of this research aimed to verify the moderating effect of social support in the job demand–WLB relationship. This moderating effect is partially confirmed for physical demands in the presence of supervisor support; that is, the negative effect of physical demands on WLB is mitigated when supervisor support is available. In conclusion, the physical demands (handling potentially infectious materials, moving patients, maintaining painful positions) that nursing professionals face generate problems with WLB, but these problems are reduced if nurses have the support of their immediate supervisors. A similar conclusion was reached by Abdul-Rashid et al. (2017), who applied a structural equations model in a sample of nurses from public hospitals in Malaysia [122]. Social support is decisive in an occupation in which teamwork, specifically cooperative work, occupies a leading role [123,124]. The creation of a work environment based on open communication and social support from co-workers and supervisors necessarily increases WLB [125]. Professionals in nursing units face complex problems that require very specific skills, support, and a great capacity for adaptation [126]. In this sense, support from both co-workers and supervisors can moderate the harmful effects of nursing demands on WLB. The studies of Tucker et al. (2018), Somers et al. (2018), and Jennings (2007) confirm that positive interpersonal relationships with supervisors improve safety, mutual respect, and positive feelings, which translate to greater WLB [127–129]. The results of our research support the cushioning effect of social support (at least in terms of supervisor support) in the job demands–WLB relationship, thus supporting Hypothesis 3.

7. Conclusions and Limitations

This study yields important theoretical and practical implications for the nursing profession in Europe. At the theoretical level, understanding how the JDCS model works in a sector such as nursing, where complex and dynamic tasks are performed, can decisively contribute to improving the WLB of professionals subjected to intense work demands. From a practical perspective, the findings of this study corroborate the idea that job demands are not the only variables that affect WLB, particularly when employees perceive job control and/or social support from their organizations. Consequently, the industry must analyze the workplace factors that affect WLB. Human resource managers should explore new tools to provide employees with control over their daily activities, especially in an occupation such as nursing, which involves direct contact with patients and in which the quality of the services provided is conditioned by the workers' decision-making capacity and freedom of actions. All progress in this regard (for example, modifying action protocols) will lead to greater autonomy, which should translate into better WLB. In addition, managers should promote a cooperative work environment based on an organizational culture of support, and teamwork should be encouraged. Investing in the training of work teams will improve aspects such as the organizational climate and social support, which will translate into improvements within the organization (for example, in the organization of work shifts) and in the attitude towards patient service. These strategies should reduce job stress and, as a result, increase the WLB of workers.

As is often the case in empirical research conducted in the field of social sciences, the results obtained should be interpreted with caution. First, a causal relationship between variables cannot be established since this is a cross-sectional study. Second, the study of the JDCS model is based on self-assessed measures and is therefore susceptible to bias; however, Pelfrene et al. (2002) corroborated that studies based on self-assessed measures support the strain hypothesis of the model to a greater extent than studies that use more objective evaluations [130]. Third, the research was developed in a specific socio-geographic scenario (Europe) where very different health systems and labor codes coexist that condition the fundamental variables of the JDCS model. Fourth, no control variables have been introduced, despite being a highly feminized profession. Therefore, it would not be prudent to generalize these assumptions and ideas to other work environments. Future studies should investigate other groups in the health industry (for example, doctors or hospital managers) and analyze the influence of different geographic areas to allow comparisons among different cultural environments.

Author Contributions: "Conceptualization, V.N-R and A.A.-M.; Methodology, A.A.-M. and F.H-P.; Software, F.H.-P. Validation, V.N-R and A.A.-M.; Formal Analysis, V.N.-R. and A.A.-M; Investigation, V.N.-R. and A.A.-M.; Resources, F.H.-P. and A.A.-M.; Data Curation, A.A.-M. Writing—Original Draft Preparation, V.N.-R. and F.H.-P.; Writing—Review & Editing, A.A.-M. and V.N.-R.; Visualization, F.H.-P. and A.A.-M.; Supervision, A.A.-M. and F.H.-P.; Project Administration, V.N.-R. All authors have read and agreed to the published version of the manuscript.

Acknowledgments: We thank Eurofound for providing the data set for this research. Reference [9], European Working Conditions Survey Integrated Data File, 1991–2015, [data collection], UK Data Service. SN: 7363, https://doi.org/10.5255/UKDA-SN-7363-4.

References

1. Babatunde, A.; Mordi, C.; Simpson, R.; Adisa, T.; Oruh, E. Time Biases: Exploring the Work-Life Balance of Single Nigeria Managers and Professionals. *J. Manag. Psychol.* **2019**, *35*, 35–70. [CrossRef]
2. Lee, D.J.; Sirgy, M.J. Work-Life Balance in the Digital Workplace: The Impact of Schedule Flexibility and Telecommuting on Work-Life Balance and Overall Life Satisfaction. *Thriving Digit. Work.* **2019**, 355–384. [CrossRef]
3. Kowitlawkul, Y.; Yap, S.F.; Makabe, S.; Chan, S.; Takagai, J.; Tam, W.W.S.; Nurumal, M.S. Investigating nurses' quality of life and work-life balance statuses in Singapore. *Int. Nurs. Rev.* **2019**, *66*, 61–69. [CrossRef] [PubMed]
4. Casper, W.J.; Vaziri, H.; Wayne, J.H.; DeHauw, S.; Greenhaus, J. The jingle-jangle of work–nonwork balance: A comprehensive and meta-analytic review of its meaning and measurement. *J. Appl. Psychol.* **2018**, *103*, 182. [CrossRef] [PubMed]
5. Duxbury, L.E.; Higgins, C.A. Gender differences in work-family conflict. *J. Appl. Psychol.* **1991**, *76*, 60. [CrossRef]
6. Williams, L.J.; Bozdogan, H.; Aiman-Smith, L. Inference problems with equivalent models. In *Advanced Structural Equation Modeling: Issues and Techniques*; Erlbaum: Mahwah, NJ, USA, 1996; pp. 279–314.
7. Ozer, E.M. The impact of childcare responsibility and self-efficacy on the psychological health of professional working mothers. *Psychol. Women Q.* **1995**, *19*, 315–355. [CrossRef]
8. Crompton, R.; Lyonette, C. Work-life 'balance' in Europe. *Acta Sociol.* **2006**, *49*, 379–393. [CrossRef]
9. Parent-Thirion, A.; Fernandez Macias, E.; Hurley, J.; Vermeylen, G. *Fourth European Working Conditions Survey*; European Foundation for the Improvement of Living and Working Conditions: Dublin, Ireland, 2007.
10. Lee, J.M.; Choi, H.G. Influence of organizational culture supporting work-life balance on well-being and depression mediated by work-life balance. *Korean J. Ind. Organ. Psychol.* **2019**, *32*, 1–27. [CrossRef]
11. Niessen, C.; Müller, T.; Hommelhoff, S.; Westman, M. The impact of preventive coping on business travelers' work and private life. *J. Organ. Behav.* **2018**, *39*, 113–127. [CrossRef]
12. Rodríguez González, S. Desigualdad por causa de género en la Seguridad Social: Carreras de cotización y prestaciones. *Lan Harremanak. Rev. Relac. Laborales* **2017**, *38*, 93–125.

13. Cramer, E.; Hunter, B. Relationships between working conditions and emotional wellbeing in midwives. *Women Birth.* **2019**, *32*, 521–532. [CrossRef] [PubMed]
14. Hayes, B.; Prihodova, L.; Walsh, G.; Doyle, F.; Doherty, S. Doctors don't Do-little: A national cross-sectional study of workplace well-being of hospital doctors in Ireland. *BMJ Open* **2019**, *9*, e025433. [CrossRef] [PubMed]
15. Nielsen, M.B.; Einarsen, S.V. What we know, what we do not know, and what we should and could have known about workplace bullying: An overview of the literature and agenda for future research. *Aggress. Violent Behav.* **2018**, *42*, 71–83. [CrossRef]
16. Karasek, R. Job demands, job decision latitude, and mental strain: Implications for job redesign. *Adm. Sci. Q.* **1979**, *24*, 285–308. [CrossRef]
17. Karasek, R. *Healthy Work: Stress, Productivity, and the Reconstruction of Working Life*; Basic Books: New York, NY, USA, 1990.
18. Johnson, V.J.; Hall, E.M. Job strain, work place social support, and cardiovascular disease: A cross-sectional study of a random sample of the Swedish working population. *Am. J. Public Heal.* **1988**, *78*, 1336–1342. [CrossRef]
19. Salin, D. Risk factors of workplace bullying for men and women: The role of the psychosocial and physical work environment. *Scand. J. Psychol.* **2015**, *56*, 69–77. [CrossRef]
20. Ariza-Montes, A.; Arjona-Fuentes, J.M.; Han, H.; Law, R. Work environment and well-being of different occupational groups in hospitality: Job Demand–Control–Support model. *Int. J. Hosp. Manag.* **2018**, *73*, 1–11. [CrossRef]
21. Asif, F.; Javed, U.; Janjua, S.Y. The job demand-control-support model and employee wellbeing: A meta-analysis of previous research. *Pak. J. Psychol. Res.* **2018**, *33*, 1.
22. Mivšek, P.; Äimälä, A.M.; Žvanut, B.; Tuomi, J. Midwifery students' well-being among undegraduates in Slovenia: A pilot study. *Midwifery* **2018**, *61*, 63–65. [CrossRef]
23. Rong, Y.; Guo, K.R.; Yin, H.F.; Wu, Y.F.; Li, S.; Sun, D.Y. Evaluating the level of occupational stress and its influence factors among traffic police in a district in Shanghai. *Chin. J. Ind. Hyg. Occup. Dis.* **2019**, *37*, 352–356. [CrossRef]
24. Schernhammer, E.S.; Feskanich, D.; Liang, G.; Scott, A.J.; Singh, R.B.; Anjum, B.; Takahashi, M. Stress and Burnout in Doctors. *Camb. Handb. Psychol. Health Med.* **2019**, *27*, 361.
25. Schilling, R.; Colledge, F.; Ludyga, S.; Pühse, U.; Brand, S.; Gerber, M. Does cardiorespiratory fitness moderate the association between occupational stress, cardiovascular risk, and mental health in police officers? *Int. J. Environ. Res. Public Health* **2019**, *16*, 2349. [CrossRef] [PubMed]
26. Chambel, M.J.; Carvalho, V.S.; Cesário, F.; Lopes, S. *The Work-to-Life Conflict Mediation between Job Characteristics and Well-Being at Work, Career Development International*; Emerald Publishing Limited: Bingley, UK, 2017.
27. Ibrahim, R.Z.A.R.; Saputra, J.; Bakar, A.A.; Dagang, M.M.; Nazilah, S.; Ali, M.; Yasin, M.A.S.M. Role of Supply Chain Management on the Job Control and Social Support for Relationship between Work-Family Conflict and Job Satisfaction. *Int. J. Sup. Chain* **2019**, *8*, 907.
28. Goller, M.; Harteis, C.; Gijbels, D.; Donche, V. Engineering students' learning during internships: Exploring the explanatory power of the job demands-control-support model. *J. Eng. Educ.* **2020**, 1–18. [CrossRef]
29. Ogunyemi, A.O.; Babalola, S.O.; Akanbi, S.O. Job Demands and Mental Strain Relationship: The Moderating Effect of Perceived Organizational Support on the Mediating Role of Job Decision Latitude among Nigerian Immigration Officers. *KIU J. Soc. Sci.* **2019**, *5*, 141–150.
30. Rana, F.A.; Javed, U. Psychosocial job characteristics, employee well-being, and quit intentions in Pakistan's insurance sector. *Glob. Bus. Organ. Excel.* **2019**, *38*, 38–45. [CrossRef]
31. Vassos, M.; Nankervis, K.; Skerry, T.; Lante, K. Can the job demand-control-(support) model predict disability support worker burnout and work engagement? *J. Intellect. Dev. Disabil.* **2019**, *44*, 139–149. [CrossRef]
32. Park, H.; Oh, H.; Boo, S. The Role of Occupational Stress in the Association between Emotional Labor and Mental Health: A Moderated Mediation Model. *Sustainability* **2019**, *11*, 1886. [CrossRef]
33. Schmitt, H. Job Demands, Job Control, and Social Support on Burnout: Why Type Matters. Ph.D. Thesis, Alliant International University, Alhambra, CA, USA, 2019.
34. Ding, G.; Liu, H.; Huang, Q.J. Enterprise social networking usage as a moderator of the relationship between work stressors and employee creativity: A multilevel study. *Inf. Manag.* **2019**, *56*, 103165. [CrossRef]
35. Grzywacz, J.G.; Frone, M.J.; Brewer, C.S.; Kovner, C.T. Quantifying work–family conflict among registered nurses. *Res. Nurs. Heal.* **2006**, *29*, 414–426. [CrossRef]

36. Cortese, C.G.; Ghislieri, C.; Colombo, L. Determinants of nurses' job satisfaction: The role of work–family conflict, job demand, emotional charge and social support. *J. Nurs. Manag.* **2010**, *18*, 35–43. [CrossRef] [PubMed]
37. Russo, M.; Buonocore, F. The relationship between work–family enrichment and nurse turnover. *J. Manag. Psychol.* **2012**, *27*, 216–236. [CrossRef]
38. Tummers, L.G.; Den Dulk, L. The effects of work alienation on organisational commitment, work effort and work-to-family enrichment. *J. Nurs. Manag.* **2013**, *21*, 850–859. [CrossRef]
39. Lecca, L.I.; Finstad, G.L.; Traversini, V.; Lulli, L.G.; Gualco, B.; Taddei, G. The Role of Job Support as a Target for the Management of Work-Related Stress: The State of Art. *Qual. Access Success* **2020**, *21*, 174.
40. Liu, Y.; Zhang, J.; Hennessy, D.A.; Zhao, S.; Ji, H. Psychological strains, depressive symptoms, and suicidal ideation among medical and non-medical staff in urban china. *J. Affect. Disord.* **2019**, *245*, 22–27. [CrossRef] [PubMed]
41. Henson, J.S. The Effectiveness of a Robotic Seal on Compassion Satisfaction in Acute Care Nurses: A Mixed Methods Approach. Ph.D. Thesis, The University of Texas at Tyler, Tyler, TX, USA, 2019.
42. Papastavrou, E.; Andreou, P.; Tsangari, H.; Schubert, M.; De Geest, S. Rationing of nursing care within professional environmental constraints: A correlational study. *Clin. Nurs. Res.* **2014**, *23*, 314–335. [CrossRef] [PubMed]
43. Schwarzer, R.; Knoll, N. Functional roles of social support within the stress and coping process: A theoretical and empirical overview. *Clin. Nurs. Res.* **2007**, *42*, 243–252. [CrossRef]
44. McGinnity, F.; Russell, H.; Watson, D.; Kingston, G.; Kelly, E. *Winners and Losers? The Equality Impact of the Great Recession in Ireland*; Economic and Social Research Institute (ESRI): Redlands, CA, USA, 2014; ISBN 978-1-908275-67-7.
45. Lahana, E.; Tsaras, K.; Kalaitzidou, A.; Galanis, P.; Kaitelidou, D.; Sarafis, P. Conflicts management in public sector nursing. *Int. J. Health Manag.* **2019**, *12*, 33–39. [CrossRef]
46. Russo, M.; Shteigman, A.; Carmeli, A. Workplace and family support and work–life balance: Implications for individual psychological availability and energy at work. *J. Posit. Psychol.* **2016**, *11*, 173–188. [CrossRef]
47. Haar, J.M.A.; Sune, A.; Russo, M.; Ollier-Malaterre, A. A cross-national study on the antecedents of work–life balance from the fit and balance perspective. *Soc. Indic. Res.* **2019**, *142*, 261–282. [CrossRef]
48. Cheng, S.Y.; Lin, P.C.; Chang, Y.K.; Lin, Y.K.; Lee, P.H.; Chen, S.R. Sleep quality mediates the relationship between work–family conflicts and the self-perceived health status among hospital nurses. *J. Nurs. Manag.* **2019**, *27*, 381–387. [CrossRef] [PubMed]
49. Neeson, J. Nurses are human beings too. *Nurs. Stand.* **2017**, *31*, 32. [CrossRef] [PubMed]
50. Lu, H.; Zhao, Y.; While, A. Job satisfaction among hospital nurses: A literature review. *Int. J. Nurs. Stud.* **2019**, *94*, 21–31. [CrossRef] [PubMed]
51. World Health Organization. *World Health Statistics: Monitoring Health for the SDGs Sustainable Development Goals*; World Health Organization: Geneva, Switzerland, 2018.
52. Lemieux-Cumberlege, A.; Taylor, E.P. An exploratory study on the factors affecting the mental health and well-being of frontline workers in homeless services. *Health Soc. Care Community* **2019**, *27*, e367–e378. [CrossRef]
53. Maslach, C.; Schaufeli, W.B.; Leiter, M.P. Job burnout. *Annu. Rev. Psychol.* **2001**, *52*, 397–422. [CrossRef]
54. Barnett, M.D.; Martin, K.J.; Garza, C.J. Satisfaction with work–family balance mediates the relationship between workplace social support and depression among hospice nurses. *J. Nurs. Sch.* **2019**, *51*, 187–194. [CrossRef]
55. Griffith, R. The elements of negligence liability in nursing. *Br. J. Nurs.* **2020**, *29*, 176–177. [CrossRef]
56. Harrod, M.; Petersen, L.; Weston, L.E.; Gregory, L.; Mayer, J.; Samore, M.H.; Drews, A.; Krein, S.L. Understanding workflow and personal protective equipment challenges across different healthcare personnel roles. *Clin. Infect. Dis.* **2019**, *69*, 185–191. [CrossRef]
57. Bureau of Labor Statistics Nonfatal Occupational Injuries and Illnesses Requiring Days Away From Work. *Industry Injury and Illness Data–2015*; Bureau of Labor Statistics, US Department of Labor: Washington, DC, USA, 2015; pp. 1–28.
58. Khan, S.A.; Waqas, M.; Siddiqui, M.; Ujjan, B.U.; Khan, M.; Bari, M.E.; Azeem, M.A. Work-life balance amongst residents in surgical and non-surgical specialties in a tertiary care hospital in Karachi. JPMA. *J. Pak. Med. Assoc.* **2020**, *70*, 252. [CrossRef]

59. Daxini, S.; Mehta, N. A Study on Impact of Work Stress on Work-Life balance Among Full Time Women Faculties in Self Financing Courses in Mumbai Suburban. *Adv. Innov. Res.* **2019**, *29*, 130–139.
60. Lin, Y.L.; Tomasi, J.; Guerguerian, A.M.; Trbovich, P. Technology-mediated macrocognition: Investigating how physicians, nurses, and respiratory therapists make critical decisions. *J. Crit. Care* **2019**, *53*, 132–141. [CrossRef] [PubMed]
61. Fukumori, T.; Miyazaki, A.; Takaba, C.; Taniguchi, S.; Asai, M. Traumatic Events Among Cancer Patients That Lead to Compassion Fatigue in Nurses: A Qualitative Study. *J. Pain Symptom Manag.* **2020**, *59*, 254–260. [CrossRef] [PubMed]
62. Hysong, S.J.; Amspoker, A.B.; Hughes, A.M.; Woodard, L.; Oswald, F.L.; Petersen, L.A.; Lester, H.F. Impact of team configuration and team stability on primary care quality. *Implement. Sci.* **2019**, *14*, 22. [CrossRef] [PubMed]
63. Hussain, I.R.; Mujtaba, B.G. The relationship between work-life conflict and employee performance: A study of national database and registration authority workers in Pakistan. *J. Knowl. Manag. Econ. Inf. Technol.* **2012**, *2*, 1–11.
64. Dobber, J.; Latour, C.; Snaterse, M.; van Meijel, B.; terRiet, G.; Scholte op Reimer, W.; Peters, R. Developing nurses' skills in motivational interviewing to promote a healthy lifestyle in patients with coronary artery disease. *Eur. J. Cardiovasc. Nurs.* **2019**, *18*, 28–37. [CrossRef]
65. Ulrich, B.; Barden, C.; Cassidy, L.; Varn-Davis, N. Frontline nurse manager and chief nurse executive skills: Perceptions of direct care nurses. *Nurse Leader* **2019**, *17*, 109–112. [CrossRef]
66. Dello Russo, S.; Mascia, D.; &Morandi, F. Individual perceptions of HR practices, HRM strength and appropriateness of care: A meso, multilevel approach. *Int. J. Hum. Resour. Manag.* **2018**, *29*, 286–310. [CrossRef]
67. Ronquillo, C.; Boschma, G.; Wong, S.T.; Quiney, L. Beyond greener pastures: Exploring contexts surrounding Filipino nurse migration in Canada through oral history. *Nurs. Inq.* **2011**, *18*, 262–275. [CrossRef]
68. Labrague, L.J.; McEnroe-Petitte, D.M.; Tsaras, K. Predictors and outcomes of nurse professional autonomy: A cross-sectional study. *Int. J. Nurs. Pr.* **2019**, *25*, e12711. [CrossRef]
69. Olmedo, G.R. Medicalización, psiquiatrización ... żdespsiquiatrización? *Con-Cienc. Soc. Anu. Didáctica Geogr. Hist. Cienc. Soc.* **2009**, *13*, 17–40.
70. Azizi, S.; Jafari, S.; Ebrahimian, A. Shortage of Men Nurses in the Hospitals in Iran and the World: A Narrative Review. *Sci. J. Nurs. Midwifery Paramed. Fac.* **2019**, *5*, 6–23.
71. White, E.M.; Aiken, L.H.; Sloane, D.M.; McHugh, M.D. Nursing home work environment, care quality, registered nurse burnout and job dissatisfaction. *Geriatr. Nurs.* **2019**, 52. [CrossRef] [PubMed]
72. McGilton, K.S.; Tourangeau, A.; Kavcic, C.; Wodchis, W.P. Determinants of regulated nurses' intention to stay in long-term care homes. *J. Nurs. Manag.* **2013**, *21*, 771–781. [CrossRef] [PubMed]
73. Ropponen, A.; Koskinen, A.; Puttonen, S.; Härmä, M. Exposure to working-hour characteristics and short sickness absence in hospital workers: A case-crossover study using objective data. *Int. J. Nurs. Stud.* **2019**, *91*, 14–21. [CrossRef]
74. Van Der Heijden, B.I.; Peeters, M.C.; Le Blanc, P.M.; Van Breukelen, J.W.M. Job characteristics and experience as predictors of occupational turnover intention and occupational turnover in the European nursing sector. *J. Vocat. Behav.* **2018**, *108*, 108–120. [CrossRef]
75. De Jonge, J.; Mulder, M.J.; Nijhuis, F.J. The incorporation of different demand concepts in the job demand-control model: Effects on health care professionals. *Soc. Sci. Med.* **1999**, *48*, 1149–1160. [CrossRef]
76. Scanlan, J.N.; Still, M. Relationships between burnout, turnover intention, job satisfaction, job demands and job resources for mental health personnel in an Australian mental health service. *BMC Health Serv. Res.* **2019**, *19*, 62. [CrossRef]
77. Yamaguchi, Y.; Inoue, T.; Harada, H.; Oike, M. Job control, work-family balance and nurses' intention to leave their profession and organization: A comparative cross-sectional survey. *Int. J. Nurs. Stud.* **2016**, *64*, 52–62. [CrossRef]
78. Mark, G.; Smith, A.P. Occupational stress, job characteristics, coping, and the mental health of nurses. *Br. J. Health Psychol.* **2012**, *17*, 505–521. [CrossRef]
79. Smith, J.H.; Sweet, L. Becoming a nurse preceptor, the challenges and rewards of novice registered nurses in high acuity hospital environments. *Nurse Educ. Pr.* **2019**, *36*, 101–107. [CrossRef]
80. Sigurdardottir, A.O.; Svavarsdottir, E.K.; Juliusdottir, S. Family nursing hospital training and the outcome on job demands, control and support. *Nurse Educ. Today* **2015**, *35*, 854–858. [CrossRef] [PubMed]

81. Chiu, Y.L.; Tsai, C.C.; Chiang, C.Y.F. The relationships among nurses' job characteristics and attitudes toward web-based continuing learning. *Nurse Educ. Today* **2013**, *33*, 327–333. [CrossRef] [PubMed]
82. Nabirye, R.C.; Brown, K.C.; Pryor, E.R.; Maples, E.H. Occupational stress, job satisfaction and job performance among hospital nurses in Kampala, Uganda. *J. Nurs. Manag.* **2011**, *19*, 760–768. [CrossRef] [PubMed]
83. Sheridan, P.; Carragher, L.; Carragher, N.; Treacy, J. Development and validation of an instrument to measure stress among older adult nursing students: The Student Nurse Stressor-15 (SNS-15) Scale. *J. Clin. Nurs.* **2019**, *28*, 1336–1345. [CrossRef]
84. Kelly, L.A.; Lefton, C.; Fischer, S.A. Nurse Leader Burnout, Satisfaction, and Work-Life Balance. *JONA: J. Nurs. Adm.* **2019**, *49*, 404–410. [CrossRef]
85. Xanthopoulou, D.; Bakker, A.B.; Demerouti, E.; Schaufeli, W.B. Work engagement and financial returns: A diary study on the role of job and personal resources. *J. Occup. Organ. Psychol.* **2009**, *82*, 183–200. [CrossRef]
86. McVicar, A. Scoping the common antecedents of job stress and job satisfaction for nurses (2000–2013) using the job demands–resources model of stress. *J. Nurs. Manag.* **2016**, *24*, E112–E136. [CrossRef]
87. Hochwälder, J. The psychosocial work environment and burnout among Swedish registered and assistant nurses: The main, mediating, and moderating role of empowerment. *Nurs. Health Sci.* **2007**, *9*, 205–211. [CrossRef]
88. Sundin, L.; Hochwälder, J.; Bildt, C.; Lisspers, J. The relationship between different work-related sources of social support and burnout among registered and assistant nurses in Sweden: A questionnaire survey. *Int. J. Nurs. Stud.* **2007**, *44*, 758–769. [CrossRef]
89. Rugulies, R.; Aust, B.; &Pejtersen, J.H. Do psychosocial work environment factors measured with scales from the Copenhagen Psychosocial Questionnaire predict register-based sickness absence of 3 weeks or more in Denmark? *Scand. J. Public Health* **2010**, *38*, 42–50. [CrossRef]
90. Widerszal-Bazyl, M. Copenhagen psychosocial questionnaire (copsoq). *Medycynapracy* **2017**, *68*, 329–349.
91. Van Smeden, M.; Moons, K.G.; de Groot, J.A.; Collins, G.S.; Altman, D.G.; Eijkemans, M.J.; Reitsma, J.B. Sample size for binary logistic prediction models: Beyond events per variable criteria. *Stat. Methods Med Res.* **2019**, *28*, 2455–2474. [CrossRef] [PubMed]
92. Debray, T.P.; Damen, J.A.; Riley, R.D.; Snell, K.; Reitsma, J.B.; Hooft, L.; Collins, G.; Moons, K.G. A framework for meta-analysis of prediction model studies with binary and time-to-event outcomes. *Stat. Methods Med Res.* **2019**, *28*, 2768–2786. [CrossRef] [PubMed]
93. Birolim, M.M.; Mesas, A.E.; González, A.D.; Santos, H.G.D.; Haddad, M.D.C.F.L.; Andrade, S.M.D. Job strain among teachers: Associations with occupational factors according to social support. *Cienc. Saudecoletiva* **2019**, *24*, 1255–1264. [CrossRef]
94. Tam, J.Z.; Mohamed, Z.; Puteh, S.E.W.; Ismail, N.H. A systematic review on identifying associated factors in deciding work-relatedness of chronic back pain among employee. *Malays. J. Public Health Med.* **2019**, *19*, 1–14.
95. Nguyen Ngoc, A.; Le ThiThanh, X.; Le Thi, H.; Vu Tuan, A.; Nguyen Van, T. Occupational Stress Among Health Worker in a National Dermatology Hospital in Vietnam, 2018. *Frontiers in Psychiatry.* **2020**, *10*, 950. [CrossRef]
96. Wesołowska, K.; Elovainio, M.; Gluschkoff, K.; Hietapakka, L.; Kaihlanen, A.M.; Lehtoaro, S.; Heponiemi, T. Psychosocial work environment and cross-cultural competence among native and foreign-born registered nurses. *Res. Nurs. Health* **2019**, *42*, 349–357. [CrossRef]
97. BagheriHosseinabadi, M.; Ebrahimi, M.H.; Khanjani, N.; Biganeh, J.; Mohammadi, S.; Abdolahfard, M. The effects of amplitude and stability of circadian rhythm and occupational stress on burnout syndrome and job dissatisfaction among irregular shift working nurses. *J. Clin. Nurs.* **2019**, *28*, 1868–1878. [CrossRef]
98. Arnetz, J.; Sudan, S.; Goetz, C.; Counts, S.; Arnetz, B. Nurse work environment and stress biomarkers: Possible implications for patient outcomes. *J. Occup. Environ. Med.* **2019**, *61*, 676–681. [CrossRef]
99. Karatepe, O.M.; Uludag, O. Conflict, exhaustion, and motivation: A study of frontline employees in Northern Cyprus hotels. *Int. J. Hosp. Manag.* **2007**, *26*, 645–665. [CrossRef]
100. Ghislieri, C.; Gatti, P.; Molino, M.; Cortese, C.G. Work–family conflict and enrichment in nurses: Between job demands, perceived organisational support and work–family backlash. *J. Nurs. Manag.* **2017**, *25*, 65–75. [CrossRef] [PubMed]
101. Voydanoff, P. The effects of work demands and resources on work-to-family conflict and facilitation. *J. Nurs. Manag.* **2004**, *66*, 398–412. [CrossRef]

102. Hussain, A.; Rivers, P.A.; Glover, S.H.; Fottler, M.D. Strategies for dealing with future shortages in the nursing workforce: A review. *Health Serv. Manag. Res.* **2012**, *25*, 41–47. [CrossRef] [PubMed]
103. Mc Carthy, V.J.; Wills, T.; Crowley, S. Nurses, age, job demands and physical activity at work and at leisure: A cross-sectional study. *Appl. Nurs. Res.* **2018**, *40*, 116–121. [CrossRef]
104. Nam, S.; Lee, S.J. Occupational factors associated with obesity and leisure-time physical activity among nurses: A cross sectional study. *Int. J. Nurs. Stud.* **2016**, *57*, 60–69. [CrossRef]
105. Qureshi, M.A.; Ab Hamid, K.B.; Jeihoony, P.; Ali, R.; Brohi, N.A.; Magsi, R.; Shah, S.M.M. Is Supervisor Support Matter in Job Satisfaction? A Moderating Role of Fairness Perception among Nurses in Pakistan. *Acad. Strateg. Manag. J.* **2018**, *17*, 1–10.
106. Greenglass, E.R.; Burke, R.J.; Fiksenbaum, L. Workload and burnout in nurses. *J. Community Appl. Soc. Psychol.* **2001**, *11*, 211–215. [CrossRef]
107. Garrett, D.K.; McDaniel, A.M. A new look at nurse burnout: The effects of environmental uncertainty and social climate. *JONA J. Nurs. Adm.* **2001**, *31*, 91–96. [CrossRef]
108. Haluza, D.; Schmidt, V.M.; Blasche, G. Time course of recovery after two successive night shifts: A diary study among Austrian nurses. *J. Nurs. Manag.* **2019**, *27*, 190–196. [CrossRef]
109. Vedaa, Ø.; Harris, A.; Erevik, E.K.; Waage, S.; Bjorvatn, B.; Sivertsen, B.; Moen, B.E.; Pallesen, S. Short rest between shifts (quick returns) and night work is associated with work-related accidents. *Int. Arch. Occup. Environ. Health* **2019**, *92*, 829–835. [CrossRef]
110. Mahendran, A.V.; Panatik, S.A.; Rajab, A.; Nordin, N. The Influence of Work-life Balance on Burnout among Nurses. *Indian, J. Public Health Res. Dev.* **2019**, *10*, 3338. [CrossRef]
111. Bae, J.; Jennings-McGarity, P.; Hardeman, C.P.; Kim, E.; Lee, M.; Littleton, T.; Saasa, S. Compassion Satisfaction Among Social Work Practitioners: The Role of Work–Life Balance. *J. Soc. Serv. Res.* **2019**, 1–11. [CrossRef]
112. Pisarski, A.; Brook, C.; Bohle, P.; Gallois, C.; Watson, B.; Winch, S. Extending a model of shift-work tolerance. *Chronobiol. Int.* **2006**, *23*, 1363–1377. [CrossRef] [PubMed]
113. Chunta, K.S. New Nurse Leaders: Creating a Work-Life Balance and Finding Joy in Work. *J. Radiol. Nurs.* **2020**. [CrossRef]
114. Dousin, O.; Collins, N.; Kaur Kler, B. Work-Life Balance, Employee Job Performance and Satisfaction Among Doctors and Nurses in Malaysia. *Int. J. Hum. Resour. Stud.* **2019**, *9*, 306–319. [CrossRef]
115. Fuentes, R. Implementing a Self-Scheduling Model to Decrease Nurse Turnover in Medical-Surgical Nursing. Ph.D. Thesis, Walden University, Minneapolis, MI, USA, 2019.
116. Ahmed, J.; Saleem, N.; Fatima, K. Factors Influencing Work Life Balance of Women Entrepreneurs: A Case of Quetta (Pakistan). *Dialogue* **2019**, *14*, 93.
117. Zaghini, F.; Fiorini, J.; Piredda, M.; Fida, R.; Sili, A. The relationship between nurse managers' leadership style and patients' perception of the quality of the care provided by nurses: Cross sectional survey. *Int. J. Nurs. Stud.* **2020**, *101*, 103446. [CrossRef]
118. De Souza, B.; Ramsay, R. Medical Women's Federation celebrates its long history. *BMJ* **2019**, *336*, 90. [CrossRef]
119. Hirschman, A.O. *Exit, Voice, and Loyalty: Responses to decline in Firms, Organizations, and States*; Harvard University Press: Cambridge, MA, USA, 1970; Volume 25.
120. Mushfiqur, R.; Mordi, C.; Oruh, E.S.; Nwagbara, U.; Mordi, T.; Turner, I.M. The impacts of work-life-balance (WLB) challenges on social sustainability: The experience of Nigerian female medical doctors. *Empl. Relat.* **2018**, *40*, 868–888. [CrossRef]
121. Adisa, T.A.; Gbadamosi, G.; Osabutey, E.L. What happened to the border? The role of mobile information technology devices on employees' work-life balance. *Pers. Rev.* **2017**, *46*, 1651–1671. [CrossRef]
122. Abdul-Rashid, S.H.; Sakundarini, N.; Raja Ghazilla, R.A.; Thurasamy, R. The impact of sustainable manufacturing practices on sustainability performance: Empirical evidence from Malaysia. *Int. J. Oper. Prod. Manag.* **2017**, *37*, 182–204. [CrossRef]
123. Kim, J.H.; Kim, M.Y. Factors affecting organizational commitment of general hospital nurses in small and medium sized cities. *J. Korean Acad. Nurs. Adm.* **2019**, *25*, 14–24. [CrossRef]
124. Tabriz, A.A.; Birken, S.A.; Shea, C.M.; Fried, B.J.; Viccellio, P. What is full capacity protocol, and how is it implemented successfully? *Implement. Sci.* **2019**, *14*, 73. [CrossRef]

125. Wallace, A.S.; Pierce, N.L.; Davisson, E.; Manges, K.; Tripp-Reimer, T. Social resource assessment: Application of a novel communication tool during hospital discharge. *Patient Educ. Couns.* **2019**, *102*, 542–549. [CrossRef] [PubMed]
126. Baris, V.K.; Seren Intepeler, S. Cross-cultural adaptation and psychometric evaluation of the Turkish version of the Self-Efficacy for Preventing Falls-Nurse. *J. Nurs. Manag.* **2019**, *27*, 1791–1800. [CrossRef] [PubMed]
127. Tucker, M.K.; Jimmieson, N.L.; Bordia, P. Supervisor support as a double-edged sword: Supervisor emotion management accounts for the buffering and reverse-buffering effects of supervisor support. *Int. J. Stress Manag.* **2018**, *25*, 14. [CrossRef]
128. Somers, M.J.; Birnbaum, D.; Casal, J. Supervisor support, control over work methods and employee well-being: New insights into nonlinearity from artificial neural networks. *Int. J. Hum. Resour. Manag.* **2018**, 1–23. [CrossRef]
129. Jennings, K.N. In the balance: Work/life balance of senior development professionals within higher education. Ph.D. Thesis, Iowa State University, Ames, IA, USA, 2007.
130. Pelfrene, E.; Vlerick, P.; Kittel, F.; Mak, R.P.; Kornitzer, M.; Backer, G.D. Psychosocial work environment and psychological well-being: Assessment of the buffering effects in the job demand–control (–support) model in BELSTRESS. *Stress Health* **2002**, *18*, 43–56. [CrossRef]

14

Prevalence of Comorbidities in Individuals Diagnosed and Undiagnosed with Alzheimer's Disease in León, Spain and a Proposal for Contingency Procedures to Follow in the Case of Emergencies Involving People with Alzheimer's Disease

Macrina Tortajada-Soler [1], Leticia Sánchez-Valdeón [2,*], Marta Blanco-Nistal [3], José Alberto Benítez-Andrades [4], Cristina Liébana-Presa [2] and Enrique Bayón-Darkistade [2]

1 Facultad de Ciencias de la Salud, Campus de Vegazana, Universidad de León, s/n, C.P. 24071 León, Spain; macrina-96@hotmail.com
2 SALBIS Research Group, Facultad de Ciencias de la Salud, Campus de Ponferrada, Universidad de León, Avda/ Astorga s/n, C.P. 24402 Ponferrada (León), Spain; cristina.liebana@unileon.es (C.L.-P.); jebayd@unileon.es (E.B.-D.)
3 Complejo Asistencial Universitario de León, C/ Altos de nava s/n, C.P. 24001 León, Spain; mblancon@saludcastillayleon.es
4 SALBIS Research Group, Department of Electric, Systems and Automatics Engineering, University of León, s/n, 24071 León, Spain; jbena@unileon.es
* Correspondence: lsanv@unileon.es

Abstract: *Background*: Alzheimer's disease (AD) which is the most common type of dementia is characterized by mental or cognitive disorders. People suffering with this condition find it inherently difficult to communicate and describe symptoms. As a consequence, both detection and treatment of comorbidities associated with Alzheimer's disease are substantially impaired. Equally, action protocols in the case of emergencies must be clearly formulated and stated. *Methods:* We performed a bibliography search followed by an observational and cross-sectional study involving a thorough review of medical records. A group of AD patients was compared with a control group. Each group consisted of 100 people and were all León residents aged ≥65 years. *Results:* The following comorbidities were found to be associated with AD: cataracts, urinary incontinence, osteoarthritis, hearing loss, osteoporosis, and personality disorders. The most frequent comorbidities in the control group were the following: eye strain, stroke, vertigo, as well as circulatory and respiratory disorders. Comorbidities with a similar incidence in both groups included type 2 diabetes mellitus, glaucoma, depression, obesity, arthritis, and anxiety. We also reviewed emergency procedures employed in the case of an emergency involving an AD patient. *Conclusions:* Some comorbidities were present in both the AD and control groups, while others were found in the AD group and not in the control group, and vice versa.

Keywords: Alzheimer's disease; comorbidity; older adults; elderly

---

1. Introduction

A general increase in life expectancy has caused an aging population and a resulting rise in the incidence of diseases that were less prevalent a few years ago such as neurodegenerative disorders [1]. At present, Alzheimer's disease (AD) is the most common type of dementia [2–17]. It was first described in 1907 [9] by the German physician Alois Alzheimer [1], who diagnosed it in a 51-year-old woman. It was described as a disease characterized by an impaired memory, disorientation, and hallucinations leading to death [1]. Currently, AD is considered to be a neurodegenerative disease [1,9,11–13,15,17–20] that is progressive [4,11,12,17–20] and results in mental or cognitive dysfunctions [1,5,11,17].

AD has become a major world health problem affecting a continuously increasing number of people. In Spain, 500,000–800,000 people suffer from AD, a number expected to double by 2050 [2,3]. More specifically, it is calculated that 10% of the population aged ≥65 years and 50% of that ≥85 years will suffer from AD [18]. Aging, therefore, greatly increases the risk of AD [6,9,21], which by now has become a social and public health issue [1].

The main symptom of AD is the loss of episodic memory [4,9,10,14]. This is accompanied by other characteristic "warning signs" [4,6,9,20,22] namely:

1. Failures or memory loss, which make everyday activities difficult;
2. Difficulty to face and/or solve problems;
3. Disorientation;
4. Difficulty understanding visual images and spoken language;
5. Problems with oral and/or written language;
6. Placing objects out of place;
7. Diminished and absent capacity of judgment;
8. Loss of initiative;
9. Personality changes, including apathy and depression;
10. Higher anxiety levels, restlessness, and sleep disorders;
11. Development of a state of increased dependency.

1.1. Pathophysiology of AD

The pathophysiology of AD is characterized by the occurrence of neurofibrillary tangles and neuritic plaques [2,3,5,10,12,17]. Several theories try to explain its onset [2–5,7,8,12,16,23,24] as follows:

Amyloid theory The essential element of extracellular deposits is the protein β-amyloid, which forms fibrils that aggregate and cause the development of diffuse and neuritic plaques. The β-amyloid protein is produced by an abnormal cleavage of the amyloid precursor protein (APP). Normally, the product of secretase α action is a soluble peptide that can be easily removed from the body. In AD, the cleavage is performed by β- and γ-secretases producing insoluble peptides that are removed from neurons. Microglial cells unsuccessfully attempt their removal, and this results in inflammation and nerve damage.

Tau protein theory The tau protein is the main component of intracellular deposits in neurons. It is a microtubule-associated protein, with microtubules being cytoplasmic structures involved in the assembly and function of the cytoskeletal network of cells including neurons. Tau acts as a microtubule stabilizer. In AD, Tau hyper-phosphorylation prevents its binding to tubulin and results in autoaggregation and formation of neurotoxic intraneuronal precipitates.

Cholinergic theory A decrease in the levels of the neurotransmitter acetylcholine in patients with AD causes a diminished performance of neural connections.

In addition to the three theories mentioned above, several other hypotheses have attempted to explain the etiology of AD, such as oxidative stress and glutamate-mediated excitotoxicity [7,12].

1.2. Risk and Protective Factors

AD is associated with a series of risk and protective factors. A risk factor is understood as one that increases the probability that an individual will develop a health problem or disease; while a protective factor is one that reduces such probability. We present a list of such factors that are associated with AD as follows:

Risk factors [4,19,21,23,25–31]

- Non-modifiable factors include age, gender, genetics-related (karyotype alterations, gene mutations, etc.), parental education, family background;
- Modifiable factors include low educational or socioeconomic level, obesity, type II diabetes mellitus, cardiovascular diseases (hypertension, atherosclerosis, heart disease, atrial fibrillation, and dyslipidemia), smoking, stroke, depression, alcohol abuse, and pneumonia;
- Environmental factors [24] include aluminum, pesticides, pollution.

Protective factors [21]

- physical, educational, intellectual and social activities, moderate consumption of alcoholic beverages, and a Mediterranean diet.

Establishing which factors are protective or risk-linked for AD patients is made difficult by these patients' inherent inability to communicate consistently. One way to approach this problem is by detecting comorbidities associated with AD and developing possible action protocols to be employed in emergency cases. The present study compared the comorbidities in a population of individuals aged ≥65 years and diagnosed with AD with those in an undiagnosed (control) population of similar characteristics, in the city of León, during 2019. In brief, the objectives of this work are as follows:

- To compare the sociodemographic characteristics of the individuals in the two populations under scrutiny;
- To establish and compare the comorbidities associated with the individuals of each of the two populations;
- To know, if any, the protocols of action employed by the Alzheimer Center of León or the León University Hospital in emergency situations concerning people with AD.

The cognitive or mental impairment that people with Alzheimer's disease present increases the difficulty they have in expressing themselves and manifesting their symptoms. Therefore, there is a need to study the comorbidities associated with Alzheimer's, and to examine possible protocols for action in the case of an emergency with these patients who have difficulty with expression and communication. This proposal for action protocols would facilitate emergency situations (such as triage in the emergency department) for these patients with other people, despite their difficulty with expression and communication.

2. Materials and Methods

2.1. Population Study

We performed an observational and cross-sectional study of the medical records of the populations under comparison. This involved a preliminary search strategy from primary and secondary bibliographic sources. A total of 200 individuals were analyzed, 100 from each of the 2 populations.

A significance study was conducted using GPower software to estimate the sample size [32], then, two groups were established, i.e., control and AD, each consisting of 100 subjects, which provided a confidence level of 90%, on the basis of a total population with AD estimated in 7000 individuals, in the León region of Spain [33]. The Alzheimer's Center León register contains 370 patients, with a proportion of them diagnosed with dementias other than Alzheimer's (fluctuating percentage of about 20% diagnosed with other types of dementia, primarily frontotemporal dementia, Parkinson's, and Lewy body dementia).

2.2. Literature Search

The bibliographic search connected with the present study included the PUBMED, WOS, and CUIDEN PLUS databases. A number of inclusion criteria were considered as follows:

- Publications from 2014 to 2019;
- Publications in English or Spanish;
- Data concerning the adult population aged ≥65 years diagnosed with AD;
- Both primary (original articles) and secondary (systematic reviews) sources;
- Full texts accessible through the University of León Library;
- Keywords employed (combined with Boolean operators AND and OR), in English included Alzheimer's disease, comorbidity, elderly, and aged and, in Spanish, "Enfermedad de Alzheimer", "comorbilidad", "adulto mayor", and "anciano".

2.3. Data Collection

The current study was complied with the rules of the Helsinki Declaration of 1975. It was approved by the Ethics Committee of León University Hospital according to Resolution #1929 of 26 February 2019.

The criteria for inclusion in the AD study group were:

- Alzheimer's disease diagnosis (this diagnosis has been previously identified by the Psychiatric Service of the León University Hospital);
- Age ≥65 years;
- Residency in the city of León, Spain;

The selection of subjects meeting these criteria was random.

The criteria for inclusion in the control group were:

- Not diagnosed with AD;
- Age ≥65 years;
- Residency in the city of León, Spain.

2.3.1. Alzheimer's Disease (AD) Group

Data were obtained from the Alzheimer's Comprehensive Care Center of León of the León Alzheimer Center. Each subject was identified by a code number to protect anonymity and confidentiality. This procedure was approved by the León Alzheimer Center and supported by signed agreements. Medical records were reviewed at random, reached the maximum number of individuals possible from the total number of people registered at the center, and met the inclusion criteria.

2.3.2. Control Group

Data corresponding to the undiagnosed population were collected from the León University Hospital.

Subjects who were undiagnosed in the general population with Alzheimer's disease, were randomly selected among those attending the Emergency Department of León University Hospital, for a few days, using the Gacela® computer program (León University Hospital, León, Spain), considering the following characteristics: age, sex, reason for admission, and medical history number. We used the Jimena® software (León University Hospital, León, Spain) to review and collect data, which included the pathologies suffered and the list of drugs taken by each individual. Each subject was identified by a code number to protect anonymity and confidentiality. This procedure was approved by the León Alzheimer Center and supported by signed agreements.

2.3.3. Data Processing

Data were stored and analyzed using an Office Excel® spreadsheet processor (2019 version) (University of León, Spain). The data analyzed for both groups included age, sex, comorbidities, and number of drugs taken. It is important to mention that diagnoses of comorbidities were uniformly identified by both primary care and continuing care physicians. They were entered into an SPSS version 24 computer statistical program (University of León, Spain), which was followed by analysis of the variables for each of the 2 populations to be compared with each other.

Additionally, action protocols to be used in the case of an emergency involving a patient with Alzheimer's disease were obtained.

2.4. Significance Studies

Data significance level was calculated with Pearson's Chi-square, and a value of $p \leq 0.1$ was considered to be satisfactory. As mentioned in Section 2.1., the 2 populations of 100 individual analyzed, in the present study, provided a confidence level of 90% and $p = 0.1$.

3. Results

3.1. Sociodemographics

3.1.1. Gender Distribution

The entire sample of 200 individuals comprising both the control and AD groups consisted of 61% women and 39% men. Figure 1 shows that the control group was composed of 47% males and 53% females; whereas the AD group consisted of 31% males and 69% females.

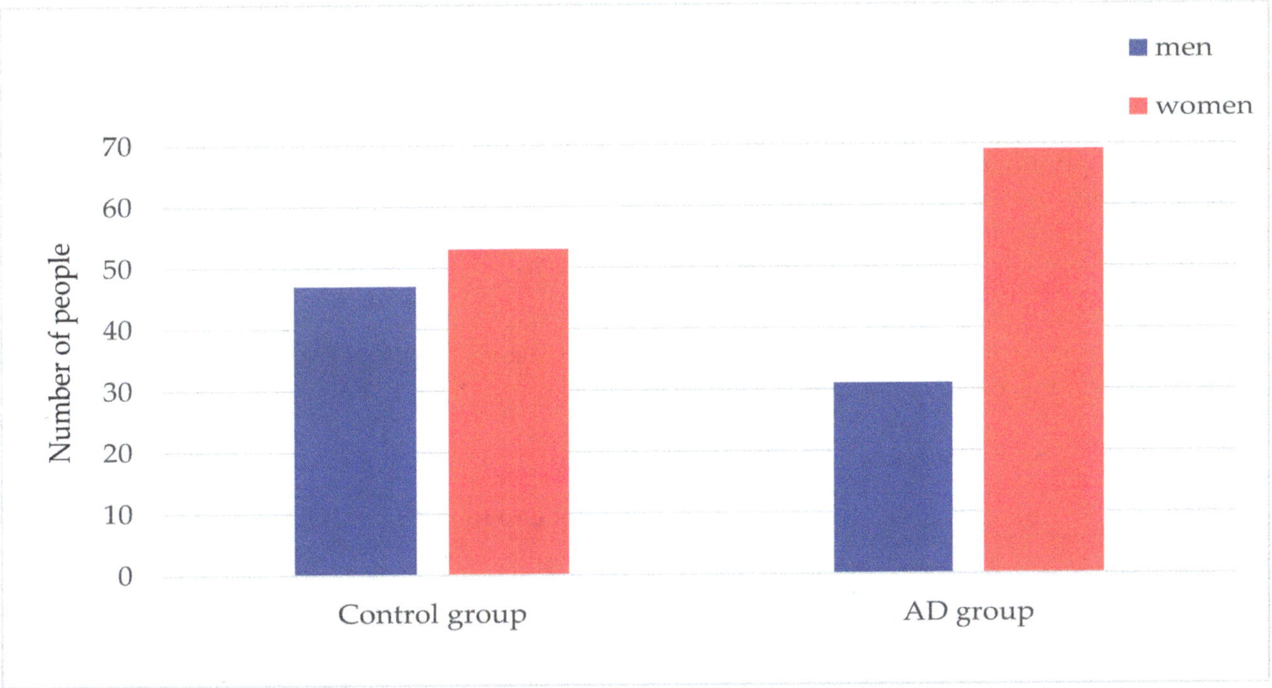

Figure 1. Alzheimer's disease and gender. This figure shows the number of men and women that make up both the control group and the Alzheimer's disease (AD) group.

3.1.2. Age Distribution

Figure 2 shows the comparative age analysis of the AD and control groups. This cohort study indicates that the number of subjects within the age interval 76–85 years is the largest in both groups. The age distribution of the AD and control groups clearly differs. The AD population shows an uneven pattern, with the >85 years group placed second after 76–85 years and a clearly smaller 66–75-year-old group. Instead, the distribution is rather symmetrical in the control population. In brief, the age interval in the AD group is shifted to older ages as compared with the control population.

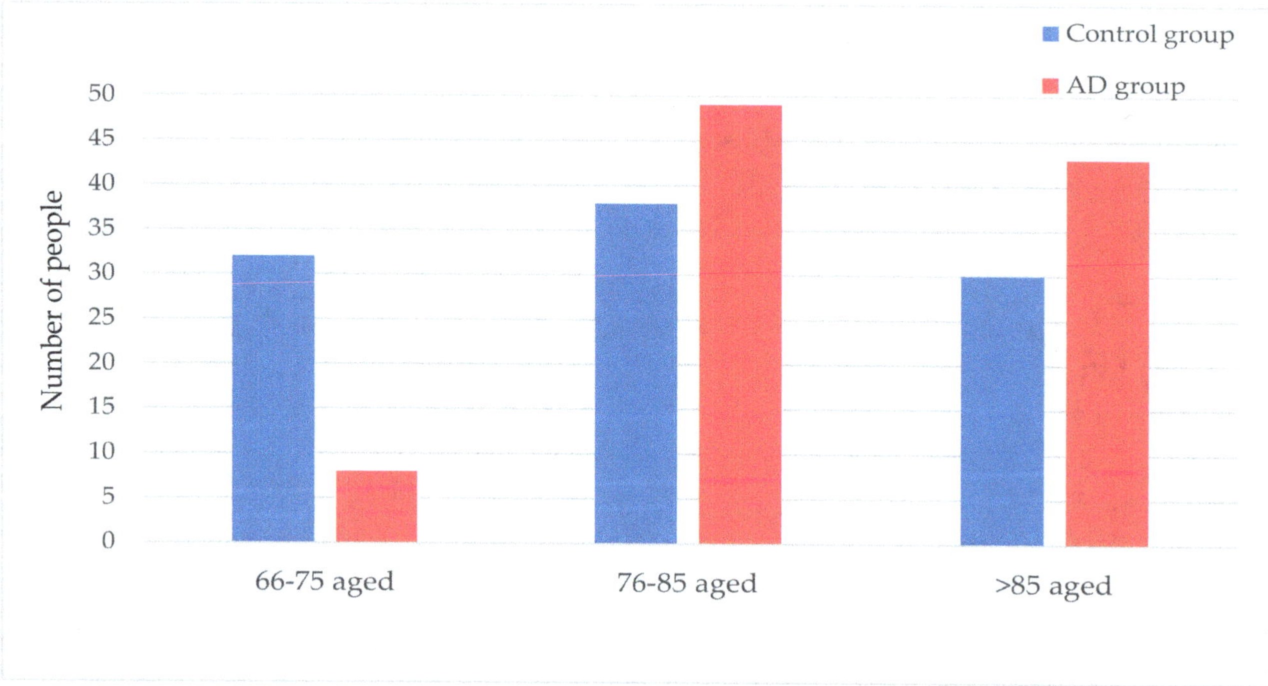

Figure 2. Age range distributions of the AD and controls. This figure shows the distribution of both the control group and the AD group, into three age range groups.

3.2. *Pathologies*

The comparison of the AD group with the control group and the analysis of the pathologies observed in the populations under study shows three clear age range groups according to their higher, similar, or lower incidence of pathologies.

3.2.1. Pathologies with a Higher Incidence in the AD Group

Table 1 shows the percentages of individuals with comorbidities more abundant in the AD group than in the controls. The pathologies in question are cataracts, urinary incontinence, vitamin D deficiency, osteoarthritis, hearing loss, osteoporosis, and personality disorders.

Table 1. Presence of comorbidities with higher incidence in the AD group.

	Control Group	AD Group
Medical condition	%	%
Cataract	12.0%	21.0%
Urinary incontinence	16.0%	38.0%
Vitamin D deficiency	5.0%	11.0%
Osteoarthritis	9.0%	26.0%
Hypoacusis	1.0%	13.0%
Osteoporosis	1.0%	20.0%
Personality disorders	1.0%	12.0%

The percentage of individuals not affected by these comorbidities are the remaining quantities up to 100, since in each group there are a total of 100 individuals.

Cataracts, urinary incontinence, and vitamin D deficiency affect 21%, 38%, and 11% of the individuals in the AD group, respectively, doubling the values observed in the control group, which are

12%, 16% and 5%, respectively. The difference is even more pronounced for osteoarthritis, which was present in 26% of the individuals in the AD group as compared with 9% in the control group. Strikingly, only 1% of individuals (one subject) was affected by hypoacusis, osteoporosis, or personality disorder in the control group, while the values were 13%, 20%, and 12% in the AD group, respectively.

In particular, emphasis is placed on the relationship between osteoporosis and gender.

Figure 3 shows the difference in prevalence of osteoporosis between men and women in the control and AD groups. As indicated in Table 1, 1% of women in the control group have osteoporosis while there are no cases of men. In the AD group, a total of 17% of women and 3% of men have osteoporosis.

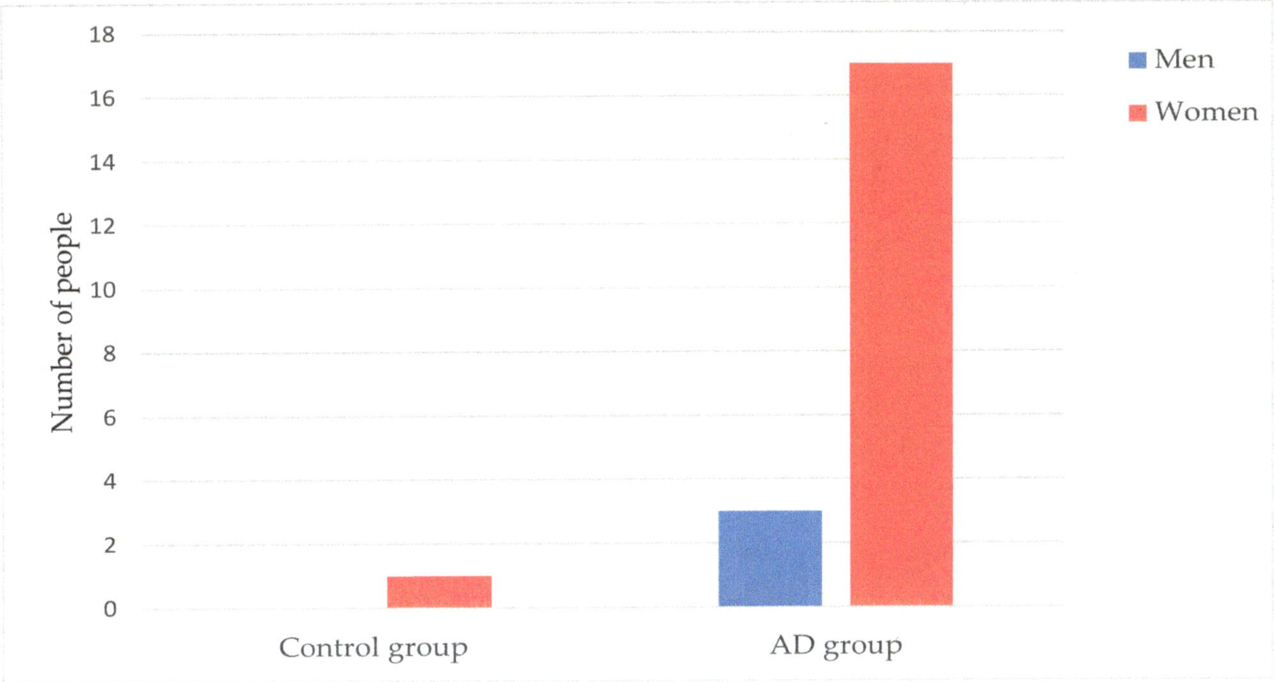

Figure 3. Osteoporosis' disease and gender. This figure shows the percentage of men and women who have osteoporosis, differentiated into the two groups under study.

Table 2 indicates the Pearson's Chi-square values and significance levels for the comorbidities shown in Table 1.

Table 2. Chi-square data and significance values for cataracts, urinary incontinence, vitamin D deficiency, osteoarthritis, hypoacusis, osteoporosis, and personality disorders.

Medical Condition	Chi-Square	df	Sig.
Cataracts	2.940	1	0.086 *
Urinary Incontinence	12.278	1	0.000 *
Vitamin D deficiency	2.446	1	0.118
Degenerative joint disease	10.009	1	0.002 *
Hearing loss	11.060	1	0.001 *
Osteoporosis	19.207	1	0.000 *
Personality disorders	9.955	1	0.002 *

* The Chi-square statistic is significant at the level 1.

The significance levels of cataracts, urinary incontinence, osteoarthritis, hypoacusis, osteoporosis, and personality disorders were 0.086, <0.00, 0.002, 0.001, <0.00, and 0.002, respectively. These values were lower than the p-value of 0.1. Instead, vitamin D deficiency showed a significance level value of 0.118, i.e., higher than the *p*-value. Therefore, we can say that the differences observed for the conditions listed on Table 2 are significant, except for vitamin D deficiency.

3.2.2. Pathologies with a Lower Incidence in the AD Group

Table 3 shows the percentages of individuals with comorbidities less abundant in the AD group as compared with the control group. The comorbidities which were analyzed included eye strain (increase in intraocular pressure), stroke, vertigo, hyperuricemia, circulatory insufficiency, atrial fibrillation, and respiratory insufficiency.

Table 3. Presence of comorbidities with lower incidence in the AD group.

	Control Group	AD Group
Medical condition	%	%
Eye strain	9.0%	2.0%
Ictus	5.0%	1.0%
Vertigo	11.0%	2.0%
Hyperuricemia	14.0%	9.0%
Circulatory insufficiency	34.0%	21.0%
Atrial fibrillation	11.0%	7.0%
Respiratory failure	25.0%	4.0%

The percentage of individuals not affected by these comorbidities are the remaining numbers up to 100, since in each group there is a total of 100 individuals.

The AD group shows 2%, 1%, and 2% of individuals affected by eye strain, stroke, and vertigo, respectively; whereas the values in the control group are higher, i.e., 5%, 11%, and 14%, respectively.

The percentages of control individuals affected by hyperuricemia (increased uric acid in the blood), circulatory failure, and atrial fibrillation are 14%, 34%, and 11%, respectively. In the AD group, those percentages are 9%, 21%, and 7%, respectively; all of them lower than in the undiagnosed population. The percentage of individuals with respiratory failure is 25% in the control and 4% in the AD group, indicating an incidence five times higher in the control group.

Table 4 shows the Pearson's Chi-square values corresponding to the comorbidities listed on Table 3.

Table 4. Chi-square data and significance values for eye strain, stroke, vertigo, hyperuricemia, circulatory failure, atrial fibrillation, and respiratory failure.

Medical Condition	Chi-Square	df	Sig.
Eye strain	4.714	1	0.030 *
Ictus	2.749	1	0.097 *b
Vertigo	6.664	1	0.010 *
Hyperuricemia	1.228	1	0.268
Circulatory insufficiency	4.238	1	0.040 *
Atrial fibrillation	0.977	1	0.323
Respiratory failure	17.786	1	0.000 *

* The Chi-square statistic is significant at the level 10. [b] More than 20% of the cells in this subtable had predicted cell counts less than 5. The Chi-square results may not be valid.

The significance levels of the comorbidities eye strain, stroke, dizziness, circulatory insufficiency, and respiratory insufficiency are all below the p-value of 0.10. In contrast, the comorbidities hyperuricemia and atrial fibrillation have a significance level of 0.268 and 0.323, respectively, i.e., higher than the p-value of 0.10. Thus, we can say that the differences observed for the conditions listed on Table 4 are significant except for hyperuricemia and atrial fibrillation.

3.2.3. Pathologies with a Similar Incidence in both Populations

Table 5 shows the comorbidities that do not show significant differences based on a comparison of the control and AD populations.

Table 5. Presence of comorbidities that do not show significant differences in both groups.

	Control Group	AD Group
Medical condition	%	%
Type 2 diabetes mellitus	20.0%	19.0%
Glaucoma	6.0%	6.0%
Depression	26.0%	27.0%
Obesity	7.0%	7.0%
Arthritis	9.0%	8.0%
High blood pressure	64.0%	51.0%
Dyslipidemia	39.0%	45.0%
Anxiety	12.0%	14.0%
Heart disease	26.0%	31.0%

The percentage of individuals not affected by these comorbidities are the remaining numbers up to 100, since in each group there is a total of 100 individuals.

The proportions of individuals affected by type 2 diabetes mellitus, glaucoma, depression, obesity, arthritis, anxiety, and heart disease in the AD group are 19%, 6%, 27%, 7%, 8%, 14%, and 31%, respectively. In the control group, these values are 20%, 6%, 26%, 7%, 9%, 12%, and 26%, respectively. The figures show a similar incidence of these comorbidities in both the AD and control groups. The comorbidities arterial hypertension and dyslipidemia present a relatively high incidence in both the control and AD groups; with values, in the AD group, of 51% and 45%, respectively and, in the control group, the corresponding percentages are 64% and 39%, respectively.

Table 6 shows the significance levels of the comorbidities type 2 diabetes mellitus, glaucoma, depression, obesity, arthritis, dyslipidemia, anxiety, and heart disease are all well above the p-value of 0.10. Instead, hypertension shows a significance level of 0.063, which is lower than the p-value of 0.10. Thus, we can say that only the differences observed for hypertension are significant.

Table 6. Chi-square data and significance values for type 2 diabetes mellitus, glaucoma, depression, obesity, arthritis, hypertension, dyslipidemia, anxiety, and heart disease.

Medical Condition	Chi-Square	df	Sig.
Type 2 diabetes mellitus	0.032	1	0.858
Glaucoma	0.000	1	1.000
Depression	0.026	1	0.873
Obesity	0.000	1	1.000
Arthritis	0.064	1	0.800
High blood pressure	3.458	1	0.063*
Dyslipidemia	0.739	1	0.390
Anxiety	0.177	1	0.674
Heart disease	0.613	1	0.434

* The Chi-square statistic is significant at the level, 10.

3.3. Medication

The number of medications taken by individuals from both study populations shows an average number of seven for each group, with the most abundant range being 6–10 medications.

Figure 4 shows that individuals in the control group took a larger number of drugs as compared with the AD group, with no one in the AD group taking >15 drugs. Nonetheless, the average number of drugs taken by each individual is the same ($n = 7$) in both groups.

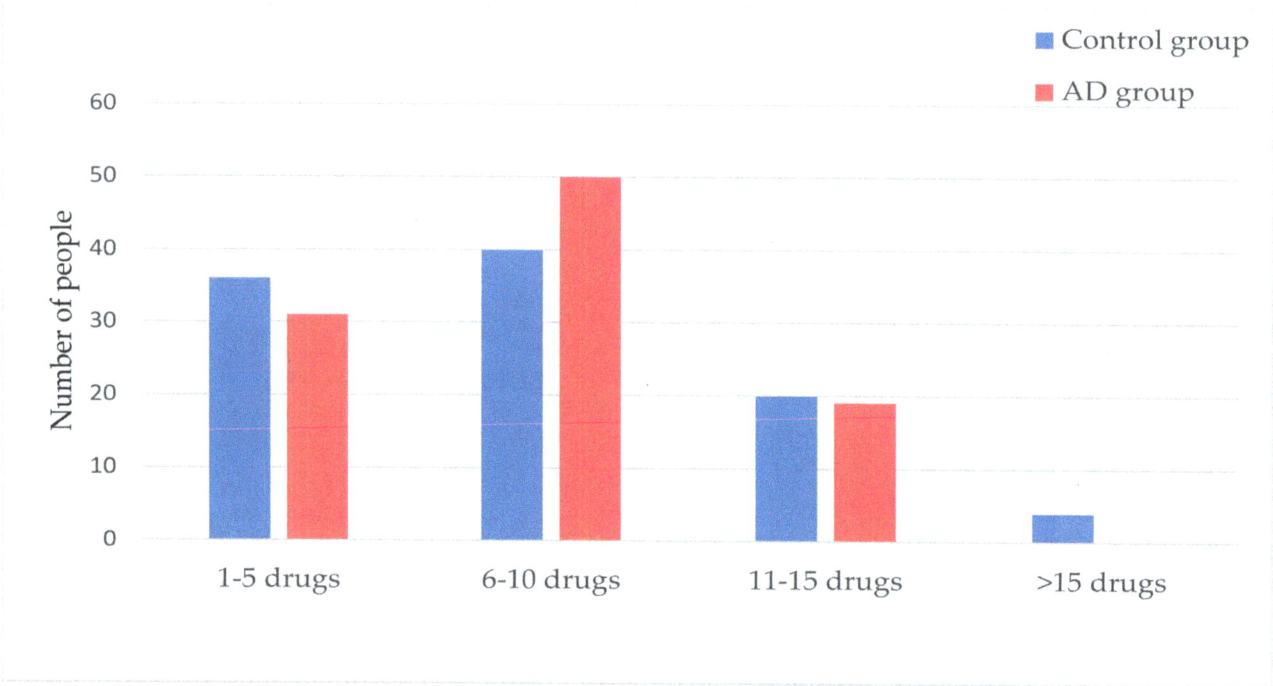

Figure 4. Number of medicines prescribed in the control and AD populations. This figure shows the amount of medication taken by subjects belonging to both the control and AD groups.

4. Operating Procedures in the Case of Emergencies

This section outlines the analyses of possible courses of action in the case of emergencies involving AD patients. We re-examined the standard operating procedures employed in the two centers from which the data presented here were collected, namely the Alzheimer's Comprehensive Care Center and the León University Hospital (León, Spain) (Table 7).

Table 7. Comparative table of the action protocols of León University Hospital and Alzheimer's Comprehensive Care Center of León.

	Comprehensive Care Center of León	León University Hospital
Target	Prevention and response in case of falls in patients with Alzheimer's disease	Activities to be performed by the nursing staff according to the different nursing diagnosis lists of the NANDA that the individual with Alzheimer's disease has
Coincidences	-Use of specific support measures for wandering, i.e., walking sticks or support rails -Specific protocol for physical restraint, if necessary, under medical order (with information to relatives) -Specific nursing care monitoring skin integrity or reassessment of the need for restraints -Increase environmental safety by avoiding slippery floors and architectural barriers, placing objects more easily accessible, positioning beds at a lower height and with handrails to prevent falls	
The differences	-Directed to all employees	-Directed only to the nursing staff
Key points	-The use of the J.H. Downton scale -It assesses the presence of certain intrinsic factors (age, drugs, or associated comorbidities) and extrinsic factors (of an environmental nature as inappropriate soil or equipment in each case) -There is an action protocol in case of falls -1st aid + 2nd reassures and secures the rest -Evaluate general condition and emergency equipment needs, report on the fall (questionnaire)	-Individualized protocol for the nursing staff
Lacks	-Lack of personalized care by the employees because there is a single protocol for all	-The J.H. Downton scale is not used -It does not take into account both intrinsic and extrinsic factors -There is no protocol for intervention in the event of a fall -Lack of protocols for the rest of the professional staff members working in the hospital

This table compares different points between the Protocol of the Alzheimer's Center León and the Protocol of the University Hospital of León

The protocol for the Alzheimer's Comprehensive Care Center regarding patients with Alzheimer's disease is focused on the prevention of falls and an action plan should a fall occur; whereas the protocol for the León University Hospital refers to the activities the nursing staff should perform according to the different nursing diagnosis lists of the NANDA (North American Nursing Diagnosis Association), for individuals with AD. The main difference between these two action protocols is that while that for the León University Hospital is exclusively directed to the nursing staff, the Alzheimer's Comprehensive Care Center's protocol is aimed at all its workers. Each of these approaches has different characteristics. A protocol of action, exclusively in the hands of the nursing staff, is based on their qualifications and competence to handle AD patients, and is standardized and excludes individual initiatives, thus, eliminating additional variables. An action plan aimed at all the workers dealing with AD patients has to be centered on the needs of such patients and must contemplate the fact that less qualified workers should seek professional advice whenever in doubt or when faced with unexpected events.

Fall prevention can require the physical restraint of AD patients, which must only be performed by medical order. In this respect, both centers have a specific protocol. When restraint requires the use of straps, the patient's skin integrity is first assessed. Importantly, the subjects in question and their relatives must be informed. Furthermore, the Alzheimer's Comprehensive Care Center's protocol contains a scale of evaluation of fall risks according to the J.H. Downton scale [34]. This evaluation has been applied to all the individuals in this center, who are professionally supervised depending on their individual risks. The reliability of the risk scale must be regularly reassessed. The León University Hospital's protocol does not use any scale to assess the risk of falls and simply considers the nature of the mental state alteration of each AD patient, for example, dementia, delirium, etc.

The Alzheimer Comprehensive Care Center also considers some intrinsic and extrinsic factors that affect fall risks. Classical intrinsic factors are age, medicines taken or associated comorbidities; while extrinsic factors are of an environmental nature, for example, inappropriate floor surfaces, lack of appropriate equipment, among others.

Procedures in the Event of a Fall

Intervention in the case of a fall is protocolized in the Alzheimer Comprehensive Care Center but not in the León University Hospital.

The first step of the intervention is to help the person who fell, as well as reassure other individuals in the vicinity who witnessed the event. The latter is essential since AD patients are particularly sensitive to traumatic situations even if not personally involved, and their behavior can be altered. The second step is a professionally conducted evaluation of the fallen patient's condition, with the help of an emergency team if necessary. It is extremely important to examine in detail why the fall occurred, in order to detect its possible causes, and therefore prevent other falls. It is equally important to consider the associated comorbidities of the patient, which may impinge on the action protocol to be used.

5. Discussion

The purpose of this work was to study the prevalence of comorbidities in an AD population as compared with a control population. First, we confirmed that the probability of developing AD is associated with an older population and is more frequent in females, in agreement with previous studies [26]. Presently, there is a debate as to whether AD is more prevalent among women due to genetic reasons or as a result of their longer life expectancy, which would make them more susceptible during later years.

Østergaard et al. (2015) [19] and Gallego and Guerrero (2017) [21] proposed that certain cardiovascular factors could facilitate the appearance of Alzheimer's disease. Among them, they mentioned high blood pressure, type 2 diabetes mellitus, heart disease, dyslipidemia, and obesity. This view was shared by Dugger et al. [25]. Our results do not fully support these suggestions. In fact, we detected a lower incidence of arterial hypertension in the AD group as compared with the control group, which was significant (Tables 5 and 6). No differences were observed between the AD group and the control group regarding the incidence of type 2 diabetes mellitus and obesity (Table 5). On the contrary, the incidence values for dyslipidemia and cardiopathy, although non-significant ($p \geq 0.1$), indicate a higher prevalence in the AD group.

In our study, the incidence of glaucoma, depression, anxiety, and arthritis was similar, though not significant, in both the AD and control populations. Xu et al. [35] claimed, in 2019, that the correlation between glaucoma and Alzheimer's disease was due to an enhanced susceptibility of AD patients to glaucoma. Depression and anxiety were described as AD predisposing factors by Ehrenberg et al., in 2019 [36]. Kao et al. [37] proposed that the correlation between arthritis and AD was actually an inverse relationship. According to our observations, there is a higher incidence of a history of stroke in the control group as compared with the AD group. The difference was significant and disagrees with previous studies by Nucera and Hachinski [27] and Hachinski [38], published in 2018, which showed that a previous history of stroke predisposed AD.

The comorbidities that we observed to be less prevalent in the AD group are ocular tension, vertigo, hyperuricemia, circulatory insufficiency, atrial fibrillation, and respiratory insufficiency. They are all significant except for hyperuricemia and atrial fibrillation. Lu et al. [39] reported, in 2017, a lack of a clear relationship between hyperuricemia and AD. No clear link between atrial fibrillation and AD was found by Ihara et al., in 2018 [40], while a positive correlation with AD was observed for vascular dementia.

The following comorbidities were found to be much more prevalent within the AD group as compared with the control group: cataracts, urinary incontinence, vitamin D deficiency, osteoarthritis, hearing loss, osteoporosis, and personality disorders. With the exception of vitamin D deficiency, their incidence values were all significant. In particular, in Figure 3 it is possible to see that there is a higher prevalence of osteoporosis in women than in men. This fact causes us to consider whether this comorbidity is associated with sex rather than a diagnosis of Alzheimer's disease. For this reason, it is necessary to go deeper into the relationship between osteoporosis and Alzheimer's disease and to see the factors that cause this comorbidity in patients with Alzheimer's. The vitamin D deficiency results, though not significant, agree with those of Annweiler et al. [41] and Chen et al. [42]. The latter also found, similar to our findings, that osteoporosis appears to be associated with Alzheimer's disease. Similarly, Lee et al. [43], Swords et al. [44], and Rouch et al. [45] reported the association of AD with urinary incontinence, hearing loss, and personality disorders. The fact that the AD group consists of more women (69%) than the control group (53%) may explain the higher incidence of osteoarthritis for the AD group [46]. Similarly, the fact that it is composed of an older population could also explain that this group of subjects has a greater number of associated comorbidities, not incidents in the same way as for the control group [46].

Altogether, our results show a satisfactory number of coincidences, as well as some discrepancies with those from other investigations. The discrepancies found could be due, among other possible aspects, to the difference between the sample size of our study with that of the other investigations or to the subjects chosen at random in one study or another.

6. Future Research

The observations reported, here, encourage further studies. First, an extension of the present research involving a greater number of patients and controls would be advisable. Secondly, longitudinal follow-up studies would allow the analysis of the existing and developing comorbidities of AD patients over long periods of time. As far as the Alzheimer's-free population is concerned, longitudinal studies would enable the detection of people that develop AD related to ageing. It would be possible to document whether the comorbidities they already suffered from were affected or not after the onset of AD, or whether the comorbidities were in any way related to the onset of AD itself. Such retrospective studies would obviously require a thorough analysis of medical records over long periods of time.

Author Contributions: Conceptualization, M.T.-S., L.S.-V., M.B.-N., C.L.-P., and E.B.-D.; Formal analysis, M.T.-S., J.A.B.-A., and E.B.-D.; Investigation, M.T.-S., L.S.-V., M.B.-N., and C.L.-P.; Methodology, M.T.-S., L.S.-V., M.B.-N., J.A.B.-A., and C.L.-P.; Software, J.A.B.-A.; Supervision, E.B.-D.; Validation, M.T.-S. and L.S.-V.; Visualization, J.A.B.-A.; Writing—original draft, M.T.-S., L.S.-V., and E.B.-D.; Writing—review & editing, L.S.-V., J.A.B.-A., and E.B.-D. All authors have read and agreed to the published version of the manuscript.

Acknowledgments: The authors would like to thank each of the people who participated in this project, all of them in a selfless way. Especially, Flor de Juan, Director, and Laura Fuentes, Neuropsychologist, both from the Alzheimer's Day Care Centre of León, for providing us access to the Centre and collecting data. To Beatriz Abad, nurse of the León University Hospital, who helped in the collection of data from the control group, and finally, to Rodolfo Garcia for the exhaustive review of the manuscript.

References

1. Custodio, N.; Montesinos, R. Enfermedad de Alzheimer Conociendo a la Enfermedad, que Llegó para Quedarse; 2015; p. 274. Available online: https://www.alzheimeruniversal.eu/wp-content/uploads/2015/09/libroenfermedaddealzheimer-150925020156-lva1-app7263.pdf (accessed on 23 April 2020).
2. Valenti, R.; Pantoni, L.; Markus, H.S. Treatment of vascular risk factors in patients with a diagnosis of Alzheimer's disease: A systematic review. *BMC Med.* **2014**, *12*, 160. [CrossRef] [PubMed]
3. Durazzo, T.C.; Mattsson-Carlgren, N.; Weiner, M.W.; Initiative, A.D.N. Smoking and increased Alzheimer's disease risk: A review of potential mechanisms. *Alzheimer's Dement.* **2014**, *10*, S122–S145. [CrossRef]
4. Alzheimer's Association; Chételat, G.; Villemagne, V.; Villain, N.; Jones, G.; Ellis, K.; Ames, D.; Martins, R.; Head, R.; Masters, C.; et al. Alzheimer's disease facts and figures. *Alzheimer's Dement.* **2011**, *7*, 208–244. [CrossRef]
5. Miranda, A.; Gómez-Gaete, C.; Mennickent, S. Dieta mediterránea y sus efectos benéficos en la prevención de la enfermedad de Alzheimer. *Revista Médica Chile* **2017**, *145*, 501–507. [CrossRef]
6. Cabrera-Pivaral, C.E.; Báez-Báez, M.G.L.; Rosa, A.D.J.C.-D.L. Mortalidad por enfermedad de Alzheimer en México de 1980 a 2014. *Gac. Med. Mex* **2018**, *154*, 550–554. [CrossRef] [PubMed]
7. Ashraf, G.M.; Tarasov, V.V.; Makhmutova, A.; Chubarev, V.N.; Avila-Rodriguez, M.; Bachurin, S.O.; Aliev, G. The Possibility of an Infectious Etiology of Alzheimer Disease. *Mol. Neurobiol.* **2018**, *56*, 4479–4491. [CrossRef]
8. Mancino, R.; Martucci, A.; Cesareo, M.; Giannini, C.; Corasaniti, M.T.; Bagetta, G.; Nucci, C. Glaucoma and Alzheimer Disease: One Age-Related Neurodegenerative Disease of the Brain. *Curr. Neuropharmacol.* **2018**, *16*, 971–977. [CrossRef]
9. Alzheimer's Association 2018 Alzheimer's disease facts and figures. *Alzheimer's Dement.* **2018**, *14*, 367–429. [CrossRef]
10. Garcez, M.L.; Falchetti, A.C.B.; Mina, F.; Budni, J. Alzheimer´s Disease associated with Psychiatric Comorbidities. *Anais Academia Brasileira Ciências* **2015**, *87*, 1461–1473. [CrossRef]
11. Haaksma, M.L.; Vilela, L.R.; Marengoni, A.; Calderón-Larrañaga, A.; Leoutsakos, J.-M.S.; Rikkert, M.G.M.O.; Melis, R.J.F. Comorbidity and progression of late onset Alzheimer's disease: A systematic review. *PLoS ONE* **2017**, *12*, e0177044. [CrossRef]
12. Butterfield, D.A.; Di Domenico, F.; Barone, E. Elevated risk of type 2 diabetes for development of Alzheimer disease: A key role for oxidative stress in brain. *Biochim. Biophys. Acta (BBA) Bioenerg.* **2014**, *1842*, 1693–1706. [CrossRef] [PubMed]
13. Richardson, J.; Roy, A.; Shalat, S.L.; Von Stein, R.T.; Hossain, M.M.; Buckley, B.; Gearing, M.; Levey, A.I.; German, D.C. Elevated serum pesticide levels and risk for Alzheimer disease. *JAMA Neurol.* **2014**, *71*, 284–290. [CrossRef] [PubMed]
14. Cervantes, C.M.; Mimenza, A.J.; Navarro, S.A.; Ávila, P.A.; Gutiérrez, L.G.; Arellano, S.J.; Avila-Funes, J.A. Factores asociados a la demencia mixta en comparación con demencia tipo Alzheimer en adultos mayores mexicanos. *Neurología* **2017**, *32*, 309–315. [CrossRef]
15. Monzani, F.; Pasqualetti, G.; Tognini, S.; Calsolaro, V.; Polini, A. Potential drug–drug interactions in Alzheimer patients with behavioral symptoms. *Clin. Interv. Aging* **2015**, *10*, 1457–1466. [CrossRef] [PubMed]

16. Yildiz, D.; Pekel, N.B.; Kiliç, A.K.; Tolgay, E.N.; Tufan, F. Malnutrition is associated with dementia severity and geriatric syndromes in patients with Alzheimer disease. *Turk. J. Med. Sci.* **2015**, *45*, 1078–1081. [CrossRef] [PubMed]
17. Podcasy, J.L.; Epperson, C.N. Considering sex and gender in Alzheimer disease and other dementias. *Dialog Clin. Neurosci.* **2016**, *18*, 437–446.
18. Borrell, F. Enfermedad de Alzheimer y Factores de Riesgo Ambientales|Armenteros Borrell|Revista Cubana de Enfermería. Available online: http://www.revenfermeria.sld.cu/index.php/enf/article/view/1024/239 (accessed on 21 April 2020).
19. Oosterveld, S.M.; Kessels, R.P.; Hamel, R.; Ramakers, I.H.G.B.; Aalten, P.; Verhey, F.R.J.; Sistermans, N.; Smits, L.L.; Pijnenburg, Y.A.; Van Der Flier, W.M.; et al. The Influence of Co-Morbidity and Frailty on the Clinical Manifestation of Patients with Alzheimer's Disease. *J. Alzheimer's Dis.* **2014**, *42*, 501–509. [CrossRef]
20. Marfany, A.; Sierra, C.; Camafort, M.; Domenech, M.; Coca, A. High blood pressure, Alzheimer disease and antihypertensive treatment. *Panminerva Med.* **2018**, *60*, 8–16.
21. Muñoz, C.G.; Navarro, N.G. Manejo de pacientes con enfermedad de Alzheimer: ¿cambio en el paradigma actual? *Revista Científica Sociedad Española Enfermería Neurológica* **2017**, *45*, 30–31. [CrossRef]
22. Kumar, A.; Sidhu, J.; Goyal, A.; Tsao, J.W. Alzheimer Disease–PubMed. Available online: https://pubmed.ncbi.nlm.nih.gov/29763097/ (accessed on 21 April 2020).
23. Attems, J.; Jellinger, K.A. The overlap between vascular disease and Alzheimer's disease–lessons from pathology. *BMC Med.* **2014**, *12*, 206. [CrossRef]
24. Culqui, D.R.; Linares, C.; Ortiz, C.; Carmona, R.; Diaz, J. Association between environmental factors and emergency hospital admissions due to Alzheimer's disease in Madrid. *Sci. Total. Environ.* **2017**, *592*, 451–457. [CrossRef] [PubMed]
25. Dugger, B.N.; Malek-Ahmadi, M.H.; Monsell, S.E.; Kukull, W.A.; Woodruff, B.K.; Reiman, E.M.; Beach, T.G.; Wilson, J. A Cross-Sectional Analysis of Late-Life Cardiovascular Factors and Their Relation to Clinically Defined Neurodegenerative Diseases. *Alzheimer Dis. Assoc. Disord.* **2016**, *30*, 223–229. [CrossRef] [PubMed]
26. Andrew, M.K.; Tierney, M.C. The puzzle of sex, gender and Alzheimer's disease: Why are women more often affected than men? *Women's Health* **2018**, *14*, 174550651881799. [CrossRef]
27. Nucera, A.; Hachinski, V. Cerebrovascular and Alzheimer disease: Fellow travelers or partners in crime? *J. Neurochem.* **2018**, *144*, 513–516. [CrossRef] [PubMed]
28. Ringman, J.M.; Sachs, M.C.; Zhou, Y.; Monsell, S.E.; Saver, J.L.; Vinters, H.V. Clinical predictors of severe cerebral amyloid angiopathy and influence of APOE genotype in persons with pathologically verified Alzheimer disease. *JAMA Neurol.* **2014**, *71*, 878–883. [CrossRef] [PubMed]
29. Campdelacreu, J. Enfermedad de Parkinson y enfermedad de Alzheimer: Factores de riesgo ambientales. *Neurología* **2014**, *29*, 541–549. [CrossRef]
30. Domínguez, R.; Pagano, M.; Marschoff, E.; González, S.; Repetto, M.; Serra, J. Enfermedad de Alzheimer y deterioro cognitivo asociado a la diabetes mellitus de tipo 2: Relaciones e hipótesis. *Neurología* **2014**, *29*, 567–572. [CrossRef]
31. Jefferson, A.L.; Beiser, A.; Himali, J.J.; Seshadri, S.; O'Donnell, C.J.; Manning, W.J.; Wolf, P.A.; Au, R.; Benjamin, E.J. Low cardiac index is associated with incident dementia and Alzheimer disease: The Framingham Heart Study. *Circulation* **2015**, *131*, 1333–1339. [CrossRef]
32. Cunningham, J.B.; McCrum-Gardner, E. Power, effect and sample size using GPower: Practical issues for researchers and members of research ethics committees Joseph. *Evid. Based Midwifery* **2007**, *5*, 132.
33. Alzheimer León Alza su Voz el 21 de Septiembre|Leonoticias. Available online: https://www.leonoticias.com/leon/alzheimer-leon-alza-20180915185052-nt.html (accessed on 21 April 2020).
34. Escala de Downton—Enfermería Creativa. Available online: https://enfermeriacreativa.com/2019/07/08/escala-de-downton/ (accessed on 22 April 2020).
35. Xu, X.; Zou, J.; Geng, W.; Wang, A. Association between glaucoma and the risk of Alzheimer's disease: A systematic review of observational studies. *Acta Ophthalmol.* **2019**, *97*, 665–671. [CrossRef]
36. Ehrenberg, A.J.; Suemoto, C.K.; Resende, E.D.P.F.; Petersen, C.; Leite, R.E.P.; Rodriguez, R.D.; Ferretti-Rebustini, R.E.D.L.; You, M.; Oh, J.; Nitrini, R.; et al. Neuropathologic Correlates of Psychiatric Symptoms in Alzheimer's Disease. *J. Alzheimer's Dis.* **2018**, *66*, 115–126. [CrossRef] [PubMed]

37. Kao, L.; Kang, J.-H.; Lin, H.-C.; Huang, C.-C.; Lee, H.-C.; Chung, S.-D. Rheumatoid Arthritis Was Negatively Associated with Alzheimer's Disease: A Population-Based Case-Control Study. *PLoS ONE* **2016**, *11*, e0168106. [CrossRef] [PubMed]
38. Hachinski, V. The convergence of stroke and dementia TT—A convergência do acidente vascular cerebral e da demência. *Arq. Neuropsiquiatr.* **2018**, *76*, 849–852. [CrossRef] [PubMed]
39. Lu, N.; Dubreuil, M.; Zhang, Y.; Neogi, T.; Rai, S.K.; Ascherio, A.; Hernan, M.; Choi, H.K. Gout and the risk of Alzheimer's disease: A population-based, BMI-matched cohort study. *Ann. Rheum. Dis.* **2015**, *75*, 547–551. [CrossRef] [PubMed]
40. Ihara, M.; Washida, K. Linking Atrial Fibrillation with Alzheimer's Disease: Epidemiological, Pathological, and Mechanistic Evidence. *J. Alzheimer's Dis.* **2018**, *62*, 61–72. [CrossRef]
41. Annweiler, C.; Dursun, E.; Féron, F.; Gezen-Ak, D.; Kalueff, A.V.; Littlejohns, T.; Llewellyn, D.J.; Millet, P.; Scott, T.; Tucker, K.L.; et al. 'Vitamin D and cognition in older adults': Updated international recommendations. *J. Intern. Med.* **2014**, *277*, 45–57. [CrossRef]
42. Lo, R.Y.; Chen, Y.-H. Alzheimer's disease and osteoporosis. *Tzu Chi Med. J.* **2017**, *29*, 138–142. [CrossRef]
43. Lee, H.-Y.; Li, C.-C.; Juan, Y.-S.; Chang, Y.-H.; Yeh, H.-C.; Tsai, C.-C.; Chueh, K.-S.; Wu, W.-J.; Yang, Y.-H. Urinary Incontinence in Alzheimer's Disease. *Am. J. Alzheimer's Dis. Other Dementiasr* **2016**, *32*, 51–55. [CrossRef]
44. Swords, G.; Nguyen, L.; Mudar, R.A.; Llano, D.A. Auditory system dysfunction in Alzheimer disease and its prodromal states: A review. *Ageing Res. Rev.* **2018**, *44*, 49–59. [CrossRef]
45. Rouch, I.; Dorey, J.-M.; Boublay, N.; Henaff, M.-A.; Dibie-Racoupeau, F.; Makaroff, Z.; Harston, S.; Benoit, M.; Barrellon, M.-O.; Fédérico, D.; et al. Personality, Alzheimer's disease and behavioural and cognitive symptoms of dementia: The PACO prospective cohort study protocol. *BMC Geriatr.* **2014**, *14*, 110. [CrossRef]
46. Verbrugge, L.M. Women, men, and osteoarthritis. *Arthritis Rheum.* **1995**, *8*, 212–220. [CrossRef] [PubMed]

15

Experiences of Homeless Families in Parenthood

Filipa Maria Reinhardt Andrade [1,*], Amélia Simões Figueiredo [2], Manuel Luís Capelas [2], Zaida Charepe [2] and Sérgio Deodato [2]

1 Institute of Health Sciences, Doctorate Student of the Doctorate Degree in Nursing, Universidade Católica Portuguesa, 1649-023 Lisbon, Portugal

2 Institute of Health Sciences, Centre for Interdisciplinary Research in Health (CIIS), Universidade Católica Portuguesa, 1649-023 Lisbon, Portugal; simoesfigueiredo@ics.lisboa.ucp.pt (A.S.F.); luis.capelas@ics.lisboa.ucp.pt (M.L.C.); Zaidacharepe@ics.lisboa.ucp.pt (Z.C.); sdeodato@ics.lisboa.ucp.pt (S.D.)

* Correspondence: fandrade@ics.lisboa.ucp.pt

Abstract: The objective of this systematic review was to identify the available qualitative data and to develop a framework to address the life experiences of homeless families in parenthood. The research was performed in the PubMed and CINAHL Complete databases, for works published in Portuguese, English, French and Spanish. Studies that included qualitative data, or both qualitative and quantitative data, were considered for this research. A total of 358 articles were obtained, of which 37 were assessed for eligibility, and 26 were rejected. In the end, 11 studies were selected. The Joanna Briggs Institute Critical Appraisal Checklist for Qualitative Research was used. These studies were conducted mostly in the United States, in temporary/transitional shelters for nuclear or single-parent families (led by women) in a homeless situation. In this context, the area which arose as the more relevant one was mental health, followed by the social studies. Two types of dimensions emerged from the results: mediating dimensions (which include the categories "Insecurity", "Lack of Privacy", "Isolation", "Stigma" and "Disempowerment") that are responsible for difficulties related to education, and behavioural changes in both the parents and the children; and supporting dimensions (which include the categories "Context as a Facilitator", "Relationship with Others" and "Parents' and children's Self") that lead to motivation, as well as the acquisition of strategies by the parents, to resolve parenting issues. This research helps expand nursing knowledge and presents a synthesis of the life experiences of homeless families in parenthood. Nursing can respond to the vulnerable population, due to its predominant role in promoting their health.

Keywords: family; homeless; nursing; parenting; parents; vulnerable population

---

1. Introduction

Parenthood is considered "the recognition of a mother's/father's responsibilities, the assumption of behaviours that promote the children's growth and development, as well as the internalisation of expectations expressed by individuals, families, friends and society, regarding the parental role's appropriate or inappropriate behaviours"(own translation, from: Ordem dos Enfermeiros) [1] (p. 66). Parenthood is understood as a transition [2–4]. Life transitions correspond to periods of greater vulnerability and increased health risk, which is why they have been increasingly considered a central concept for nursing [2,5]. Nurses are aware of the needs and changes brought upon by transitions, and they prepare the patient/family to better cope with such events, through learning and acquiring new skills [2].

The transition experience requires, as outcome indicators: the incorporation of new knowledge; the change of behaviours; the redefinition of the meanings associated with the occurred events; and, consequently, the redefinition of oneself within the social context [5]. Concerning possible constraints to the transition process, the author refers that, although community resources are able to create conditions which facilitate transition (family support, relevant information, referral, decision-making support), they may also create transition-inhibiting conditions (inappropriate counselling, insufficient information, etc.). The author points out that the society's development stage has a similar dual effect on transition—it may either facilitate the process, through the creation of laws and regulations, or inhibit it, through stigma, stereotypes, and marginalization [3].

In this regard, parenthood is considered to be an important, complex, challenging and highly responsible task for the human being, since it concerns the preparation of another human being for the challenges of development, namely physical, economical and psycho-social adversities [6]. While being an activity that usually involves the children, the parents and other family members in an interaction throughout life, it is not exclusive for these players and may involve other people, such as nurses, teachers, friends, partners, and even strangers [7]. In this sense, any person that participates in the care and development of a child is part of the parenthood process [8]. This concept emphasises that, in order to acquire the sense of being a father, or a mother, and to meet all the relevant requirements, it is not enough to just become a parent. It is necessary to go through a complex, conscious—and sometimes unconscious—process of role appropriation. Although parenthood is a subjective concept, because it is influenced by cultural beliefs, the dimensions and structural tasks of the parent-child relationship tend to remain similar, thus allowing its assessment (i.e., the evaluation of parental skills and competences) and producing data adequate for research purposes [6]. In this sense, Cruz considers five assessable parental functions: (1) Satisfaction of the basic survival and health needs—Where he emphasizes that the inability to assume this function may be related to socio-economic constraints, natural disasters, drug addiction, or parents' disease; (2) Providing of an organized and predictable physical world for the child—Which includes safety-promoting routines (severely dysfunctional families reveal a great difficulty in performing this function); (3) Responding to the needs of cognitive understanding with respect to extra-family realities—Stresses the difficulty of families that are more isolated or less permeable in ensuring this function; (4) Satisfaction of the needs of affection, trust and safety—This function is associated with the construction of attachment, which has proved to be a fundamental predictor of personal adaptation throughout life; (5) Satisfaction of the child's social interaction needs—The family should perform this function because, as the original nucleus of the child's socialization, it influences the future integration of the child in broader social contexts [9].

Furthermore, Figueiredo uses the life cycle stages ("Family with young children", "Family with children at school", and "Family with adolescent children") to define several assessment categories with respect to the parental role's competence. The aforesaid categories differ in terms of knowledge dimension, as well as adhesion behaviour. This author relates the knowledge of the role with the available information and the ability to learn skills, in order to identify the need to acquire new knowledge conducive to behavioural changes. She also relates the adhesion behaviour dimension to those aspects which highlight the parents' actions that reflect the full incorporation of parenthood through the identity of the role. That incorporation is evidenced by trust and competence in the role's performance. The evaluative categories of knowledge and adhesion behaviour are related to: physical care (which includes nourishment, elimination, personal hygiene and physical exercise); leisure activities; health surveillance; safety and prevention of accidents; attachment; cognitive, psychosexual, emotional and social development; structuring rules; a positive interaction with the child; adaptation to school; and the parents' involvement in education [10].

When we observe the different conditions that should be involved in the parental process/activity, the complexity associated with the process of educating a child becomes evident. In this sense, family plays a key role: it constitutes the most immediate space for the child's care, affections, dependence and socialization; it defines habits, health care routines, education, and the contexts to which the child is exposed (friends, school, neighbourhood, etc.); and it influences the present, the future and the development of the child. However, the family is not always able to provide a homogeneous environment and can have a negative impact on the child's well-being [11].

Within the family, there may be risk factors (internal or external), which represent a deficit in the children's development potential. On the other hand, the existence of protective factors (internal or external) that encourage the full development of the child can also occur. The internal protection factors relate to the quality of the interactions between family members. or to the involvement in stimulant activities. The external protective factors are associated with socioeconomic patterns, such as the family's structure, the parents' adequate working conditions, or the social support provided by public policies. As for external risk factors, they are related to demographic variables (e.g., having a single/adolescent mother, father's absence, separations and divorces) and to socioeconomic patterns (e.g., poverty, inequalities, mother's lack of education, violence, lack of social support, and restricted access to public policies regarding health and education). In contrast, the internal risk factors are associated with parental practices and parent-child interaction styles (e.g., abuse, neglect, negative communication, inconsistent discipline) [11]. In homeless families, many of those internal and external risk factors are simultaneously present, which accounts for their greater vulnerability [12]. From a nursing care perspective, vulnerability has always been considered a priority. As such, these families are a focus of interest for the nursing practice, often being the target of the aforementioned care [13].

A homeless person is an individual who, "regardless of his/her nationality, racial or ethnic origin, religion, age, sex, sexual orientation, socio-economic status, and physical and mental health status, is: homeless, living in a public space, in an emergency shelter, or in a precarious location; or homeless, living in a temporary accommodation destined for that purpose" (own translation, from: Ministério do Trabalho, Solidariedade e Segurança Social) [14] (p. 3925).

The reasons for the families' homelessness are different from those that lead to homelessness in adults. Most families are left homeless by: domestic violence [15–17]; repeated episodes of trauma and violence throughout life; child abuse; relationship breakups [15,16]; neighbourhood harassment; mental health problems involving parents and/or children [15,16,18]; special educational needs [15,16]; lack of family and social support networks; lack of access to statutory services [15–17,19]; social and emotional problems [17,20]; chronic instability; compromised health [19]; family head with a physical disability, with chronic health problems or with mental health problems [17]; poor financial situations and/or low income streams [21]; precarious housing situations; financial problems due to underemployment or unemployment; past mistakes (e.g., high school or college dropouts); and premature responsibilities, such as assuming a parental role at a young age [19]. The characteristics of these homeless families are heterogeneous. The most common are single-parent families led by (single) women [16,17,22]; with two children, generally under 11 years of age [16].

The lack of housing brings high social costs [23] and in families, has profound consequences, including the risk of health deterioration in family members [24,25]; the disruption of family dynamics, and the separation of parents and children [25]. Homeless families present multiple problems and needs that are interrelated (e.g., social, educational and health care) [15]. Homelessness is rarely an isolated event. Children from homeless families are prone to have a history of: low birth weight; anaemia; tooth decay; delayed immunizations; growth deficits; increased accident frequency, mainly injuries and burns [16]; developmental deficits; mental health problems [16,24,26,27]; behaviour disorders (e.g., sleep disorders, eating disorders, aggression and hyperactivity in young children); anxiety and post-traumatic stress [16]. A combination of multiple adverse childhood experiences may weaken their resilience [28] and they may become homeless as adults [28,29].

The protective factors for children belonging to homeless families include: school, due to its social stability, its routines and the parents' sense of achievement when they are capable of maintaining their child in the same school [16]; and the positive relationships between parents and children, which can mitigate the negative effects of homelessness in childhood, by helping the children to better manage their emotions, by promoting self-regulation, by forming positive relationships and by improving the children's functioning [30].

Homeless families face unique conditions that can affect the health and well-being of both the parents and the children. They may also affect parental practices, a better understanding of the homeless parents' life experiences being necessary in order to increasingly meet the real needs of this population. The Canadian Homeless Press Observatory argues that the support given to families, through the strengthening of relationships, is essential to avoid situations of homeless youth [29].

The European Federation of National Organisations Working with the Homeless (*Fédération Européenned' Associations Nationales Travaillant avec les Sans-Abri*—FEANTSA) suggests future research, highlighting the importance of studies in the following areas: homeless families, in order to further unveil the existing challenges and the strategies to be implemented, concerning the relationship with these families; parenting, in order to identify the constraints and strategies that homeless women (and men) face in their parental roles, as well as in the construction of their parental identities [31].

A preliminary search in the PubMed and CINAHL databases revealed the inexistence of systematic reviews on this topic and that none is currently in progress. Hence the necessity of aggregating knowledge to better comprehend the parental experiences of homeless individuals, and to identify useful factors for the monitoring of these vulnerable families. This will contribute to the understanding of how professionals can support families in managing their situation.

It is important to highlight the importance of this work for the scientific area of nursing, since nurses are considered the health professionals closest to the population, playing a fundamental role in health promotion and disease prevention, especially among the vulnerable population, as is the case of homeless families. This work is part of the Special Issue of the International Journal of Environmental Research and Public Health, since it emphasizes the importance of nursing for society as promoters of the population's health.

In this sense, we decided to conduct this systematic review, in order to better recognize the main research lines that have been explored up to this date, and to respond to the challenge proposed by the FEANTSA. For that purpose, we employed a scientific methodology which follows the Joanna Briggs Institute (JBI) protocol for systematic reviews of qualitative evidence [32].

The objective of this systematic review was to identify available qualitative evidence and to develop a framework to address the life experiences of homeless families in parenthood. We intended to answer the following research question, formulated according to the PICo acronym, [32] (Population, phenomenon of Interest and Context): What are the parenthood (I) experiences of the homeless (C) family (P)?

2. Methods

This systematic review adopts the method suggested by Moher, Liberati, Tetzlaff, Altman and the PRISMA group [33].

2.1. Inclusion Criteria

Population—This review considered all the studies that focus on homeless families constituted by adult parents (over 18 years of age) and their children (under 18 years of age). The parents and/or family correspond to the individuals who are responsible for providing care to the child/adolescent [32]. The following types of family were included: nuclear family (a man and a woman, who may or may not be legally married, with one or more biological/adopted children); reconstructed family (a couple in which at least one of the elements had a previous marital relationship and has a child who resulted from that relationship); single-parent family (a single parent and one or more children, being identified the gender of the person who represents the parental figure); extended family (a nuclear family, plus other relatives, or people who share with them bonds other than kinship) [10].

Phenomenon of interest—This review considered all the studies that address the parenthood experiences of homeless families, with parenthood being based on the evaluative categories of the parental role proposed by Figueiredo [10], and also the five parental functions of Cruz [9].

Context—This review considered studies conducted with homeless families. To that end, we employed the definition of "Homeless" recommended by the ENIPSSA [14].

Type of studies—Primary studies, of mixed or qualitative nature, published in Portuguese, French, English and Spanish, without a previously defined time span.

2.2. Exclusion Criteria

We excluded text (review) articles, opinion articles, letters to the editor, response letters, dissertations and reports, since priority was given to the numerous original research articles.

2.3. Search Strategy

The research strategy that was used aimed to find published studies indexed in certain databases. It comprised three stages. The first stage included an initial search in the PubMed and CINAHL databases, to analyse the keywords; it also encompassed the analysis of the MeSH Health Sciences descriptors in the respective query platform, as well as in CINAHL. The MeSH terms were then used in the PubMed database, while the corresponding MeSH headings were used in the CINAHL database. After selecting the relevant Boolean operators, descriptors, and indexed terms used to describe them, a second search was conducted in all the included databases—PubMed and CINAHL Complete (through EBSCOhost). The keywords which were used corresponded to the ones defined according to the PICo acronym (**P**opulation, phenomenon of **I**nterest and **C**ontext). The research strategy was sensitive to the specific characteristics of each selected database (Table 1).

Table 1. Search strategy.

Database	Search Strategy
PubMed	(((((((((((((((parenting) OR parenting styles) OR parenting practices) OR parent education) OR childrearing) OR family practice) OR parenting education) OR parenting education) OR parental behaviour) OR parent* behaviour) OR parent* education) OR parent* attitudes) OR altered parenting) OR parent* roll) OR parenthood)) AND ((((homeless persons) OR homeless people) OR homelessness) OR vulnerable populations)) AND ((((((((((((parent* OR biological parents) OR child of impaired parents) OR marriage) OR spouses) OR mothers) OR fathers) OR parents) OR only child) OR nuclear family) OR single parent) OR single parent family) OR family)
CINAHL	(parent* OR biological parents OR child of impaired parents OR marriage OR spouses OR mothers OR fathers OR parents OR only child OR nuclear family OR single parent OR single parent family OR family) AND (homeless persons OR homeless people OR homelessness OR vulnerable populations) AND ((MH "Parenting") OR "parenting" OR (MH "Altered Parenting (NANDA)") OR (MH "Parenting (Iowa NOC)") OR (MH "Parenting Alteration (Saba CCC)") OR (MH "Parenting Education") OR (MH "Risk for Altered Parenting (NANDA)" OR parenting styles OR parenting practices OR child-rearing OR family practice OR parental behaviour OR parent* behaviour OR parent* education OR parent* attitudes OR parent* role OR parenthood)

The searches were carried out between January 9th and January 30th, 2019. Duplicates were removed and, subsequently, two independent reviewers performed an analysis of the terms and descriptors found in the titles and abstracts of the articles. Studies that did not meet the inclusion criteria were excluded. Afterwards, the selected articles were read in full. Those that did not satisfy the inclusion criteria, or corresponded to the exclusion criteria, were eliminated. Finally, in a third stage, the selected articles' bibliographic references were analysed, in order to identify additional relevant studies. This review was not recorded in any systematic review database.

Before their integration in the final sample, all the selected articles were subjected to a methodological quality assessment.

2.4. Evaluation of the Methodological Quality

The methodological quality evaluation was conducted by two independent reviewers, using the JBI Critical Appraisal Checklist for Qualitative Research [32]. Disagreements between the reviewers were resolved through debating. The evaluation's purpose was to analyse the strengths and weaknesses of each selected work. The reviewers critically appraised the articles, which were accepted for inclusion if there was congruence between the research methodology, the research's objectives, and the methods used for data collection, representation and analysis.

2.5. Data Extraction

Data was extracted from all the works included in the review, using the JBI-QARI standardized data extraction tool [32]. The extracted data encompassed specific details about each research's objectives, scientific area, type of study (design and data collection method), population, context, phenomena of interest, and significant findings for our research question and objective.

2.6. Data Synthesis

The qualitative research's results were grouped and categorized based on the similarity of meaning, with at least two findings per category, using the JBI-QARI tool [32]. The different categories were created through a process of consensus between the reviewers. Data was then aggregated and subjected to synthesis, resulting in a single comprehensive set of findings that can provide a basis for evidence-based practice. The findings were classified as "credible" or "unquestionable" (according to their credibility level), using the JBI-QARI tool.

3. Results

We obtained a preliminary total of 358 articles through the database search. After duplicate removal, 349 works were subjected to relevance assessment based on their title and abstract. Of these, 248 were excluded after title evaluation and 64 were excluded after abstract evaluation, because they did not meet the established inclusion criteria. The remaining 37 studies were subjected to an eligibility assessment, and 26 were rejected, since they did not meet the inclusion criteria. Thus, a total of 11 articles were subjected to critical evaluation, with none being excluded. Figure 1 shows a PRISMA flowchart of the studies' identification and selection process for inclusion in the review.

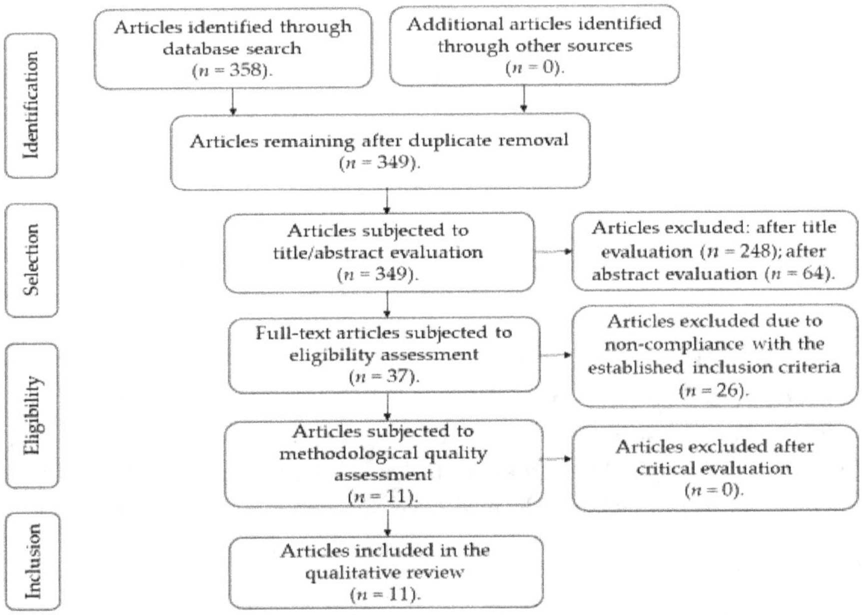

Figure 1. PRISMA flowchart detailing the search's results and the studies' selection/inclusion process (based on the method suggested by Moher, Liberati, Tetzlaff, Altman and the PRISMA group) [33].

3.1. *Methodological Quality*

All the 11 selected works were included in the analysis. These studies met the inclusion criteria and were considered methodologically rigorous, regarding the evaluation criteria. They offered useful descriptions of the daily life of homeless families. They also showed congruence between the research methodology, the research's objectives, the methods used for data collection, representation and analysis, and the methods employed to interpret the results. Most of the data represented the participants' opinions adequately. Despite the high quality of the selected articles, there was a lack of information in some of them. For instance, only 18% presented a statement contextualising the researchers' cultural and/or theoretical background. Furthermore, only 54.55% of the reported conclusions were derived from data interpretation. Prior to the critical evaluation, the reviewers decided that these shortcomings were not essential criteria that needed to be met for the article's inclusion. Table 2 presents the final assessment of the included works, specifying the research design's accuracy, as well as the quality of the resulting reports.

Table 2. Final evaluation of the included studies (according to the method used by Lockwood) [32].

Quote	Q1	Q2	Q3	Q4	Q5	Q6	Q7	Q8	Q9	Q10
Anderson et al. 2006 [15]	Y	Y	Y	Y	Y	N	Y	Y	N	Y
Anthony et al., 2017 [34]	Y	Y	Y	Y	Y	N	Y	Y	Y	Y
Cosgrove and Flynn, 2005 [35]	N	Y	Y	NC	Y	N	Y	Y	N	NC
Haskett et al., 2018 [36]	Y	Y	Y	Y	Y	Y	Y	Y	Y	Y
Holtrop et al., 2015 [37]	Y	Y	Y	Y	Y	N	Y	Y	Y	NC
Lindsey, 1997 [38]	Y	Y	Y	Y	Y	N	N	Y	N	NC
Morris and Butt, 2003 [39]	N	Y	Y	Y	Y	N	Y	Y	Y	Y
Roche et al., 2018 [40]	Y	Y	Y	Y	Y	N	Y	Y	Y	Y
Sylvestre et al., 2018 [25]	Y	Y	Y	Y	Y	Y	Y	Y	Y	Y
Tischler et al., 2004 [41]	Y	Y	Y	NC	Y	N	Y	NC	Y	N
Vanleit et al., 2006 [42]	Y	Y	Y	Y	Y	N	Y	Y	Y	N
% Yes	81.82	100	100	81.82	100	18.18	90.91	90.91	72.73	54.55

N: No; NC: Not Conclusive; Y: Yes.

Q1. Is there congruence between the declared philosophical perspective and the research methodology? Q2. Is there consistency between the research methodology and the research's question(s)/objective(s)? Q3. Is there consistency between the research methodology and the data collection methods? Q4. Is there congruence between the research methodology and the data's representation and analysis? Q5. Is there congruence between the research methodology and the results' interpretation? Q6. Is there a statement that contextualises the researcher from a cultural or theoretical point of view? Q7. Are the researcher's influence in the research and the inverse phenomenon addressed? Q8. Are the participants and their opinions adequately represented? Q9. Is the research considered ethical, according to the current criteria, or, for recent studies, is there evidence of ethical approval by an appropriate committee? Q10. Do the conclusions drawn in the research report derive from the data's analysis/interpretation? Note: Q1, Q2, Q3, etc., refer to the questions included in the JBI Critical Appraisal Checklist for Qualitative Research [32].

Regarding the CONQual results, most of the selected studies obtained a moderate score [37–40,42], four reached a high score [15,25,34,36], one obtained a low score [35], and one achieved a very low score [41]. Despite their low classification, these last two articles were not eliminated, because their findings were unique and contributed to the knowledge of the phenomenon. Additional details can be seen in Tables S1 and S2, which are available in electronic format.

3.2. *Results of the Extracted Data*

Concerning the research design, the studies are mostly qualitative in nature [15,25,34,35,38–40,42]. Only three works present a mixed nature, with qualitative and quantitative approaches [36,37,41].

Two of the articles are grounded in theory [38,39], while the remaining did not declare any specific methodology, merely stating that they used a qualitative approach. The methods applied in the 11 articles were diverse, namely: qualitative individual interviews, family interviews, focus groups with parents, participant observation, diaries and reflection activities.

The works are scattered over time (from 1997 to 2018). After the first article, which appears in 1997, there is a large gap, whilst the remaining articles were published between the time period 2003 to 2018. The first article that appears after this gap is the nursing study. They were mainly conducted in the United States, except for two studies that were performed in the United Kingdom [15,41] and one study that was carried out in Australia [40]. The context of the studies corresponded to temporary/transitional shelters for nuclear families [15,25,34,36,37,41] or single-parent families led by homeless women [35,38,42]. Only one study was conducted in multiple contexts (shelters, motels and transition houses) for homeless nuclear families [39]. Another research was carried out with single-parent families led by homeless men, who were recruited for the study by agencies that provide support to the homeless [40].

As for the number of families interviewed, the majority were single-parent families led by women, with a total of 506 families, and in two studies the number of interviews was not mentioned [35,38]. Next, the largest number of records were single-parent families led by men with a total of 51 interviews, 40 of whom were part of the same study [40]. Finally, there were 22 nuclear families (couple with children) in two of the studies [15,41], and five interviews that were represented by relatives in one of the studies [39].The most frequent research field was mental health [15,25,35–37,41], followed by social sciences [34,38,40], occupational therapy [42], education (in one of the psychology studies) [35], and nursing [39]. Further details about the included studies are presented in Table S3 that will be available in electronic form.

3.3. Synthesis of the Qualitative Research's Results

Taking into account the objective of the study, which sought to develop a structure to address the experiences of homeless families in parenthood, we extracted a total of 74 results from the 11 studies. Those findings were combined to form 12 categories based on similarity of meaning. The categories were grouped into two dimensions: "Parenthood Mediating Dimensions" and "Parenthood Supporting Dimensions". As mediating dimensions, we considered situations of transition to a higher parenthood stage, where the transition's inhibiting factors are highlighted. As supporting dimensions, we considered situations which reveal the transition process, emphasising the facilitating resources for that transition. The mediating dimensions include the categories "1—Insecurity", "2—Lack of Privacy", "3—Isolation", "4—Stigma", and "5—Disempowerment", which support the categories "6—Education Difficulties", "7—Changes in Parents' Behaviour", and "8—Changes in Children's Behaviour". On the other hand, the supporting dimensions include the categories "9—Context as a Facilitator", "10—Relationship with Others", and "11—Parents' and Children's Self", which lead to the additional category "12—Parenting Motivation and Strategies" that addresses parenting issues.

Next, we will present the synthesis of our findings, in the form of a narrative text, followed by an overview of the obtained results associated with the aforesaid findings and the established categories.

3.4. Synthesis of the Findings

3.4.1. Parenthood Mediating Dimensions

This synthesis derives from 53 findings and the following eight categories: "Insecurity", "Lack of Privacy", "Isolation", "Stigma", "Disempowerment", "Education Difficulties", "Changes in Parents' Behaviour", and "Changes in Children's Behaviour".

The mediating dimension of the "Insecurity" category is sustained by the following findings: lack of security; lack of hygiene; racism; intimidation; attacks from shelter residents; and negative influences from others. In the "Lack of Privacy" category, it is supported by: space limitations;

restrictive environment; and the need for privacy to play. In the "Isolation" category, it is sustained by: shelters located far from family, school and city centre; separation from friends and family; distancing from children; and the existence of loneliness feelings. In the "Stigma" category, it is supported by: feelings of stigmatization, humiliation, disrespect, and judgment. The "Disempowerment" category is divided into 3 subcategories: "Routine Change", sustained by the changes in the shelter's routines, the difficulty in maintaining routines, and the involvement of other adults; "**Rule Enforcement**", supported by shelter rules not consistent with previous parenthood options, as well as by the imposition of external rules; and "Parents' Needs", sustained by the need for practical, material and financial help, employment, education, transport, housing assistance, mental health promotion, pregnancy support, and time for oneself and one's children, as well as by the inability to play the role of provider and guide. The "Changes in Children's Behaviour" category includes: mental health problems; disobedience; mood swings; disrespect for authority; aggression; feelings of anguish, boredom and confusion; eating disorders; development regressions; concerns; and hiding the reality of living in shelters. The "Changes in Parents' Behaviour" category encompasses the lack of availability and conditions to meet the child's needs, as well as the dependence on the shelter's resources. Finally, the "Education Difficulties" category includes: difficulty in establishing discipline; the need for help when dealing with school; difficulty in integrating the school's community; difficulty in identifying school absenteeism as a problem; inability to help the child with school tasks, to maintain the child in a single school system throughout the year, and to identify academic problems; abdication of the responsibilities concerning school; absence of regular school attendance; and education barriers related to communication.

3.4.2. Parenthood Supporting Dimensions

This synthesis derived from 21 findings and 4 categories: "Context as a Facilitator", "Relationship with Others", "Parents' and Children's Self", and "Parenting Motivation and Strategies". It demonstrates that the homeless situation experienced in temporary/transitional shelters seems to enhance parenthood issues in some families, since they lead to motivation and acquisition of strategies by the parents, in order to deal with those issues. Some parents perceive this "Context as a Facilitator", because: it gives them access to services and resources; it is a safe place; it strengthens family practices and cohesion; and it is a stabilising experience that highlights the parental role. Additionally, they consider that it promotes the "Relationship with Others", defending that: it is a social opportunity; it provides a sense of community and of collective parenting; it provides supportive relationships, positive encounters with community service providers, and social support from family and friends. In addition, it seems to encourage the "Children's Self", since a young person demonstrated having resilience and perseverance, despite being homeless. It also seems to promote the "Parents' Self", since they reveal: the ability to help their children to deal with emotions; the ability to identify academic problems; optimism; hope for the future; perseverance; self-efficacy; resilience; resistance; the ability to set goals; and that they can do without help. Despite the homelessness situation, in some families parenthood seems to be enhanced, and it is even verified that the children function as a source of "Motivation", leading parents to seek improvement regarding their life situation and employment status, as well as to seek help to promote their mental health and maintain their morale. Parenthood also appears to feed the desire to move forward, in order to provide a better life for the respective children. Furthermore, to cope with the various challenges, the parents seek "Strategies", such as: reading; writing a diary; keeping focus; attending church; and talking to the respective support team, friends and family.

Figure 2 shows the relationship between the categories and the synthesised findings, to illustrate the general synthesis process.

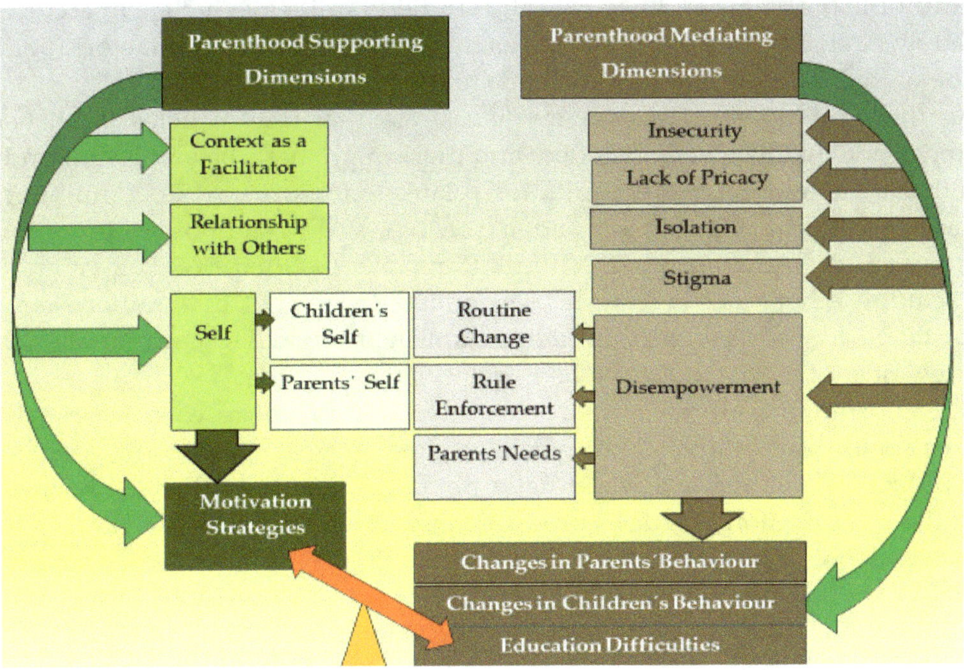

Figure 2. Overview of the synthesised findings.

4. Discussion

This systematic review sought to gather the best available evidence on the parenthood experiences of homeless families. As stated previously, the aggregation of 11 qualitative research articles resulted in the finding of two types of parenthood dimensions. On the one hand, we found "Parenthood Mediating Dimensions" (corresponding to transitional states), which include: "Insecurity", "Lack of Privacy", "Isolation", "Stigma", and "Disempowerment" (the latter pertaining to routine changes, rule enforcement and the multiple needs of the parents). On the other hand, we found "Parenthood Supporting Dimensions", which encompass: "Context as a Facilitator" (of access to services and resources, by acting as a stabilising experience for the family, and by highlighting the parental role), "Relationship with Others", and finally the "Parents' and Children's Self". In their turn, these categories led to relevant findings. The "Parenthood Mediating Dimensions" sustain changes in the parents' and children's behaviour, but, above all, they are associated with difficulties in education. Conversely, the "Parenthood Supporting Dimensions" lead to motivation and to the acquisition of strategies by the parents, with respect to parenting issues.

We found that some of the considered dimensions fit into the concept of parenthood recommended by the International Council of Nurses [1], as well as into the one suggested by Figueiredo [10]. Nevertheless, most of the dimensions corresponded to experiences, or feelings, reported by the parents. Some reflected difficulties in exercising the parental role, while others revealed protective factors related to the homelessness situation. This was one of the limitations we encountered in this study. In the "Parenthood Supporting Dimensions", the transition process is revealed through: the need of establishing relationships with others, as sources of support and information; the interaction with others; and the use of resources and coping strategies, to deal with the situation. This is in line with the findings presented by Meleis [3].

We encountered another limitation in this study, related to the context of the included works (all were conducted in temporary or transitional shelters). The research should be extended to other contexts of homelessness, such as: the street/public spaces, precarious locations, pensions, and rooms paid for by the social services.

We also found that the families identified in the study fit the characteristics of the different types of homeless families, such as single-parent families led by (single) women [16,17]. Additionally, we identified multiple problems and needs in the studied families, which is in accordance with the results obtained by Anderson et al. [15], as well as multiple risk/protection factors (both internal and external), in line with the findings of Macana and Comim [11].

Regarding the limitations of this review, we stress that only articles published in English, Portuguese, French and Spanish were included, and there might have been relevant findings in works published in other languages. Another limitation relates to the use of a small number of databases, since its extension would have led to a broader research, and to the possibility of including other significant contributions. Another possible limitation concerns the priority given to the search for articles, thus excluding other kinds of text, such as opinion documents, dissertations and reports. Since the literature available for inclusion was limited to published original research articles, there is always the risk that relevant studies may not have been identified.

Despite the effort to find all relevant articles, some significant research works may have been overlooked. There is the possibility that both reviewers may have neglected important studies, during the screening process of the 358 articles initially obtained. On the other hand, the bibliographic search allowed the identification of articles produced in various professional fields, such as psychiatry, psychology, social sciences, occupational therapy, and nursing. This provided a broader picture of the homeless parents' experiences.

Some of the obtained articles corresponded to secondary findings related to the parenthood experiences of homeless families, being thus included in the review. For instance, the purpose of one of the selected articles was to identify the parents' and the employees' perceptions, regarding their experience with the family support team, and also to recognise ways of improving this service in the future [15]. Although the focus was on the experience with the family support team, some of this study's findings were considered relevant to the objective of the present systematic review, being, therefore, included in it. This would not have been possible using a more restrictive bibliographic search strategy.

When we critically evaluated the 11 included articles, they revealed a variety of strengths and limitations. All works showed coherence between the research methodology and the research's question(s)/objective(s), the data collection methods and the results' interpretation. Nonetheless, two of the studies did not present congruence between the stated philosophical perspective and the research methodology [35,39], and there were two articles that did not present congruence between the research methodology and the data's representation and analysis [35,41].

The absence of an appropriate statement enhanced the complexity of evaluating the congruence between the philosophical perspective and the research methodology. Additionally, the inexistence of congruence, regarding the data's presentation and analysis, increased the difficulty of the data's evaluation. Although the reviewers did not consider these phenomena a reason for exclusion, the congruence between the philosophical perspective and the research methodology, as well as between the research methodology and the data's representation and analysis, would have been preferable, to strengthen the studies' credibility.

Data were collected through participant observation, individual interviews, written diaries, reflection activities, and group interviews/focus groups. The fathers' perspectives were under-represented, because most of the interviewees belonged to single-parent families led by women, thus highlighting the perspective of homeless mothers. However, in one of the studies, it was possible to analyse exclusively the male perspective, since it encompassed single-parent families led by men [40]. This unequal representation might be considered a limitation, because homeless fathers may have different experiences from homeless mothers. Even so, it may provide a realistic picture of homeless families.

Most of the studies were conducted in the United States, except for two which were carried out in the United Kingdom [15,41], and one that was performed in Australia [39]. This geographical distribution can result in limitations related to cultural differences, concerning the way homeless parenthood is viewed. It is important to note that these results can also refer to refugee families, which are becoming more important today. Such divergences may be relevant, since they can have implications for the practice in various settings and cultures. Nonetheless, we consider the studies' heterogeneity a strength, because it represents the complexity and diversity of the parenthood experiences in homelessness situations.

5. Conclusions

This review's findings contributed to the scientific knowledge about the complexities of homeless families/fathers/mothers and the challenges faced by them. Homeless parents living in temporary or transitional shelters are confronted with the intricacy of parental experiences influenced by insecurity, lack of privacy, isolation, stigma and disempowerment. On the other hand, to some families, the homelessness experience lived in temporary or transitional shelters seems to enhance parenthood, since they regard that context as a facilitator of the parental role, which promotes family cohesion, the relationships within the family and with others, as well as the parents' and the children's self. During the complicated journey of homeless parenthood, the parents use coping strategies and see their children as a great source of motivation, where they find strength to fight against the multiple difficulties they experience.

This review adds scientific knowledge on the experiences of homeless families, by revealing several parenthood mediating and parenthood supporting dimensions. However, the specific knowledge about parental experiences is still limited. The concept of homeless parenthood is scarcely researched; there exists a need for further studies in other homeless contexts, and in the field of Nursing, in order to adapt nursing responses to those families. While conducting this review, we found a reduced number of articles about the studied topic, which justifies the presented need and encourages additional research in the area of homeless parenthood. We stress the need for further research on paediatric nursing care, in the above-mentioned area. Regarding our methodological approach, we conclude that it was appropriate, since it allowed answering the research question.

Author Contributions: Conceptualization, F.M.R.A. and A.S.F.; methodology, F.M.R.A., A.S.F., M.L.C. and Z.C.; software, F.M.R.A., A.S.F. and M.L.C.; validation, F.M.R.A., A.S.F.; formal analysis, F.M.R.A., A.S.F.; investigation, F.M.R.A., A.S.F., M.L.C., Z.C. and S.D.; resources F.M.R.A., A.S.F., M.L.C., Z.C. and S.D.; data curation, F.M.R.A., A.S.F., M.L.C. and Z.C.; writing—original draft preparation, F.M.R.A. and A.S.F.; writing—review and editing, F.M.R.A. and A.S.F.; visualization, F.M.R.A., A.S.F., M.L.C., Z.C. and S.D.; supervision, F.M.R.A., A.S.F., M.L.C., Z.C. and S.D.; project administration, F.M.R.A. and A.S.F.; funding acquisition, S.D. All authors have read and agreed to the published version of the manuscript.

References

1. Ordem dos Enfermeiros. *CIPE®Versão2—Classificação Internacional Para a Prática de Enfermagem*; Ordem Dos Enfermeiros: Lisboa, Portugal, 2011.
2. Meleis, A.I.; Sawyer, L.M.; Im, E.O.; Messias, D.K.H.; Schumacher, K. Experiencing transitions: An emerging middle-range theory. *Adv. Nurs. Sci.* **2000**, *23*, 2–28. [CrossRef] [PubMed]
3. Meleis, A.I. *Transitions Theory: Middle Range and Situation Specific Theories in Nursing Research and Practice*; Springer Publishing Company: New York, NY, USA, 2010.
4. Meleis, A.I. *Theoretical Nursing: Development and Progress*, 5th ed.; Wolters Kluwer Health/Lippincott Williams & Wilkins: Philadelphia, PA, USA, 2012.
5. Meleis, A.I. *Theoretical Nursing: Development and Progress*, 4th ed.; Lippincott Williams & Wilkins: Philadelphia, PA, USA, 2007.
6. Barroso, R.G.; Machado, C. Definições, dimensões e determinantes da parentalidade. *Psychologica* **2010**, *52*, 211–229. [CrossRef]
7. Hoghughi, M. Parenting: An introduction. In *Handbook of Parenting: Theory and Research for Practice*; Hoghughi, M., Long, N., Eds.; SAGE Publications Ltd.: London, UK, 2004.
8. Ordem dos Enfermeiros. *Guia Orientador de Boa Prática: Adaptação à Parentalidade Durante a Hospitalização*; Ordem dos Enfermeiros: Lisboa, Portugal, 2015.
9. Cruz, O. *Parentalidade*; LivPsic: Porto, Portugal, 2005.

10. Figueiredo, M.H. *Modelo Dinâmico de Avaliação e Intervenção Familiar: Uma Abordagem Colaborativa em Enfermagem de Família*, 1st ed.; Lusociência—Edições Técnicas e Científicas, Lda: Loures, Portugal, 2012.
11. Macana, E.C.; Comim, F. O papel das práticas e estilos parentais no desenvolvimento da primeira infância. In *Fundamentos da Família Como Promotora do Desenvolvimento Infantil: Parentalidade em Foco*; Pluciennik, G.A., Lazzari, M.C., Chicaro, M.F., Eds.; Fundação Maria Cecilia Souto Vidigal: São Paulo, Brasil, 2015.
12. Nichiata, L.Y.I.; Bertolozzi, M.R.; Takahashi, R.F.; Fracolli, L.A. The use of the "Vulnerability" concept in the nursing area. *Rev Latino Am. Enferm.* **2008**, *16*, 923–928. [CrossRef] [PubMed]
13. Meleis, A.I. *Theoretical Nursing: Development and Progress*, 6th ed.; Wolters Kluwer: Philadelphia, PA, USA, 2018.
14. Ministério do Trabalho, Solidariedade e Segurança Social. Estratégia Nacional para a Integração das Pessoas em Situação de Sem-Abrigo (ENIPSSA) 2017-2023. In Presidência do Conselho de Ministros, Resolução do Conselho de Ministros n.° 107/2017, Diário da República n.° 142/2017—Série, I. Available online: https://data.dre.pt/eli/resolconsmin/107/2017/07/25/p/dre/pt/html (accessed on 5 January 2019).
15. Anderson, L.; Stuttaford, M.; Vostanis, P. A family support service for homeless children and parents: User and staff perspectives. *Child Fam. Soc. Work* **2006**, *11*, 119–127. [CrossRef]
16. Vostanis, P. Mental health of homeless children and their families. *Adv. Psychiatr. Treat* **2002**, *8*, 463–469. [CrossRef]
17. Kim, K.; Garcia, I. Why Do Homeless Families Exit and Return the Homeless Shelter? Factors Affecting the Risk of Family Homelessness in Salt Lake County (Utah, USA) As a Case Study. *Int. J. Environ. Res. Public Health* **2019**, *16*, 4328. [CrossRef]
18. Simões Figueiredo, A.; Seabra, P.; Sarreira-Santos, A.; Vollrath, A.; Medeiros Garcia, L.; Vidal, T.; Neves Amado, J. Nursing consultation in a public bathhouse: A community resource for the vulnerable population in a European capital. *Issues Ment. Health Nurs.* **2019**, *40*, 28–32. [CrossRef]
19. Gultekin, L.; Brush, B.L. In their own words: Exploring family pathways to housing instability. *J. Fam. Nurs.* **2017**, *23*, 90–115. [CrossRef]
20. Simões Figueiredo, A.; Vidal, T.; Sarreira-Santos, A.; Medeiros-Garcia, L.; García-Padilla, F.; Seabra, P. Nursing consultation in public showers: What lies beyond the results? *Issues Ment. Health Nurs.* **2019**, *40*, 535–536. [CrossRef]
21. Grant, R.; Gracy, D.; Goldsmith, G. Twenty-five years of child and family homelessness: Where are we now? *Am. J. Public Health* **2013**, *103*, e1–e10. [CrossRef]
22. Pleace, N. Family Homelessness in Europe. In *Homeless in Europe. Family Homelessness in Europe*; Feantsa: Brussels, Belgium, 2019; Available online: https://www.feantsa.org/public/user/Resources/magazine/2019/Autumn/Homeless_in_Europe_Magazine_Autumn2019_final.pdf (accessed on 18 November 2019).
23. Baptista, I.; Marlier, E. *Fighting Homelessnes Sand Housing Exclusion in Europe: A Study of National Policies*; European Commission: Brussels, Belgium, 2019.
24. Martin-Fernandez, J.; Lioret, S.; Vuillermoz, C.; Chauvin, P.; Vandentorren, S. Food Insecurity in Homeless Families in the Paris Region (France): Results from the ENFAMS Survey. *Int. J. Environ. Res. Public Health* **2018**, *15*, 420. [CrossRef]
25. Sylvestre, J.; Kerman, N.; Polillo, A.; Lee, C.M.; Aubry, T.; Czechowski, K. A qualitative study of the pathways into and impacts of family homelessness. *J. Fam. Issues* **2018**, *39*, 2265–2285. [CrossRef]
26. Bassuk, E.L.; Richard, M.K.; Tsertsvadze, A. The prevalence of mental illness in homeless children: A systematic review and meta-analysis. *J. Am. Acad. Child Adoles. Psychiatr.* **2015**, *54*, 86–96. [CrossRef] [PubMed]
27. Haskett, M.E.; Armstrong, J.M.; Tisdale, J. Developmental status and social-emotional functioning of young children experiencing homelessness. *Early Child. Educ. J.* **2015**, *44*, 19–125. [CrossRef]
28. Mzwandile, A.; Mabhala, M.A.; Yohannes, A. Being at the Bottom Rung of the Ladder in an Unequal Society: A Qualitative Analysis of Stories of People without a Home. *Int. J. Environ. Res. Public Health* **2019**, *16*, 4620. [CrossRef]
29. Gaetz, S.; O'grady, B.; Kidd, S.; Schwan, K. Without a Home: The National Youth Homelessness Survey. Available online: https://homelesshub.ca/sites/default/files/WithoutAHome-final.pdf (accessed on 21 January 2019).

30. Perlman, S.; Sheller, S.; Hudson, K.M.; Wilson, C.L. Parenting in the face of homelessness. In *Supporting Families Experiencing Homelessness. Current Practices and Future Directions*; Haskett, M., Perlman, S., Cowan, B.A., Eds.; Springer: New York, NY, USA, 2014.
31. Baptista, I. Women and homelessness. In *Homelessness Research in Europe: Festschrift for Bill Edgar and Joe Doherty*; O'Sullivan, E., Busch-Geertsema, V., Quilgars, D., Pleace, N., Eds.; Feantsa: Brussels, Belgium, 2010.
32. Lockwood, C.; Porrit, K.; Munn, Z.; Rittenmeyer, L.; Salmond, S.; Bjerrum, M.; Loveday, H.; Carrier, J.; Stannard, D. Chapter 2: Systematic reviews of qualitative evidence. In *Joanna Briggs Institute Reviewer's Manual*; Aromataris, E., Munn, Z., Eds.; The Joanna Briggs Institute: Adelaide, Australia, 2017; Available online: https://reviewersmanual.joannabriggs.org/ (accessed on 30 January 2019).
33. Moher, D.; Liberati, A.; Tetzlaff, J.; Altman, D.G. The PRISMA Group. Preferred Reporting Items for Systematic Reviews and Meta-Analyses: The PRISMA Statement. *PLoS Med.* **2009**, *6*, e1000097. [CrossRef]
34. Anthony, E.R.; Vincent, A.; Shin, Y. Parenting and child experiences in shelter: A qualitative study exploring the effect of homelessness on the parent-child relationship. *Child. Fam. Soc. Work* **2017**, *23*, 8–15. [CrossRef]
35. Cosgrove, L.; Flynn, C. Marginalized mothers: Parenting without a home. *Anal. Soc. Issues Public Policy* **2005**, *5*, 127–143. [CrossRef]
36. Haskett, M.E.; Armstrong, J.; Neal, S.C.; Aldianto, K. Perceptions of triple P-positive parenting program seminars among parents experiencing homelessness. *J. Child Fam. Stud.* **2018**, *27*, 1957–1967. [CrossRef]
37. Holtrop, K.; McNeil, S.; McWey, L.M. It's a struggle but I can do it. I'm doing it for me and my kids: The psychosocial characteristics and life experiences of at-risk homeless parents in transitional housing. *J. Marital Fam. Ther.* **2015**, *41*, 177–191. [CrossRef]
38. Lindsey, E.W. The process of restabilization for mother-headed homeless families: How social workers can help. *J. Fam. Soc. Work* **1997**, *2*, 49–72. [CrossRef]
39. Morris, R.I.; Butt, R.A. Parents' perspectives on homelessness and its effects on the educational development of their children. *J. Sch. Nurs.* **2003**, *19*, 43–50. [CrossRef] [PubMed]
40. Roche, S.; Barker, J.; McArthur, M. 'Performing' fathering while homeless: Utilising a critical social work perspective. *Br. J. Soc. Work* **2018**, *48*, 283–301. [CrossRef]
41. Tischler, V.; Karim, K.; Rustall, S.; Gregory, P.; Vostanis, P. A family support service for homeless children and parents: Users' perspectives and characteristics. *Health Soc. Care Community* **2004**, *12*, 327–335. [CrossRef] [PubMed]
42. Vanleit, B.; Starrett, R.; Crowe, T.K. Occupational concerns of women who are homeless and have children: An occupational justice critique. *Occup. Ther. Heal. Care* **2006**, *20*, 47–62. [CrossRef] [PubMed]

16

Nurse Manager Core Competencies: A Proposal in the Spanish Health System

Alberto González García [1], Arrate Pinto-Carral [2,*], Jesús Sanz Villorejo [3] and Pilar Marqués-Sánchez [4]

1. Department of Nursing and Physiotherapy, Universidad de León, 24401 Ponferrada, Spain; agong@unileon.es
2. SALBIS Research Group, Department of Nursing and Physiotherapy, Universidad de León, 24001 Ponferrada, Spain
3. Director of the University Dental Clinic, European University of Madrid, 28670 Madrid, Spain; jesus.sanz@universidadeuropea.es
4. SALBIS Research Group, Department of Nursing and Physiotherapy, Universidad de León, 24401 Ponferrada, Spain; pilar.marques@unileon.es

* Correspondence: apinc@unileon.es

Abstract: Nurses who are capable of developing their competencies appropriately in the field of management are considered fundamental to the sustainability and improvement of health outcomes. These core competencies are the critical competencies to be developed in specific areas. There are different core competencies for nurse managers, but none in the Spanish health system. The objective of this research is to identify the core competencies needed for nurse managers in the Spanish health system. The research was carried out using the Delphi method to reach a consensus on the core competencies and a Principal Component Analysis (PCA) to determine construct validity, reducing the dimensionality of a dataset by finding the causes of variability in the set and organizing them by importance. A panel of 50 experts in management and healthcare engaged in a four-round Delphi study with Likert scored surveys. We identified eight core competencies from an initial list of 51: decision making, relationship management, communication skills, listening, Leadership, conflict management, ethical principles, collaboration and team management skills. PCA indicated the structural validity of the core competencies by saturation into three components (α Cronbach >0.613): communication, leadership and decision making. The research shows that eight competencies must be developed by the nursing managers in the Spanish health system. Nurse managers can use these core competencies as criteria to develop and plan their professional career. These core competencies can serve as a guideline for the design of nurse managers' development programs in Spain.

Keywords: nurse manager; competence; core competencies; governance; leadership

---

1. Introduction

Economic and social changes have led to an adaptation of healthcare management at all levels and a change in the way in which services are provided [1–6]. The relationship between the economy and sustainability should be causes that make it necessary to develop management competencies with a high level of development, because these competencies are related to higher performance and outcomes [7–10]. To address these changes, nurses need to be part of the core of healthcare [2,4,11,12]. This claim is justified because the nurse is a professional with a high degree of leadership in many healthcare processes [13], because of their closeness to patients, families and the community [14]. Multiple research programs are led by nurses, including oncology, mental health, patient safety, palliative care and childcare, among others, which shows the importance of the nurse in the healthcare system [15–19]. For this reason, the participation of the nurse in the governance of healthcare organizations is recognized as fundamental, both for health outcomes and the sustainability of the health system [20–23].

The American Institute of Medicine, in its report entitled "The future of nursing: leading change in health", already identified nursing in 2010 as a key player in critical decision making and in the transformation of healthcare [24]. In the same way, Weber et al. [25] and McClaringan et al. [20] express themselves by stating that nursing is fundamental to the implementation of shared governance, because their commitment and participation is essential for the sustainability and improvement of health. Panayotou et al. [26] emphasizes nursing within strategic plans, so that their key actions are focused on the creation of a culture of good practice. Brooks-Cleator et al. [27], in his studies on transculturality and governance, focus on the importance of the nurse in establishing a culture of safety. The involvement of nurses in social action committees has achieved a great impact on the everyday problems of people [28], highlighting the importance of their participation in decision making [29]. When the nurse is involved in the different parts of the healthcare process (management and nursing care), better results are achieved [30], communication is enhanced, together with collaboration between the different professional groups, innovation, organizational commitment and retention of staff [23].

Nurse leaders and nurse manager are different roles, although there is a natural overlap of the required competencies [1,10,31]. To develop the role of the nurse in the governance of healthcare organizations, the Global Nursing Leadership Institute (GNLI) in the actions of Nursing Now (2020) has developed a nurse preparation program designed to promote leaders for change, focused on new policies to improve the health of the population [18,32]. Thus, to identify, mentor and train nurse leaders, the management competencies are an essential resource [31]. Furthermore, for the integration of nurses at different levels of organizational management and governance, the nurse should develop management competencies that go beyond the scope of nursing [33–35].

The nurse manager is responsible for planning and managing resources, organizing nursing care, supporting teamwork, evaluating the services provided, and contributing to the achievement of optimal results for the both the organization and the patients [36,37]. Based on the literature review, it is necessary to increase the knowledge of the role of the nurse manager [36,38–41], because the necessary competencies are often not clearly defined [35,42], which would explain this lack of conceptualization of the nurse manager's role. This same absence is evident in the Spanish context since there are no core competencies for carrying out management functions.

Core competencies are the collective learning of the organization, especially with regard to skills related to the generation of a product or service, so that all necessary knowledge and technologies are integrated [43,44]. The core competencies in nursing management are associated with the success of the healthcare organization [45]. Therefore, the core competencies for nurse managers are the set of fundamental competencies needed to ensure their work effectiveness [46]. There are three functional roles within nursing management, the operational nurse manager (performs his or her function at unit level), the logistic nurse manager (performs his or her function at the department level), and the top nurse manager (performs his or her function at the organizational level); all of them should develop the core competencies to help improve the quality of healthcare. [46].

Hence, the main objective of this study is to propose the core competencies to be developed by the nurse manager in the Spanish health system. To achieve this objective, the following specific objectives were set:

- To determine core competencies for each functional level of nursing management by expert consensus;
- To describe the level of development of competencies for each functional level of nursing management by expert consensus;
- To describe the training needed to develop each of the required competencies by expert consensus;
- To evaluate the structural validity of the proposed core competencies.

This paper is laid out as follows: first, the current state of knowledge about the nurse manager is described. The second part explains the research methods. Next, the results are presented and interpreted. Finally, the paper includes a discussion and conclusion.

2. Materials and Methods

2.1. Review Literature

Based on a scoping literature review during 2018-19 to identify existing competencies related to nurse managers, electronic databases were used (Web of Science, Scopus, PubMed and CINAHL) to conduct the search, identifying 56 competencies for nurse managers. Relevant studies were identified, such as that carried out by the American Organization of Nurse Executives (AONE) who established two competency models for nurse managers [47]. In addition, the literature review identified other important research to define competencies—for example, the Chase instrument [48] or the research carried out by Kantanen [42], DeOnna [35] or Pillay [49], among others. The results of this review are the foundation for the execution of the current Delphi study, which assesses the competencies for nurse manager positions.

2.2. Delphi Methodology

The study was carried out through four rounds of the Delphi method. The Delphi method is a method used to obtain a consensus from a group of experts [50], where the overall view will provide more solid information than that offered by a single person on an individual basis, thus reducing the subjectivity [50,51]. The questionnaires were administered through the LimeSurvey online platform. The questionnaires included an instruction form for the expert, the authorization to participate in the research and the instructions. A reminder email was sent every 4 days until a reply was received. After the survey, the researchers selected or excluded the items that received less than 80% agreement among experts.

The objective of the first Delphi round was to reach a consensus among the panel of experts about the core competencies for nurse managers. During the second round, the experts were asked individually if they wished to reconsider their opinions in light of the feedback. In the third round, the experts were asked to provide a consensus about the core competencies at each nurse manager on a functional level. The experts also agreed on the training required for each level of competence (expert, very competent, competent, novice advanced and novice). The fourth round allowed experts to reconsider their opinions in view of the feedback from the third round.

2.2.1. Consensus

In any Delphi study, the definition of consensus should be set a priori. Thus, for this research, we defined the consensus in three ways: (I) if at least 80% of the experts agreed with the competencies, responding "agree" or "complete agreement" in the questionnaires; (II) if at least 80% of the experts agreed with the degree of development of the competencies; (III) if at least 80% of the experts agreed with the type of training required. Where an agreement was not reached, items were deleted for the next Delphi round.

2.2.2. Participants

In this study, we decided to invite experts from two categories and twelve groups: experts in health management (Table 1) and experts in the health environment (Table 1), because experts in these two categories have valuable knowledge on nursing management.

Table 1. Socio-demographic data from the panel of experts.

Demographic Variable			Frequency
Gender			
		Female	32 (64%)
		Male	18 (36%)
Age			
		Mean	49.52
		Standard deviation	11.02
		<40 years	10 (20%)
		41–50 years	15 (30%)
		51–60 years	18 (36%)
		>60 years	7 (14%)
Education			
		Master's degree	34 (68%)
		Ph.D.	14 (28%)
Scope of representation			
Expert group	Group 1	Minister of Health	3 (6.1%)
	Group 2	Head of the Health Department	5 (10%)
	Group 3	General Council of Nurses	3 (6%)
	Group 4	Scientific Association	4 (8%)
	Group 5	Trade Union	3 (6%)
	Group 6	General Manager	5 (10%)
	Group 6	Medical Director	2 (4%)
	Group 6	Nurse Executive	5 (10%)
	Group 6	Management Director	1 (2%)
	Group 7	Middle Nurse manager	2 (4.1%)
	Group 8	Nursing supervisor	3 (6.1%)
	Group 9	Nurse	3 (6.1%)
	Group 9	Doctor	2 (4.1%)
	Group 9	Assistant Nursing Care Technician	2 (4.1%)
	Group 10	Nursing Degree Students	2 (4.1%)
	Group 11	Research/Teaching	4 (8.2%)
	Group 12	Lawyer	1 (2%)

Source: own elaboration.

2.2.3. Variables

The variables of the study were:

- Socio-demographic variables: To define the profile of the experts, information was collected related to age, sex, profession, university education, postgraduate education, professional role, place of study, years of professional practice, years of management experience, management functions performed and international experience;
- Competencies: From the review of the literature emerged the list of competencies to be proposed for the experts.

2.2.4. The Delphi Questionnaires

Two questionnaires were developed ad hoc as measuring instruments.

- Competencies needed for nurse managers (Appendix A): Each participant rated his/her level of agreement or disagreement with each competency according to a one to five Likert scale (1 = complete disagreement, 5 = complete agreement);
- Level of competency development for nurse managers (Appendix B): In order to reach a consensus about the level of development of the competencies at each level of management, the degree of

agreement or disagreement with each competency according to a one to five Likert scale (1 = novice, 5 = expert), and the type of training required to develop the competencies, according to a one to six Likert scale (1 = University Extension Diploma, 2 = Continuing education, 3 = University Expert, 4 = University specialization diploma, 5 = master's degree, 6 = Ph.D.) was recorded.

2.2.5. Level of Development

For this research, the term "level of development" was used to refer to the level of deepening in each competency that the nurse manager should acquire in each of the functional levels, thus the level of development would be:

- Novice: follows the rules and plans;
- Novice advanced: can provide partial solutions to unfamiliar or complex situations;
- Competent: strong demonstration of competency;
- Very competent: significant demonstration of competency;
- Expert: when demonstrating the behavior of the competency model.

2.2.6. Validity and Reliability

The validity and reliability of the questionnaires was carried out with a group of 12 people selected on the basis of the same criteria used for the panel of experts. The reliability of the questionnaires was ensured by carrying out a Cronbach's Alpha Coefficient analysis. The content validity was estimated through expert judgement, which analyzed errors and ambiguities in the formulation of the questions, excess items, proposals for improvement, suggestions for the style of the surveys.

2.3. Principal Component Analysis

The Principal Component Analysis (PCA) is a data transformation technique. The aim of the method is to reduce the dimensionality of multivariate data, while preserving as much of the relevant information as possible [52]. The factor analyses were carried out with respect to the theory of Thurstone [53,54] (3 phases): first, the assessment of the adequacy of the data for factorial analysis, second, the extraction of factors, and finally the rotation and interpretation of factors.

For determining the suitability of the data for factorial analysis, we used the Kaiser–Meyer–Olkin (KMO) test. The next step was the extraction of factors, using Kaiser's criteria, which makes the decision based on an eigenvalue greater than one [55], and a scree plot, which is a graphical representation of the eigenvalues. This graph helps to find the inflexion point and the number of factors above this point that should be retained [56]. Finally, we proceeded with the rotation and interpretation of the factors, through the varimax rotation method and Kaiser standardization, to achieve a structure as simple as possible that was easy to interpret [57].

3. Results

3.1. Demographics of the Expert Panel

A total of 50 experts consented to participate and took part in the Delphi study. Table 1 lists the demographic characteristics of the complete expert panel. The response rate for all of the Delphi rounds was 100%.

3.2. Delphi Study

During the first and second Delphi rounds, 51 competencies were agreed by consensus (more than 80%) from the proposed list. In round 1, the percentage of "total agreement" was 100% ("agreed" or "complete agreement") with the competencies decision making, communication skills, listening and conflict management. In this round, more than 80% of the experts were in "total agreement" with eight competencies (Table·2): decision making, communication skills, listening, leadership, conflict management, ethical principles, collaboration and team management skills.

Experts in round 2 were provided with individual feedback from the round 1 survey. This feedback included the complete expert panel responses. Participants were asked if they agreed or disagreed with the statements that were made in the previous round. From round 2, it appears that the experts showed a "complete agreement" with a percentage equal to 100% in the competencies identified as the core competencies (Table 2). In round 2, the competencies with less than an 80% consensus were eliminated.

Table 2. Core of competencies.

Competency	Total Agreement	
	Round 1	Round 2
Decision making	100%	100%
Relationship management	84%	100%
Communication skills	100%	100%
Listening	100%	100%
Leadership	84%	100%
Conflict Management	100%	100%
Ethical principles	80%	100%
Collaboration and team management skills	88%	100%

Source: own elaboration.

During the third and fourth Delphi rounds, the eight competencies from the core competencies were shown to be necessary for the three levels of nurse manager existing in Spain (operations, logistics and top management), differing in the level of development of the competencies at each level of management ("Expert", "very competent" and "competent"). The panel of experts in round 3 were asked about the level of development of each competency to reach a consensus. The experts in round 4 were again provided with individual feedback from round 3, and asked to indicate their agreement with statements that were made by participants in the previous round. The final consensus is shown in Table 3.

Table 3. Development of core competencies at each level of nurse manager.

Competency	Top Management	Logistics	Operations
Decision making	Expert	Very competent	Very competent
Relationship management	Very competent	Very competent	Very competent
Communication skills	Expert	Very competent	Expert
Listening	Expert	Very competent	Expert
Leadership	Expert	Competent	Expert
Conflict Management	Very competent	Very competent	Very competent
Ethical principles	Expert	Very competent	Expert
Collaboration and team management skills	Expert	Very competent	Expert

Source: own elaboration.

During the third round, the experts were asked to indicate their opinion about the appropriate training to reach the right level of competency. In round 4, experts were again provided with individualized feedback from the previous round. The final consensus is shown in Table 4.

Table 4. Training required by competency level.

Competency Level	Type of Training (Consensus)
Novice	University Extension Diploma (100%) Continuing education (98%)
Novice advanced	University Extension Diploma (90%) Continuing education (90%) University Expert (90%)
Competent	Continuing education (96%) University Expert (100%) University Specialization Diploma (96%)
Very competent	University Expert (96%) University specialization diploma (96%) Master's degree (96%)
Expert	Master's degree (96%) Ph.D. (96%)

Source: own elaboration.

3.3. *Principal Component Analysis*

The data were suitable for factoring as the correlation matrix showed a predominance of meaningful results ($p < 0.05$), Bartlett's test was significant ($p < 0.001$) and KMO value was 0.505. The integration of competency listening into the competency communication skills was appropriate for factoring (as shown in Table 5).

Table 5. Principal Component Analysis (PCA) of core competencies.

	CP 1	CP2	CP3	
Communication skills	0.851			
Relationship management	0.771			
Conflict Management	0.620			
Leadership		0.877		
Collaboration and team management skills		0.841		
Ethical principles			0.773	
Decision making			0.706	
Explained variance	28.43%	22.665%	17.576%	
Eigenvalue	1.99	1.587	1.230	
α Cronbach				0.613

Source: own elaboration. Caption: communication (CP), leadership (CP2), decision making (CP3).

The extraction of factors showed three factors that explained 68.67% of the total accumulated variance. The varimax rotation method yielded a three-factor solution: communication, leadership and decision making (Table 5). The observed convergence between the Kaiser criteria and the scree plot adds certainty to the results. The reliability of the core competencies showed a Cronbach's alpha value of 0.613, indicating a satisfactory result. (Table 5).

4. Discussion

This paper reports on the findings of the core competencies to be developed by the nurse manager in the Spanish health system. Decision making, relationship management, communication skills, listening, leadership, conflict management, ethical principles, collaboration and team management skills were seen as the core competencies for nurse managers. These findings are consistent with the findings from previous studies [47,51,52]. Kantanen et al. [42] emphasizes competency in decision making as a critical competency. McCarthy [58] highlights core competencies that are aligned with our research in communication, relationship management, ethical values and decision making. Our research is also aligned with Pillay [59] and with Gunawan [60], when he described relationship management, conflict management and collaboration and team management as basic competencies.

To emphasize the strength of the core competencies identified in this research, we should say that this were also identified through a scoping review of the literature, with the exception of the listening skills and ethical principles, which were not found among the most frequent results in the review. It should be noted that the frequency of citation in the selected articles was used as a criterion for identifying the core competencies in the literature review.

This study identified that all the core competencies are needed independent of the functional level of nurse managers (executive management, logistics and operational management). Although each functional level requires different levels of competency development to be reached. There was a consensus between the experts in Delphi rounds 3 and 4. These findings are consistent with findings from previous studies (e.g., [47,58]). McCarthy et al. [58] highlighted that core competencies should be common to all three levels of management at different degrees of development. The AONE [61] has shown shared competencies in their different models ("Nurse Manager Competency", "Nurse Executive Competencies" and "Nurse Executive Competencies: CNE system"), and in the Nurse Executive Competency Assessment Tool, which differentiates the degree of development of each competency. In another sense, the AONE also defined non-shared competencies in their models.

With regard to the development of competencies, an agreement was reached in Delphi rounds 3 and 4. The experts agreed that competencies should be developed at "competent" (this was considered to have been reached when there is a strong demonstration of competency), "very competent" (level reached when there is a significant demonstration of competency) and "expert" level (level reached when it demonstrates the behavior of the competency model). This proposal is in agreement with AONE, who use the levels competent, proficient and expert for the development of competencies, emphasizing how these levels are reached through master's degree studies or a Ph.D. [62,63]. In contrast, in other studies such as "Nurse manager competencies", the focus is on the degree to which the competencies contribute to the nurse manager's work (minimally, moderately, significantly and essentially) [48]. Furthermore, the results of the current study emphasize the need for a high level of competence development, in the same way that Crawford et al. [64] demonstrated by indicating how executive practice would require a high degree of specialization and a specific development of competencies.

During Delphi rounds 3 and 4, the expert panel achieved a consensus about the training to be developed by the nurse manager on the three competency levels ("expert", "very competent" and "competent"). The "competent" level is reached through continuing education, University Expert and University specialization diploma. With regard to the "very competent" level, the consensus was reached with University expert, University specialization diploma or master's degree. Finally, the "expert" level is reached through master's and Ph.D. studies. We should keep in mind how work experience and education significantly influence the development of competencies of nurse managers [65]. However, experience as a nurse manager does not prepare them for the wide range of skills needed, requiring specialized training and work experience in concrete situations [33,66]. Learning experientially as a nurse manager should be accompanied by prior planning and close mentoring [67]. Previous studies show that the quality and level of training are responsible for orienting nurse managers towards good governance and the acquisition of the global vision of the organization [33,68,69]. Furthermore, the results of the current study emphasize how it is possible to appreciate differences between nurse managers who have completed advanced management programs with respect to others who have not participated in this type of training program, adding evidence to previous studies [68,70]. We share the recommendations given by the Joint Commission for Accreditation of Healthcare Organizations regarding the development of different career levels for nurses according to their level of education, training and experience [71]. In addition, and just like Fralic [72] affirmed, our results suggest that the training received by nurse managers would be one of the key aspects, because they are responsible for managing the area with the largest number of people, to make decisions about resource management and other areas such as quality of care, patient safety, research, training, expenditure or investment. The present study, along with other previous studies such as the research carried out by Herrin et al. [73], support that the master's degree training allows the nurse manager to be able to carry out adequate decision making, as well as for the effective management of health processes. In the same way, Rizani et al. [74] point out that the average competence of nurses is higher when they have developed advanced studies (master's degree or Ph.D.), increasing with time their level of competency to a higher degree than those nurses who have not developed advanced training.

The PCA verified the core competencies by defining three principal components named communication (communication skills, relationship management, conflict management), leadership (leadership and team management skills) and decision making (decision making and ethical principles), which would therefore constitute the competency factors to develop the role of a nurse manager in Spain (Table 6). The strength of the eigenvalue confirms the importance of the relationship between decision making and ethical principles [75], the need for strong leadership in working groups [76] and communication as a fundamental element in conflict resolution [77]. By comparing the core competencies emerging from our research with the most relevant international studies into core competencies for nurse managers, we would find a shared factor with communication, which should indeed be presented as a shared factor [25,78,79].

Table 6. Comparison of core competencies.

Core Competencies	**Leach et al. [79]**	**Weber [25]**	**Aone [47]**
Communication	Organizational Management	Influence	Leadership
Leadership	Interpersonal effectiveness	Emotional Intelligence	Professionalism
Decision making	Systemic thinking Creative thinking	Result orientation Change Management	Communication Leadership
	Technical skills	Communication	Knowledge of the health environment
	Ability to adapt Customer Service Personal domain	Management vision	

Source: own elaboration.

The communication ability that would be expected from the nurse manager should include the ability to convey critical thinking and generate reflection in nurse teams prior to action [36]. In the same way, it should, for example, facilitate conflict resolution and shared decision making, as well as creation, participation and team management [80]. The differences that would arise between all the core competencies could be related to the different health contexts in which management practice takes place [58].

The purpose of this study was to determine the core competencies for each functional level of nursing management by expert consensus. Our research contributes strong and important evidence to the nursing management field. Firstly, we provide a baseline of competencies for nurses who intend to carry out functions as nurse managers. Secondly, our study is also useful as a tool for evaluating and detecting areas for improvement for nurse managers. Finally, the core competencies should be useful for planning the professional development of nurse managers.

With regard to the limitations of this research, we should mention the different healthcare contexts from which the body of research knowledge is derived. Nursing management has specific characteristics for each of these contexts.

5. Conclusions

This study found core competencies for nurse managers in Spain. The successful nurse manager should develop all these competencies (as relevant to their practice) in today's rapidly evolving healthcare system. In conclusion, this study yielded a consensus on eight core competencies for nurse managers in Spain: decision making, relationship management, communication skills, listening, leadership, conflict management, ethical principles, collaboration and team management skills, oriented towards leadership and good governance of health organizations, and on the basis of the social responsibility of health professionals. The nurse manager is responsible for the largest area of a healthcare organization, managing large budgets and large numbers of nurses. Therefore, a nurse should not be promoted to the role of a nurse manager without advanced management training.

Our research shows the precise level of development of each competency for the different functional levels of nurse manager. The nurse manager at any functional level should develop these core competencies before being promoted to other roles as a nurse manager.

Any nurse who wishes to develop his or her professional career as a nurse manager should first develop the core competencies shown here.

Moreover, our research shows the necessary education required to acquire the competency development necessary for each different nursing management role. Both nurses who want to be promoted to nurse managers and current nurse managers should follow the educational programs shown in order to adapt their knowledge to the requirements of the role.

These core competencies may have implications for practice, organizational policy, and education related to nursing management. The proposed core competencies may contribute to nurse manager role design, selection processes, and nurse manager curriculum design for traditional academic institutions and organizational continued professional development programs. Further understanding of core competencies is likely to inform interventions, which may improve nurses' work environment, patient care, patient safety and organizational outcomes.

The following research should develop the characteristics corresponding to each of these competencies and training situations.

Author Contributions: Conceptualization, A.G.G.; A.P.-C.; P.M.-S.; and J.S.V.; methodology, A.P.-C.; A.G.G.; validation, M.P.-S.; formal analysis, M.P.-S.; A.P.-C.; investigation, A.G.G. and P.M.-S.; resources, J.S.V.; and writing—original draft preparation, A.G.G. and P.M.-S.; writing—review and editing, A.G.G.; A.P.-C.; P.M.-S.; J.S.V. All authors have read and agreed to the published version of the manuscript.

Appendix A. Competencies Needed for Nurse Managers

Please select the appropriate answer for each concept:

Table A1. List of competencies.

Level of Agreement Competency	1	2	3	4	5
Financial skills					
Analytical Thinking					
Decision-making					
Innovation					
Strategic Management					
Human Resources Management					
Legal aspects					
Marketing					
Organizational Management					
Relationship Management					
Communication skills					

Table A1. *Cont.*

Level of Agreement Competency	1	2	3	4	5
Feedback					
Evaluation of information and its sources					
Listening					
Information systems and computers					
Technology					
Leadership					
Career planning					
Influence					
Change Management					
Delegate					
Conflict Management					
Ethical principles					
Power and Empowerment					
Critical thinking					
Collaboration and team management skills					
Interpersonal Relations					
Multi-professional management					
Team Building Strategies					
Result orientation					
Care Management Systems					
User care skills					
Health policy					
Identification and responsibility with the organization					
Knowledge of the health environment					
Quality and Safety					
Quality and improvement processes					
Clinical skills					
Infection control practices					
Standard Nursing Practice					
Nurse Research					
Nursing Theories					
Care Planning					
Nursing training planning					
Professionalism					
Integrity					
Awareness of Personal Strengths and Weaknesses					
Strategic Vision					
Personal and professional balance					
Compassionate					
Diversity					
Emotional Intelligence					
Serve as a model					
Basic Oral English					
English medium level of writing					
English medium reading level					

Caption: 1 = Complete disagreement; 2 = Disagreement; 3 = No disagreement/No agreement; 4 = Agreement 5 = Complete agreement.

Appendix B. Level of Competency Development for Nurse Managers

In this section, you should mark which functional level(s) each competency corresponds to, taking into account that the competency may be necessary for all three levels.

You should also indicate the level of development of this competence.

Table A2. Development of competencies

Competency		Novice	Novice Advancing	Competent	Very Competent	Expert
Decision-making	Operations Logistics Top managment					
Relationship Management	Operations Logistics Top managment					
Communication skills	Operations Logistics Top managment					
Listening	Operations Logistics Top managment					
Leadership	Operations Logistics Top managment					
Conflict Management	Operations Logistics Top managment					
Ethical principles	Operations Logistics Top managment					
Collaboration and team management skills	Operations Logistics Top managment					

Indicate to which degree of training each competence level should be developed:

Table A3. Type of training required

	U. Ext D	C. Edu.	U. Exp	U. Spec. D.	Master	Ph.D.
Novice						
Novice advanced						
Competent						
Very competent						
Expert						

Caption: University Extension Diploma (U. Ext D); Continuing education (C. Edu); University Expert (U. Exp); University specialization diploma (U. Spec. D.); Master's degree (Master); Ph.D (Ph.D).

References

1. Kantanen, K.; Kaunonen, M.; Helminen, M.; Suominen, T. Leadership and management competencies of head nurses and directors of nursing in Finnish social and health care. *J. Res. Nurs.* **2017**, *22*, 228–244. [CrossRef]
2. Nursing Now. Vision Nursing Now. 2019. Available online: https://www.nursingnow.org/vision/?doing_wp_cron=1577348723.0888390541076660156250 (accessed on 26 December 2019).
3. Cathcart, E.B.; Greenspan, M. A new window into nurse manager development. *J. Nurs. Adm.* **2012**, *42*, 557–561. [CrossRef] [PubMed]
4. Cummings, G.; MacGregor, T.; Davey, M.; Lee, H.; Wong, C.A.; Lo, E.; Muise, M.; Stafford, E. Leadership styles and outcome patterns for the nursing workforce and work environment: A systematic review. *Int. J. Nurs. Stud.* **2010**, *47*, 363–385. [CrossRef] [PubMed]
5. Fennimore, L.; Wolf, G. Nurse Manager Leadership Development: Leveraging the Evidence and System-Level Support. *J. Nurs. Adm.* **2011**, *41*, 204–210. [CrossRef] [PubMed]
6. Ding, B.; Liu, W.; Tsai, S.B.; Gu, D.; Bian, F.; Shao, X. Effect of patient participation on nurse and patient outcomes in inpatient healthcare. *Int. J. Environ. Res. Public Health* **2019**, *16*, 1344. [CrossRef]
7. Boyatzis, R.E. *The Competent Manager: A Model for Effective Performance*; John Wiley & Sons: Toronto, CA, Canada, 1982; ISBN 0-471-09031-X.
8. Groves, K. Talent management best practices: How exemplary health care organizations create value in a down economy. *Health Care Manag. Rev.* **2011**, *3*, 227–240. [CrossRef]
9. Kerfoot, K.M.; Luquire, R. Alignment of the system's chief nursing officer: Staff or direct line structure? *Nurs. Adm. Q.* **2012**, *36*, 325–331. [CrossRef]

10. MacMillan-Finlayson, S. Competency development for nurse executives: Meeting the challenge. *J. Nurs. Adm.* **2010**, *40*, 254–257. [CrossRef]
11. Thorne, S. Nursing now or never. *Nurs. Inq.* **2019**, *26*, e12326. [CrossRef]
12. Aiken, L.H.; Cimiotti, J.P.; Sloane, D.M.; Smith, H.L.; Flynn, L.; Neff, D.F. Effects of nurse staffing and nurse education on patient deaths in hospitals with different nurse work environments. *Med. Care* **2011**, *49*, 1047–1053. [CrossRef]
13. Savage, C.; Kub, J. Public health and nursing: A natural partnership. *Int. J. Environ. Res. Public Health* **2009**, *6*, 2843–2848. [CrossRef] [PubMed]
14. McHugh, G.A.; Horne, M.; Chalmers, K.I.; Luker, K.A. Specialist community nurses: A critical analysis of their role in the management of long-term conditions. *Int. J. Environ. Res. Public Health* **2009**, *6*, 2550–2567. [CrossRef] [PubMed]
15. McPherson, C.; Ndumbe-Eyoh, S.; Betker, C.; Oickle, D.; Peroff-Johnston, N. Swimming against the tide: A Canadian qualitative study examining the implementation of a province-wide public health initiative to address health equity. *Int. J. Equity Health* **2016**, *15*, 0419–0424. [CrossRef] [PubMed]
16. Cummings, G.; Lee, S.D.; Tate, K.C. The evolution of oncology nursing: Leading the path to change. *Can. Oncol. Nurs. J.* **2018**, *28*, 314–317.
17. Lasater, K.; Sloane, D.; McHugh, M.; Aiken, L. *End of Life Care Quality Remains a Problem–Nurses May be a Solution*; University of Pennsylvania School of Nursing: Philadelphia, PA, USA, 2019; Available online: https://www.nursing.upenn.edu/live/news/1276-end-of-life-care-quality-remains-a-problem-nurses (accessed on 27 December 2019).
18. Campbell, L. Leadership-Patients: Empowering professionalism and celebrating the future. Patient Blood Management: Challenges of Providing a State-wide Service. In Proceedings of the Nursing &Midwifery Leadership Conference, Perth, Australia, 28–29 November 2019.
19. Rogers, J.; Middleton, S.; Wilson, P.H.; Johnstone, S.J. Predicting functional outcomes after stroke: An observational study of acute single-channel EEG. *Top. Stroke Rehabil.* **2019**, *9*, 1–12. [CrossRef]
20. McClarigan, L.; Mader, D.; Skiff, C. Yes, We Can and Did: Engaging and Empowering Nurses through Shared Governance in a Rural Health Care Setting. *Nurse Lead.* **2019**, *17*, 65–70. [CrossRef]
21. Kerfoot, K. Four measures that are key to retaining nurses. *Hosp Health Netw.* 2015. Available online: https://www.hhnmag.com/articles/3253-four-measures-that-are-key-to-retaining-nurses (accessed on 27 December 2019).
22. Press Ganey. *Nursing Special Report: The Influence of Nurse Manager Leadership on Patient and Nurse Outcomes and the Mediating Effects of the Nurse Work Environment Nurse*; Press Ganey: South Bend, IN, USA, 2017; Volume 26, pp. 3–23.
23. Ho, E.; Principi, E.; Cordon, C.P.; Amenudzie, Y.; Kotwa, K.; Holt, S.; Macphee, M. The Synergy Tool: Making Important Quality Gains within One Healthcare Organization. *Adm. Sci.* **2017**, *7*, 32. [CrossRef]
24. Institute of Medicine of the National Academies. *The Future of Nursing: Leading Change, Advancing Health*; Institute of Medicine of the National Academies: Washington, DC, USA, 2010; Volume 40, pp. 1–4.
25. Weber, E.; Ward, J.; Walsh, T. Nurse leader competencies: A toolkit for success. *Nurs. Manag.* **2015**, *46*, 47–50. [CrossRef]
26. Panayotou, M.S.; Cefaratti, D.; Hanscom, H.; Petto, P.N.; Turner, R.R.; Talley, L. Shared governance strategic plan creation and implementation. *Nurs. Manag.* **2019**, *50*, 9–12. [CrossRef]
27. Brooks-Cleator, L.; Phillipps, B.; Giles, A. Culturally Safe Health Initiatives for Indigenous Peoples in Canada: A Scoping Review. *Can. J. Nurs. Res.* **2018**, *50*, 202–213. [CrossRef]
28. Kanninen, T.H.; Häggman-Laitila, A.; Tervo-Heikkinen, T.; Kvist, T. Nursing shared governance at hospitals–it's Finnish future? *Leadersh. Health Serv. (Bradf. Engl.)* **2019**, *32*, 558–568. [CrossRef]
29. Clavelle, J.; Porter O'Grady, T.; Drenkard, K. Structural empowerment and the nursing practice environment in magnet organizations. *J. Nurs. Adm.* **2013**, *43*, 566–573. [CrossRef]
30. Whitt, M.; Baird, B.; Wilbanks, P.; Esmail, P. Tracking decisions with shared governance. *Nurse Lead.* **2011**, *9*, 53–55. [CrossRef]
31. Meadows, M.T.; Dwyer, C. AONE continues to guide leadership expertise with post-acute competencies. *Nurse Lead.* **2015**, *13*, 21–25. [CrossRef]
32. Catton, H. International Council of Nurses: Putting nurses at the centre of the world's policymaking has benefits for us all. *Int. Nurs. Rev.* **2019**, *66*, 299–301. [CrossRef] [PubMed]

33. Baxter, C.; Warshawsky, N. Exploring the acquisition of nurse manager competence. *Nurse Lead.* **2014**, *12*, 46–59. [CrossRef]
34. Chase, L.K. Are you confidently competent? *Nurs. Manag.* **2012**, *43*, 50–53. [CrossRef] [PubMed]
35. DeOnna, J. Developing and Validating an Instrument to Measure the Perceived Job Competencies Linked to Performance and Staff Retention of First-Line Nurse Managers Employed in a Hospital Setting. Ph.D. Thesis, The Pennsylvania State University, College of Education, State College, PA, USA, 2006.
36. Scoble, K.B.; Russell, G. Vision 2020, part I: Profile of the future nurse leader. *J. Nurs. Adm.* **2003**, *33*, 324–330. [CrossRef]
37. AONE. AONE Nurse Executive Competencies. Available online: http://www.aone.org/resources/nurse-leader-competencies.shtml (accessed on 12 November 2019).
38. Meadows, M.T. New Competencies for System Chief Nurse Executives. *J. Nurs. Adm.* **2016**, *46*, 235–237.
39. Pihlainen, V.; Kivinen, T.; Lammintakanen, J. Management and leadership competence in hospitals: A systematic literature review. *Leadersh. Health Serv.* **2016**, *29*, 95–110. [CrossRef]
40. Shirey, M.R. Stress and coping in nurse managers: Two decades of research. *Nurs. Econ.* **2006**, *24*, 193–203. [PubMed]
41. Vance, M. Scotland the brave: Statutory supervision transformed. *Pract. Midwife* **2009**, *12*, 16–77. [PubMed]
42. Kantanen, K.; Kent, B.; Kaunonen, M.; Helminen, M.; Suominen, T. The development and pilot of an instrument for measuring nurse managers' leadership and management competencies. *J. Res. Nurs.* **2015**, *20*, 667–677. [CrossRef]
43. Tampoe, M. Exploiting the core competences of your organization. *Long Range Plan.* **1994**, *27*, 66–77. [CrossRef]
44. Higgins, J.M. Innovation: The core competence. *Plan Rev.* **1995**, *23*, 32–36. [CrossRef]
45. Garman, A.N.; Johnson, M.P. Leadership Competencies: An Introduction. *J. Healthc. Manag.* **2006**, *51*, 13–17. [CrossRef] [PubMed]
46. Prahalad, C.K.; Hamel, G. The Core Competence of the Corporation. *Harv. Bus. Rev.* **1990**, *68*, 1–15.
47. AONE. AONE Nurse Executive Competencies. *Nurse Lead.* **2015**, *3*, 15–22.
48. Chase, L. Nurse Manager Competencies. Ph.D. Thesis, University of Iowa, Iowa City, IA, USA, 2010.
49. Pillay, R. Towards a competency-based framework for nursing management education. *Int. J. Nurs. Pract.* **2010**, *16*, 545–554. [CrossRef]
50. Linstone, H.A.; Turoff, M.; Helmer, O. *The Delphi Method*; Addison-Wesley: Redeading, MA, USA, 1975; ISBN 0-201-04294-0.
51. Varela-Ruiz, M.; Díaz-Bravo, L.; García-Durán, R. Descripción y usos del método Delphi en investigaciones del área de la salud. *Investig. Educ. Méd.* **2012**, *1*, 90–95.
52. Sewell, M. *Principal Component Analysis*; University College London: London, UK, 2008.
53. Thurstone, L.L. Multiple factor analysis. *Psychol. Rev.* **1931**, *38*, 406–427. [CrossRef]
54. Thurstone, L.L. *Multiple Factor Analysis*, 5th ed.; University of Chicago Press: Chicago, IL, USA, 1957.
55. Kaiser, H.F. The Application of Electronic Computers to Factor Analysis. *Educ. Psychol. Meas.* **1960**, *20*, 141–151. [CrossRef]
56. Cattell, R.B. The scree test for the number of factors. *Multivar. Behav. Res.* **1966**, *1*, 245–276. [CrossRef] [PubMed]
57. Carroll, J.B. An analytical solution for approximating simple structure in factor analysis. *Psychometrika* **1953**, *18*, 23–38. [CrossRef]
58. McCarthy, G.; Fitzpatrick, J.J. Development of a Competency Framework for Nurse Managers in Ireland. *J. Contin. Educ. Nurs.* **2009**, *40*, 346–350. [CrossRef]
59. Pillay, R. The skills gap in nursing management in South Africa: A sectoral analysis: A research paper. *J. Nurs. Manag.* **2010**, *18*, 134–144. [CrossRef]
60. Gunawan, J.; Aungsuroch, Y.; Fisher, M.L. Factors contributing to managerial competence of first-line nurse managers: A systematic review. *Int. J. Nurs. Pract.* **2018**, *24*, 1–12. [CrossRef]
61. AONE. Competencies Assessment. Available online: http://www.aone.org/resources/online-assessments.shtml (accessed on 18 August 2019).
62. Waxman, K.T.; Roussel, L.; Herrin-Griffith, D.; D'Alfonso, J. The AONE Nurse Executive Competencies: 12 Years Later. *Nurse Lead.* **2017**, *15*, 120–126. [CrossRef]

63. Crawford, C.L.; Omery, A.; Spicer, J. An Integrative Review of 21st-Century Roles, Responsibilities, Characteristics, and Competencies of Chief Nurse Executives: A Blueprint for the Next Generation. *Nurs. Adm. Q.* **2017**, *41*, 297–309. [CrossRef]
64. Sandehang, P.M.; Hariyati, R.T.; Rachmawati, I.N. Nurse career mapping: A qualitative case study of a new hospital. *BMC Nurs.* **2019**, *18*, 1–9. [CrossRef]
65. Kuraoka, Y. Effect of an experiential learning-based programme to foster competence among nurse managers. *J. Nurs. Manag.* **2018**, *26*, 1–9. [CrossRef] [PubMed]
66. Warshawsky, N.; Cramer, E. Describing Nurse Manager Role Preparation and Competency: Findings from a National Study. *J. Nurs. Adm.* **2019**, *49*, 249–255. [CrossRef] [PubMed]
67. Kleinman, C.S. Leadership Roles, Competencies, and Education: How Prepared Are Our Nurse Managers? *J. Nurs. Adm.* **2003**, *33*, 451–455. [CrossRef] [PubMed]
68. ANA. *Nursing Administration: Scope and Standards of Practice*, 2nd ed.; Nursesbooks.org; ANA: Washington, DC, USA, 2018; ISBN 9781558106444.
69. West, M. Evaluation of a nurse leadership development programme. *Nurs. Manag.* **2016**, *22*, 26–31. [CrossRef] [PubMed]
70. Rees, S.; Glynn, M.; Moore, R.; Rankin, R.; Stevens, L. Supporting nurse manager certification. *J. Nurs. Adm.* **2014**, *44*, 368–371. [CrossRef] [PubMed]
71. Joint Comission on Accreditation of Healthcare Organizations. Health Care at the Crossroads: Strategies for Addressing the Evolving Nursing Crisis. Available online: Shorturl.at/mCDTV (accessed on 24 August 2019).
72. Fralic, M.F. Patterns of preparation. The nurse executive. *J. Nurs. Adm.* **1987**, *17*, 35–38. [CrossRef]
73. Herrin, D.; Hathaway, D.; Jacob, S.; McKeon, L.; Norris, T.; Spears, P.; Stegbauer, C. A model academic-practice partnership. *J. Nurs. Adm.* **2006**, *36*, 547–550. [CrossRef]
74. Rizany, I.; Hariyati, R.T.; Handayani, H. Factors that affect the development of nurses' competencies: A systematic review. *Enferm. Clin.* **2018**, *28*, 154–157. [CrossRef]
75. Loreggia, A.; Mattei, N.; Rossi, F.; Venable, K.B. Preferences and Ethical Principles in Decision Making. In Proceedings of the 2018 AAAI/ACM Conference on AI, Ethics and Society-AIES '18, New York, NY, USA, 2–3 February 2018.
76. Berrios Martos, P.; Lopez Zafra, E.; Aguilar Luzon, M.C.; Auguste, J.M. Relationship between leadership style and attitude toward working groups. *Int. J. Psychol.* **2008**, *43*, 444.
77. Codier, E.; Codier, D.D. Could Emotional Intelligence Make Patients Safer? Specific skills might help nurses to improve communication, conflict resolution, and individual and team performance. *Am. J. Nurs.* **2017**, *117*, 58–62. [CrossRef]
78. Carlson, E.E.; Kline, M.M.; Zangerle, C.M. AONE Competencies: Preparing Nurse Executives to Lead Population Health. *Nurse Lead.* **2016**, *14*, 108–112. [CrossRef]
79. Leach, L.S.; McFarland, P. Assessing the professional development needs of experienced nurse executive leaders. *J. Nurs. Adm.* **2014**, *44*, 51–62. [CrossRef] [PubMed]
80. Garman, A.N.; Fitz, K.D.; Fraser, M.M. Communication and relations management. *J. Healthc. Manag.* **2006**, *51*, 291–294. [PubMed]

17

Experiences of Nursing Students during the Abrupt Change from Face-to-Face to E-Learning Education during the First Month of Confinement Due to COVID-19 in Spain

Antonio Jesús Ramos-Morcillo [1], César Leal-Costa [1,*], José Enrique Moral-García [2,*] and María Ruzafa-Martínez [1]

1 Faculty of Nursing, University of Murcia, 30100 Murcia, Spain; ajramos@um.es (A.J.R.-M.); maruzafa@um.es (M.R.-M.)
2 Physical Activity and Sports Sciences, Faculty of Education, Pontifical University of Salamanca, Street Henry Collet, 52-70, 37007 Salamanca, Spain
* Correspondence: cleal@um.es (C.L.-C.); jemoralga@upsa.es (J.E.M.-G.)

Abstract: The current state of alarm due to the COVID-19 pandemic has led to the urgent change in the education of nursing students from traditional to distance learning. The objective of this study was to discover the learning experiences and the expectations about the changes in education, in light of the abrupt change from face-to-face to e-learning education, of nursing students enrolled in the Bachelor's and Master's degree of two public Spanish universities during the first month of confinement due to the COVID-19 pandemic. Qualitative study was conducted during the first month of the state of alarm in Spain (from 25 March–20 April 2020). Semi-structured interviews were given to students enrolled in every academic year of the Nursing Degree, and nurses who were enrolled in the Master's programs at two public universities. A maximum variation sampling was performed, and an inductive thematic analysis was conducted. The study was reported according with COREQ checklist. Thirty-two students aged from 18 to 50 years old participated in the study. The interviews lasted from 17 to 51 min. Six major themes were defined: (1) practicing care; (2) uncertainty; (3) time; (4) teaching methodologies; (5) context of confinement and added difficulties; (6) face-to-face win. The imposition of e-learning sets limitations for older students, those who live in rural areas, with work and family responsibilities and with limited electronic resources. Online education goes beyond a continuation of the face-to-face classes. Work should be done about this for the next academic year as we face an uncertain future in the short-term control of COVID-19.

Keywords: COVID-19; pandemics; students; nursing; teaching; education; distance; schools; Life Changing Events; qualitative research

---

1. Introduction

The fast propagation of the severe acute respiratory syndrome coronavirus 2 (SARS-CoV-2) led to its definition as a pandemic on 13 March 2020 by the WHO [1], as it met the epidemiological criteria and had infected more than 100,000 people in 100 countries [2–4]. The main public health recommendation was to remain at home and stay safe within it [5]. The world, in a globalized manner, is facing an extraordinary public health emergency in which the nurses are, as always, on the front line. Challenges are even greater in this period of pandemic [6,7], and nurses have the knowledge and aptitudes for providing the care necessary in the different clinical scenarios [5] that are emerging.

However, this pandemic is not only affecting the area of health. A great part of the nursing activity is affected as well. In Spain, as well as in other countries, the presence of nursing students in health care centers has been suspended [5]. It has been observed how, at great speeds, schools and universities have closed in the world, affecting more than 1.570 million students in 191 countries [8]. It has been necessary to decide how to continue the education of future nurses, and multiple education solutions have been deployed, all of which are based on distance learning. The professors, experts in the subjects and knowledgeable about the didactics of traditional classes, have found themselves compelled to deal with e-learning overnight, although not all of them were prepared. The same has occurred with the students, who have had to change from a model based on obligations and face-to-face learning, to a model in which the students will have to freely and voluntarily become involved in their learning [9]. All of this aside from finding themselves in a context of expectation and uncertainty.

Nursing educators (teachers, managers) must guarantee that the students meet the academic requirements, and at the same time, recognize the current conditions faced by the health services and the needs of simultaneously satisfying the demands from students, parents, brothers, partners, and the multiple roles every individual play in their day-to-day lives. Internationally and locally, a great variety of criteria for learning and evaluation, etc., have appeared, which are adapted to their national, work and social contexts. For example, and with respect to evaluation, in Berkeley (California, USA), a pass/fail grading has been proposed [10], and in Spain, the Association of Spanish Universities (CRUE) has recommended adapting the evaluation tests utilizing distance learning evaluation procedures [11].

Understanding the experiences and expectations of the students when faced with this important change, is necessary for helping the education and teaching authorities to assign sufficient resources and re-orient university education for nursing students. To be able to manage this situation in an imminent future, it is necessary to learn from these experiences and to define the strong and weak points. The objective of this study was to discover the learning experiences and the expectations about the changes in education of nursing students enrolled in the Bachelor's and Master's nursing degrees in two Spanish public universities, when faced with the abrupt change from face-to-face to e-learning education during the first month of confinement due to the COVID-19 pandemic.

2. Materials and Methods

2.1. Study Design

A qualitative approach was utilized, and an inductive thematic analysis [12] was conducted to understand the experiences and expectations of the participants.

2.2. Settings and Participants

This research study was conducted in its entirety during the first month of the state of alarm in Spain (which began on 14 March 2020). The state of alarm implied the confinement of the entire population, the closing of all the schools and universities, closing of non-essential businesses, closing of borders and ceasing all non-essential activities. The people were only allowed to go out to the street for essential matters: shopping of food, going to pharmacies, banks, and to care for older people who were dependent, etc.

In Spain, Bachelor's degree in Nursing has a duration of four years (240 European Credit Transfer System, ECTS) and it is common for a Master's degree to have a duration of one year (60 ECTS). The reference population in this study was students from every academic year in the Bachelor´s degree in Nursing, or nurses who were conducting their Master's studies, enrolled in universities in Murcia and Granada (Spain). The participants were selected through the use of a maximum variation sampling strategy [13] to obtain heterogeneous and rich information that represented the main sociodemographic variables: gender, age, academic year, rural/urban, children, Bachelor's/Master's, university of Murcia and Granada. The maximum variation strategy is utilized to find the greatest diversity of discourses possible to identify and analyze the largest volume possible of expressions/presentation of the phenomenon studied to explain conditions/contexts where each one of them takes place.

If one did not answer the request, the students themselves proposed a replacement with another participant with similar characteristics. None of the students contacted disagreed to participate.

The students were invited to participate through the Student Delegation at the university, utilizing snowball sampling. This technique allowed us to build the sample by asking each interviewee for suggestions of people who had a similar or different perspective. This is an approach for locating information-rich key informants [13]. The saturation criterion was applied to establish the number of informants needed, an accepted method to estimate the sample size [14].

2.3. Data Collection

Semi-structured interviews were conducted to obtain the information. The semi-structured interview is normally based on a script, where the subject matter and part of the questions have been planned before starting, but it also offers the possibility of changing or adding new questions as the interview and/or the research study moves forward, with new interviews conducted. It is the most common type of interview utilized in qualitative research on health. Data were collected from 25 March to 20 April 2020. This was done in the first month as it the period of time with the greatest cognitive and social impact on learning and to obtain results that could be used to support, or not, the education measures that were utilized. All the interviews were individual and were performed online through electronic resources after agreeing on a day and time. The interviews were recorded and notes were made after each interview. All the interviews were conducted by researchers who had sufficient training and experience in semi-structured interviews (A.J.R.-M., M.R.-M.). The interviewers did not have an academic relationship with the informants. The interview followed a script which shifted from general to specific matters, and dealt with general aspects of the confinement, teaching methodologies utilized, learning and expectations (Table A1). A prior pilot study of the script was conducted [15].

2.4. Data Analysis

The 6 phases proposed for the thematic analysis were followed [16]: (1) Familiarizing yourself with your data; (2) Generating initial codes; (3) Searching for themes; (4) Reviewing themes; (5) Defining and naming themes; (6) Producing the report. The recorded interviews were transcribed verbatim. Once transcribed, the interviews were imported to the MAXQDA 12 program for its posterior analysis. A.J.R.-M., M.R.-M., C.L.-C. and J.E.M.-G. coded the data. The transcriptions, coding and themes-subthemes were discussed by the research team for their verification. Finally, participants provided feedback on the findings. The study was reported according to the Consolidated Criteria for Reporting Qualitative Research (COREQ) [15].

2.5. Ethical Considerations

This research study was approved by the Research Ethics Commission from the University of Murcia (ID: 2800/2020). All the participants received an informational electronic document about the purpose and research process, which they later kept. They were advised that their participation was voluntary. They could ask and reflect prior to the interview. Each participant was given a code to maintain anonymity.

3. Results

A total of 32 interviews were conducted, and they lasted between 17 and 51 min. The shortest interviews corresponded to the more advanced academic years (3rd and 4th year students). Of these participants, 75% were women and 25% men. The age of the participants oscillated between 18–50 years old, with an average age of 25.3, and with a participation rate of 69% for the students from the University of Murcia, and 21.8% for the University of Granada students. The sample was composed by 18.75% of the students enrolled in their 1st or 2nd academic year or in the Master's program, which accounted for about 57% of the sample, and 21.8% from the 3rd and 4th academic years, for a total of about 43%. Of those interviewed, 21.8% had children and 21.8% lived in a rural setting. Some of the characteristics of the participants are found in Table 1.

Table 1. Characteristics of the participants and duration of the interviews.

N°	Gender	Age	University	Degree Year	Working	Interview Duration
1	Woman	20	Murcia	2	No	39 min
2	Woman	19	Murcia	2	No	50 min
3	Woman	21	Murcia	4	No	20 min
4	Woman	21	Murcia	4	No	20 min
5	Woman	28	Granada	1	Yes	38 min
6	Man	21	Granada	3	No	20 min
7	Woman	19	Granada	1	No	36 min
8	Woman	41	Murcia	1	Yes	38 min
9	Woman	50	Murcia	3	No	35 min
10	Woman	21	Granada	4	No	23 min
11	Woman	20	Murcia	2	No	51 min
12	Man	32	Murcia	4	Yes	23 min
13	Woman	19	Granada	2	No	37 min
14	Woman	22	Granada	4	No	19 min
15	Man	21	Murcia	4	No	17 min
16	Woman	20	Granada	1	No	28 min
17	Woman	46	Murcia	2	No	40 min
18	Woman	25	Murcia	3	No	31 min
19	Woman	20	Murcia	3	No	31 min
20	Woman	25	Murcia	1	Yes	29 min
21	Woman	26	Murcia	4	No	18 min
22	Man	24	Murcia	Master	Yes	25 min
23	Woman	23	Granada	Master	Yes	28 min
24	Man	22	Granada	Master	No	29 min
25	Woman	18	Murcia	1	No	33 min
26	Man	42	Murcia	3	No	29 min
27	Man	26	Murcia	3	No	30 min
28	Woman	24	Murcia	Master	Yes	30 min
29	Man	26	Murcia	3	No	30 min
30	Woman	20	Murcia	2	No	35 min
31	Woman	24	Granada	Master	No	26 min
32	Woman	26	Murcia	Master	No	36 min

Six major themes were defined: (1) practicing the nursing care; (2) uncertainty; (3) time; (4) teaching methodologies; (5) the context of confinement and the added difficulties; (6) face-to-face education win. A detailed description of the themes and sub-themes can be found in Table 2.

Table 2. Themes and subthemes.

Themes	Subthemes
Practicing the nursing care	The value of clinical training
	To help
Uncertainty	-
Time	Phases: 1st shock and 2nd normalization
	Time management
	The future
Teaching methodologies	Videoconference
	The rest of the methodologies
	Use profile of the methodologies by the professors
	Interaction with the teachers
The context of confinement and the added difficulties	-
Face-to-face win	Face-to-face is better ... for everything
	Older and female: face-to-face is better

3.1. *Practicing Nursing Care*

The outstandingly practical component of care in nursing education was the most emotional aspect for the students. The experiences found were differentiated according to the group of students, depending if they had or not practice-based subjects during the education period affected by the state of alarm, the proximity to ending their training as nurses, or if they were health professionals who were conducting post-graduate studies.

3.1.1. The Value of Clinical Training

For 1st and 2nd year students, the learning is normally done with courses that are eminently theoretical or theory/practical. The informants indicated that this transitory e-learning will not have a special influence on their training, as long as all the clinical training on health care institutions is present:

> *"In think that it's not something that will affect us excessively for good or bad. In my year [1st]. In other years it will, because they have clinical training" P5*

By contrast, 3rd and 4th year students whose coursework is mainly based on clinical training in health care institutions placed value on clinical training. They linked it with the acquisition of competences and referred to it as being an essential part of health sciences degrees:

> *"My education would not be good if clinical training was missing" P15; "without the clinical training, we can't acquire competences" P19; "Especially in our degree, the clinical training ... " P21*

Clinical training provides them with security in the learning of nursing care in health care services. Part of the students in their last year (4th year) indicated that they would rather not graduate in July to do all the clinical training, therefore graduating later:

> *"I don't feel prepared. My Erasmus in Italy was really bad because I was a nursing student and a foreigner. At the hospital, I don't feel confident" P10; "Some of us prefer not to graduate in June and to do the clinical training" P14*

The Master's students indicated that not being able to do the clinical training implied the loss of job opportunities:

> *"If you cannot do the clinical training, you will lose job opportunities" P22*

3.1.2. To Help

All the participants expressed their wish to help during the pandemic. They expressed their desire to be nurses to help. At the University of Granada, a list of volunteers in their 4th year was even created. The expectation was present that the government could mobilize them in case of need. Independently of the academic year, for all the students, this crisis re-enforced their wishes to become nurses:

> *"I wish I already had my degree" P17; "I wish to be a nurse already, too bad I wasn't in 4th year so I could go" P16; "If this happens in the future, I would like to be helping" P25; "I feel like left out, I can't be in the battlefield helping" P21; "Now I really feel like being a nurse. It is a shame that we cannot help. In Granada there is a list of volunteers. I really feel like helping" P14*

Master's students who work feel satisfied to be able to help (aside from being satisfied because they can work):

> *"I feel very well with myself because I can help, even though is very difficult ... " P23; "I really feel like being in the middle of it and help. I've seen that help is really needed, it is very important work, although not very much appreciated." P24*

3.2. Uncertainty

The lack of concretion about the different aspects related with their studies is mentioned by all the interviewees. This uncertainty is accompanied by unpleasant situations due to the possible outcomes. They are mainly related with matters that could not be resolved relatively fast, such as the clinical practice and the adaptation of evaluation processes:

> *"We don't know how they are going to evaluate us. They will for sure evaluate what we have done in the last month of clinical practices" P6; "We don't know what's going to happen. I hope they don't give a general pass. I want to take the exams and the other things. I don't want them to evaluate me with just one work submitted" P5; "Not knowing how things will be done. Not getting the grades I want to get because of these circumstances" P16*

This is especially important for the 4th-year students, who reported a great feeling of wasting time. They cannot go to the clinical practices and they only have, as well, one subject: the final project (TFG). One of the alternatives to not waste time completely and that is being done by the participants is to prepare for the access exam for clinical nurse specialist training (national post-graduate residency program, EIR). Some of the participants indicated that preparing for the EIR exam was a means of escape from a situation of wasting time and total paralysis:

> *"It takes my motivation away, and (finishing my degree) is getting really hard, because I don't see the end of it" P10; "I am not taking advantage of the time" P3; "I'm preparing for the EIR exam at the academy as a means of escape. With the only the TFG ... I need something else. Right now all my time is TFG and the subjects from the EIR" P4*

The 3rd-year students find themselves in the same situation but without any subjects:

> *"The 3rd years clinical training has been abandoned. They don't know if we are going to recover them" P6*

The Masters' students have a different point of view. The differences are many. The Masters' degree can provide job opportunities, the change from traditional education to e-learning practically affects an entire trimester (half of the Master's program), and in their discourse, they have fewer demands and less pressure for obtaining the degree. At the same time, they are the only ones who speak about the teaching guidelines, indicating that they are truly being followed. In comparison, only one Bachelor's degree student referred to the teaching guidelines:

> *"If the clinical training cannot be done, you miss job opportunities" P22; "I don't know how the teaching guidelines have changed" P16; "The clinical training have been postponed until September, and it bothers me some because it interferes with the summer contract for working as a nurse" P24*

3.3. Time

Time is a determinant transversal aspect. Two differentiated phases are observed as the state of alarm moved forward (1st shock and 2nd normalization). Besides, participants reflected regarding a necessary time management and the influence in the future.

3.3.1. Phases: 1st Shock and 2nd Normalization

Two well-differentiated phases are distinguished in the timeline. On the first days, the shock phase appears (1st phase), within which we find "disorientation". This first phase lasts between 7–10 days. During this first week, it is observed that mental performance decreases, along with the ability to concentrate. This is a subtle expectant phase, where the situations are not well defined:

> *"You think that the first week is for you, for resting, you take care of unfinished business and uncertainty increases" P11; "The first week was not assimilated, I didn't have routines" P19; "During the first week, I had less concentration and studies less" P5; "The timetable is different, it's more chaotic" P21*

After the first phase, the students enter a normalization phase (2nd phase) in which they acquire new routines, attend online classes and seminars. The conditions of confinement start to be assimilated and the new everyday life is normalized:

> *"Now I do more things than before, I take more notes. It is very different from the first week, now it is easier" P25; "Now I have the habits. Before I didn't do anything, and now I do everything, it is as if I'm getting used to it" P28*

The first phase, as well as the second phase also coincide with the period in which the university ensured that the online tools were fully functioning and instructions were given to the professors about how to continue with their teaching tasks:

> *"Only 2 out of 5 teachers give online classes, the rest upload presentations that we have to understand" P13; "The teachers do not agree with each other. One says one thing and another something else" P6*

3.3.2. Time Management

The 1st and 2nd year students, as well as the Masters' students, have classes. This forces them to manage their time differently. The 1st and 2nd year students interviewed indicated that time management was necessary. They indicated that this was beneficial for having good "mental health", and that having due dates helped them with managing their time:

> *"Having self-discipline and a timetable. Not rigid, but saying that the mornings were for University and the afternoons for watching T.V. series or exercising. If you don't organize your time, work accumulates" P20; "My planning is Monday to Friday mornings for work, and the afternoon for group work or leisure. I rest on the weekends. Having due dates has helped me organize" P13; "The homework is good, because they help with following the course" P11*

All of the participants, except for the ones who worked, indicated that they had changed their sleep schedule and go to bed much later, between 1:30 and 3 a.m. The main reason mentioned was that the lack of activity did not make them tired, although this argument was ambivalent, as they went to bed later and got up later as well, so they slept the same number of hours:

> *"It takes me longer to fall sleep. I'm not tired because I don't do anything during the day" P11; "I go to bed later and I get up later. I go to bed at 2–2:30 a.m. and I get up at 10" P5; "I fall sleep very late. At 2:00 a.m. The hours have changed, you sleep when you shouldn't" P19*

3.3.3. The Future

The participants indicate that this situation affects their future plans and expectations related with obtaining their degree and work. They believe that they can be singled out for being the promotion with missing education, their international training is paralyzed, and they are afraid. Their professional expectations are also affected:

> *"I'm afraid of having bad training and that the work exchange says that this year's promotion from the University of Granada do not have the competences necessary" P6; "The plans for earning money to go to an Erasmus program are cancelled . . . " P13; "The practices have been postponed to September, and yes, it bothers me because it interferes with the summer contract for working as a nurse" P24*

3.4. *Teaching Methodologies*

The participants indicate that as for the teachers, different teaching methodologies are being utilized: real-time videoconferences (including chats), lessons recorded on video and uploaded to the e-learning platform, audio podcast, chat (exclusively), homework and uploading of documents (Word, PPT, PDF). They also mention that as time goes on, the teacher's adaptation to the online resources continuously improve.

3.4.1. Videoconference

It is without a doubt the best evaluated. This is because they think it is the most similar to a traditional class (face-to-face), and allow interaction with the professor, and provides them with nearness. Another aspect they indicate as being valuable is that this methodology helps with the teacher's explanation of the subject that is more comprehensible as compared to other methodologies. The interaction is also valued, as it allows them to say that something has not been understood and that it should be explained in another way. Lastly, they would like all the videoconferences to be recorded so they could be watched again whenever needed. This last aspect was pointed out by the students who were also working:

> *"The interaction in the videoconferences is not the same, because the questions are written and it is not the same to write something than when you talk" P26; "The videoconference is where we receive feedback. You can say that you don't understand something and if it could be explained once again" P16; "It is a way to stay in touch. Doubts emerge and the teacher can resolve them" P7*

The Master's students indicate that on some occasions, the duration of the videoconference classes is excessive. It is interesting to highlight that the Bachelor's students did not state this at any time:

> *"We've had videoconferences that lasted 5 h. This can be done better. We had one who did a good summary and it lasted 2 h. This is more relaxing, and then you broaden the knowledge with the documents provided" P24*

Despite the value of the videoconferences, the discourse is ambivalent, as negative aspects are identified, especially related with the quality of interaction with the professor. The traditional classwork contributes fundamental elements in the quality of communication, and this how it is felt by the participants.

> *"It is worse. When the teacher sees you asking about a doubt, she/he knows where you are coming from. This is lost with e-learning. Information is lost and the student does not obtain the same information as in the face-to-face class. The teacher doesn't see your face." P24; "I'm much more in favor of traditional classes. I always obtain more information in them and I'm more comfortable." P24*

3.4.2. The Rest of the Methodologies

Except for the recorded lessons, the rest of the methodologies are catalogued as sub-standard. The chats (exclusively) and the homework are not attractive, although they value them as positive aspects because it lets them stay connected with the subject and the university:

"The worse thing is when they only upload class notes, no one forces you to read them" P25; "In the homework, there are questions because they are not easy to understand, with the explanation it is easy, but when you are going to do it, it is more difficult" P25

Among the limitations, they point out that in some asynchronous methodologies and with a rigid format, limited learning is obtained, interaction is needed for explanation, and a certain amount of pressure is needed. Another limitation is the lack of feedback with the homework:

"We are going to learn the minimum, but not all, because they don't explain it to you, they don't explain it in different ways. The text [from the documents] is only written in one way . . . " P7; "the works that don't have feedback give you half the knowledge" P13; "If you only upload notes, no one is forcing you to read them. It is very easy to fall into laziness when they only upload notes" P25

A limitation of e-learning that was pointed out by all the participants was that everything that was practice-related could not be learned. They identified this as a great limitation, and point out that in nursing, practice was vital:

"Many things are not understood through the computer. For example, the basic care laboratories have to be observed and practiced" P7; "The practical things not, but the theoretical yes. They can make a video, but it's not the same. They can tell us how to give a bath on a bed, but if you don't do it . . . " P5; "It is impossible to learn the practical part. Until you are not in that role, it is impossible to learn" P24

The students are not able to propose other methodologies that are distinct from the ones offered. Two students pointed out that it could be completed with gamification (kahoot):

"Gamification would be good, for example when calculating the dose" P19

3.4.3. Use Profile of the Methodologies by the Teachers

Within the methodologies, it was found that the least complex, for example, providing Word, PPT or PDF documents, were related to the older teachers. The videoconferences and recorded classes were given by younger teachers in general. At the same time, they indicated that teachers from other non-nursing departments utilized the least complex methodologies:

"It depends on the difficulty of the course. Physiology has only uploaded documents" P16; For example, Pharmacology is a very dense and complicated subject, and you need someone to explain it to you, and until now, we have not received anything, only notes. I don't think it's enough, they are too schematic and hard to understand". P1; "The younger ones (teachers) feel like doing more things" P19; "It is more difficult for some teacher, especially those who are older" P5

3.4.4. Interaction with the Teachers

They pointed out that it is good in the videoconferences. An inconvenience is that sometimes the teacher is not aware of the doubts posted on the chat if there are too many messages. In the chat, the interaction is good, but the interruptions, even though they may be short, makes it impossible to follow it. Lastly, the students are surprised about how fast the teachers answers the e-mails:

"The chat, if you miss 5 min, you get lost" P22; "There is a good reception by the teacher for communicating" P11; "[tutoring} they are good, the answer sooner. They have improved" P21

3.5. The Context of Confinement and the Added Difficulties

The context of confinement has created some limitations for following e-learning education. These are related with internet access, access to electronic devices, and work and family responsibilities.

In rural environments, situations exist where internet access is lacking, which creates problems with being up to date with the classes. Another problem indicated is that not all had internet at home, and situations exist in which a person only has the limited amount of data available from a smartphone:

"Some people do not have all the means" P25; "I don't have internet at home, I only have data from the smartphone" P27 "I live here in the countryside, and the internet does not always work well, and if my kids are connected, then I can't do anything" P17

The confinement has obliged working from home whenever possible. This implies that it is possible for a family with three children to need an internet connection at the same time and the availability of five electronic devices simultaneously to be able to work and follow the classes. This availability is not very common. Another limitation that was pointed out was working in the presence of children/siblings at home:

"With the children at home, things cannot be done [mothers]" P25; "Studying at home when the entire family is at home, it is very hard to concentrate sometimes, they make noise, I can't print, etc." P25

Part of the students pointed out that is inconvenient, as they are used to studying in public libraries and have had to study at home:

"I always study at the library, not at home" P19; "I used to go to the library to study or do homework. No one bothers me there. At home, I set the washer, put on my pajamas and go to sleep" P28

Another difficulty added by the confinement is that one is not "trained" for shifting to e-learning. One has experience with an education system that has never been 100% online and where the traditional class is the learning stage. With respect to online exams, they do not feel secure either:

"We are used to traditional classes. This has been difficult for everyone, and more for the bachelor students than the Masters ones" P23; "I supposed they will give multiple-choice exams in a short time. It is the first time it will be online and one could be tense" P13; "If I hear it from the teacher beforehand, I understand it better, and now it's different. You take notes and then you have to understand them ... " P16

3.6. Face-to-Face Win

3.6.1. Face-to-Face is Better ... for Everything

The participants clearly preferred face-to-face to e-learning education. When faced with the possibility that some percentage of online classes will be provided along with traditional classes in future academic years, they do not think it is an option that will contribute much or needed. An exception is provided by students who have family or work responsibilities, who, exclusively for the theoretical classes, prefer them to be online and recorded, in order to be able to watch them at any time. Another aspect that was underlined was that the traditional system of education is the one they know and are used to, and changing it is difficult:

"Face-to-face is better ... for everything" P17; "The University of Murcia is traditional, and we come from the same type of learning. It takes some time to adapt" P22; "Face-to-face is better in every aspect. For example, you learn the lesson and the teacher can provide examples, it can go further than the PowerPoint presentation. It is better to be face-to-face with the professor than through a screen" P23

3.6.2. Older and Female: Face-to-Face is Better

The older students seem to be the most vulnerable group, and various problems are observed. On the one hand, they have to tend to their children now that they are all at home, they have more responsibilities at home, plus certain digital competences that they have yet to incorporate. The management of their time is a great problem, which is influenced by the use of time, space and the electronic devices by the rest of the family, to which they grant them priority without being aware:

"For me the chat is not good, because I can't write that fast. I see the limitation in me. I miss the traditional classes. Face-to-face classes are better ... for everything" P17; "You have to be very alert

with the online classroom, that you do not ignore the messages. Yesterday there was a class, and did not know" P9; "Some classmates are much older, and this is difficult. They write to the group [WhatsApp] sending pictures, and asking "What do I do? Where should I click?"" P25; "I'm much more in favor of face-to-face classes. I always obtain more information in them and I'm more comfortable" P24

4. Discussions

It is necessary to underline that all the results and discussion are centered on the first month of confinement after the start of the state of alarm, and this brings with it very specific cognitive and social states that are needed for the proper understanding of the discussion of the present research study.

Although the sample included a greater number of students from the University of Murcia as compared to those from the University of Granada, and different percentages of men and women of different ages, we believe that the main sociodemographic variables were well represented through the use of maximum variation sampling.

The nurses usually become nurses due to their desire to help other people to recover and maintain optimal health, and here we find ourselves in a situation in which not many options are available to help those who are severely sick due to COVID-19 [5]. Vocation is a determinant factor for those who decided to study nursing, and the main drive is the opportunity to care for others [17]. Our results support these two ideas in two ways: (1) they indicate that this attitude towards their professional life is still true in the new generations, with the remarkable fact that all the participants are so committed and wishing to help. (2) the pandemic has positively re-enforced their wishes to become nurses, obtaining similar results as other authors [18]. Although, the state of alarm decree includes the possible mobilization of students in their last year at university, their mobilization was principally needed in a small scale in Madrid and Catalonia, the areas greatly affected by COVID-19 [19].

The fast shift to e-learning education has not ceased to be a continuation of teaching and education through online resources, although it has not been clearly planned and adapted for e-learning [10]. Our results clearly present various relevant ideas related to this. In first place, and related with the clinical training, the health science degrees and more specifically the nursing degree have an essential need to be developed in clinical context. This element clearly cannot be substituted, and is perceived by all the students as being essential. Nevertheless, at present, a discussion exists about how high-fidelity clinical simulation could substitute the clinical training in real-world environments [20,21]. This methodology, which facilitates an intermediate learning between the theoretical dimension and the practical dimension, is proposed, aspiring to construct a real environment. However, and despite it being a type of learning established and known by the student body at the University of Murcia as well as the Granada, it is striking that this type of learning has not been described as an alternative. We interpret this finding as the clinical training being indispensable for the students.

Also, it forces us to reflect if this is the new reality of health care, and if the future nursing professionals should learn how to navigate in these conditions. The debate regarding the return of the nursing students to clinical environments is open and some recommendation has been provided [22]. The question now for the universities and nursing educators is that if as soon as the resources are provided and an adequate organization and adaptation occurs, the students should return to the health care services, what is the balance between the potential risk for the students and the importance of the clinical training? In second place, and related with the teaching of theory, the students prefer face-to-face teaching as opposed to the e-learning. They believe that the interaction is higher in quality and learning is greater. At present, another debate is open, as shown by two systematic reviews that do not provide concluding results on the existence of the greater learning linked to e-learning education of health professionals and students, highlighting the poor quality of existing studies and the importance of contextual factors [23,24]. Perhaps due to these reasons, the videoconference, distance learning, but synchronous and bi-directional, is the best assessed.

Another critical aspect is that the change to the online methodology was not chosen by the students, and the expectations they have with respect to their studies have been clearly disrupted.

Their entire academic life has been marked by a specific style of teaching, and they have become organized to continue with it, but the pandemic has imposed a different one with which they do not feel comfortable yet, thereby creating uncertainty and little security. This worries a great part of the Health Science academics [25]. It therefore absolutely necessary to start to work on the adaptation to e-learning that takes into account the previously-mentioned aspects so that the student's uncertainty decreases, especially in light of the evaluations. Academics have already expressed awareness of the students' concerns that are centered on their future degree and career progression [25]. The university counted with a technological infrastructure that has been able to deal with a drastic and fast change to distance teaching. However, the urgency of adapting this type of teaching has highlighted some situations of disadvantage. Thus, the older students, as compared to the younger ones, and in great part women and mothers, do not possess the most basic digital competences. This finding is robust, as the older students themselves, as well as the younger ones, are able to point this out in agreement with each other. They also point out that there is a small percentage of students who do not have the electronic resources or a connection to the internet necessary for adequately following the teaching.

Universities are trying to provide answers to some of these problems. It could be said that the phases of shock and normalization described by the students coincided with the period of reaction and acts of implementation by the institutions. There are activities that allow for fast implementation. For example, the Universities of Murcia and Granada freely loaned laptop computers with software to 100% of the students who requested them [26], with this number being more than 300 students in Murcia alone, as well as mobile internet-access devices [27]. However, the implementation of activities related with the evaluation has required conscientious reflection and consensus that has forced their implementation later in time [11].

In any case, once this first stage has been overcome, and faced with the absence of permanent solutions for this pandemic in the short term, it is necessary to propose distance learning strategies with a robust design, with the time necessary to create study plans that are well thought-out and durable [10,28]. We should be aware that we are currently undergoing an "emergency" education, a temporary shift of instructional delivery to an alternate delivery mode due to crisis circumstances [29]. The reality is that this transition to e-learning under these circumstances has nothing to do with a design that takes the maximum advantage and possibilities of the online format. We should reflect on the differences in the rhythm, the student-instructor relationship, pedagogy, the role of the instructor, the role of the student, the synchronicity of online communication, the role of online evaluations, and the source of feedback [30].

Limitations

Among the limitations of the study, we find that a thorough discussion and comparison with the opinions of other authors has not been possible, given the novel and exceptional situation we are currently living in. On the other hand, we should be aware that the sample studied cannot be representative of the reference population, and this can evidently affect the generalization of the results.

5. Conclusions

After the first week of adaptation to the conditions of confinement and the establishment of new online teaching systems, the students begin a new normality. The imposition of e-learning brings more limitations to students who are older, with work and family responsibilities, living in a rural environment and with limited electronic resources. Online teaching has allowed substituting the teaching of theory, although face-to-face teaching is preferred, at the same time it has shown that clinical practices are indispensable for the training of the nursing students. Online education goes beyond the online continuation of the classes. The parties responsible should already be working on this for the next academic year, in light of the uncertain future of a short-term control of COVID-19.

Author Contributions: Conceptualization, A.J.R.-M., J.E.M.-G. and M.R.-M.; Data curation, A.J.R.-M.; Formal analysis, A.J.R.-M., C.L.-C. and M.R.-M.; Investigation, A.J.R.-M., C.L.-C.and M.R.-M.; Methodology, A.J.R.-M.,

C.L.-C., J.E.M.-G. and M.R.-M.; Project administration, A.J.R.-M.; Supervision, A.J.R.-M.; Validation, A.J.R.-M.; Writing—original draft, A.J.R.-M. and M.R.-M.; Writing—review & editing, A.J.R.-M., C.L.-C., J.E.M.-G. and M.R.-M. All authors have read and agreed to the published version of the manuscript.

Acknowledgments: Our most sincere thanks to the people who agreed to participate in this research.

Appendix A

Table A1. Interviews Guide.

Introductory questions. How is your . . . ?	- Leisure - Sleep - Rest - Diet - Exercise - Interrelation - Information about COVID19, where they are informed, if they have reviewed notes of any subject (handwashing, concept of prevalence, incidence...).
Online teaching methodology	- M1 Do you think that the university is providing an adequate response to the situation related to teaching? - M2 What types of tools are being proposed to you. - M3 Which one do you like best, describe advantages and disadvantages. - M4 What things/competencies cannot be learned (teaching limitations). - M5 Is it difficult to adapt to the communication channels that are used right now? - M6 Is the content given in class adequately adapted to online teaching methodologies? - M7 How is your interaction with other participants different from face-to-face? - M8 How is your interaction with the teacher? - M9 Tasks
Learning	- A1 How is time organized with this imposition - A2 Has your ability to concentrate and/or study been affected? - A3 What are the differences when studying in this manner? - A4 Do you think that this manner of learning forces a different type of learning management? Is it necessary to have more self-management? - A5 Is it possible to achieve learning in the same way as face-to-face learning, better, worse... - A6 What modalities, online methodologies do you propose for improving your online learning?
Expectations	- E1 Expectations about grades - E2 What influence do you think this way of teaching during this time will have on your training as a nurse. - E3 Do you think that after this online teaching a greater part of it will be necessary when everything returns to normal? Why? - E4 Are students prepared for this type of teaching? - E5 Do you think it is necessary to go one step further? Should this type of teaching go further?

Table A1. *Cont.*

4th year students	- AA1 What is going to happen? - AA2 What are you afraid of? - AA3 What do you think will happen with the practice? - AA4 What do you think will happen to your degree? - AA5 If you miss a practicum how good is your training?
Life expectancy	- How does the situation caused by the crisis in the professional field affect your desire to become a nurse?

References

1. World Health Organization. WHO Director-General's Opening Remarks at the Media Briefing on COVID-19-11 March 2020. Available online: https://www.who.int/dg/speeches/detail/who-director-general-s-opening-remarks-at-the-media-briefing-on-covid-19---11-march-2020 (accessed on 15 May 2020).
2. Remuzzi, A.; Remuzzi, G. COVID-19 and Italy: What next? *Lancet* **2020**, *395*, 1225–1228. [CrossRef]
3. Torri, E.; Sbrogiò, L.G.; Di Rosa, E.; Cinquetti, S.; Francia, F.; Ferro, A. Italian Public Health Response to the COVID-19 Pandemic: Case Report from the Field, Insights and Challenges for the Department of Prevention. *Int. J. Environ. Res. Public Health* **2020**, *17*, 3666. [CrossRef]
4. Choi, H.; Cho, W.; Kim, M.-H.; Hur, J.-Y. Public Health Emergency and Crisis Management: Case Study of SARS-CoV-2 Outbreak. *Int. J. Environ. Res. Public Health* **2020**, *17*, 3984. [CrossRef] [PubMed]
5. Jackson, D.; Bradbury-Jones, C.; Baptiste, D.; Gelling, L.; Morin, K.; Neville, S.; Smith, G.D. Life in the pandemic: Some reflections on nursing in the context of COVID-19. *J. Clin. Nurs.* **2020**. [CrossRef] [PubMed]
6. Tsai, J.; Wilson, M. COVID-19: A potential public health problem for homeless populations. *Lancet Public Health* **2020**, *5*, e186–e187. [CrossRef]
7. Nurchis, M.C.; Pascucci, D.; Sapienza, M.; Villani, L.; D'Ambrosio, F.; Castrini, F.; Specchia, M.L.; Laurenti, P.; Damiani, G. Impact of the Burden of COVID-19 in Italy: Results of Disability-Adjusted Life Years (DALYs) and Productivity Loss. *Int. J. Environ. Res. Public Health* **2020**, *17*, 4233. [CrossRef] [PubMed]
8. UNESCO & IESALC COVID-19 and higher education: Today and tomorrow. In *Impact Analysis, Policy Responses and Recommendations*; UNESCO: Paris, France, 2020.
9. Diez de la Cortina, S. Teaching in Times of Pandemic [Enseñar en Tiempos de Pandemia]. Available online: https://www.educaweb.com/noticia/2020/04/21/ensenar-tiempos-pandemia-19145/ (accessed on 15 May 2020).
10. Morin, K.H. Nursing Education After COVID-19: Same or Different? *J. Clin. Nurs.* **2020**. [CrossRef] [PubMed]
11. CRUE Universidades Españolas. Available online: http://www.crue.org/Documentos%20compartidos/Informes%20y%20Posicionamientos/Informe%20procedimientos%20evaluacio%CC%81n%20no%20presencial.pdf (accessed on 15 May 2020).
12. Braun, V.; Clarke, V. Using thematic analysis in psychology. *Qual. Res. Psychol.* **2006**, *3*, 77–101. [CrossRef]
13. Patton, M.Q. *Qualitative Evaluation and Research Methods*, 4th ed.; SAGE: Thousand Oaks, CA, USA, 2015; ISBN 978-1-4129-7212-3.
14. Morse, J.M. The Significance of Saturation. *Qual. Health Res.* **1995**, *5*, 147–149. [CrossRef]
15. Tong, A.; Sainsbury, P.; Craig, J. Consolidated criteria for reporting qualitative research (COREQ): A 32-item checklist for interviews and focus groups. *Int. J. Qual. Health Care* **2007**, *19*, 349–357. [CrossRef] [PubMed]
16. Kiger, M.E.; Varpio, L. Thematic analysis of qualitative data: AMEE Guide No. 131. *Med. Teach.* **2020**, 1–9. [CrossRef] [PubMed]
17. Eley, D.; Eley, R.; Bertello, M.; Rogers-Clark, C. Why did I become a nurse? Personality traits and reasons for entering nursing. *J. Adv. Nurs.* **2012**, *68*, 1546–1555. [CrossRef] [PubMed]
18. Swift, A.; Banks, L.; Baleswaran, A.; Cooke, N.; Little, C.; McGrath, L.; Meechan-Rogers, R.; Neve, A.; Rees, H.; Tomlinson, A.; et al. COVID-19 and student nurses: A view from England. *J. Clin. Nurs.* **2020**. [CrossRef] [PubMed]

19. Rodríguez Veiga, D. Nursing Students are Already Risking Their Lives Against Covid-19 with Precarious Contracts [Las Estudiantes de Enfermería ya se Juegan la Vida Contra el Covid-19 con Contratos Precarios]. Available online: https://www.elespanol.com/sociedad/20200331/estudiantes-enfermeria-juegan-vida-covid-19-contratos-basura/478703443_0.html (accessed on 23 May 2020).
20. Sullivan, N.; Swoboda, S.M.; Breymier, T.; Lucas, L.; Sarasnick, J.; Rutherford-Hemming, T.; Budhathoki, C.; Kardong-Edgren, S. (Suzie) Emerging Evidence Toward a 2:1 Clinical to Simulation Ratio: A Study Comparing the Traditional Clinical and Simulation Settings. *Clin. Simul. Nurs.* **2019**, *30*, 34–41. [CrossRef]
21. Hayden, J.K.; Smiley, R.A.; Gross, L. Simulation in Nursing Education: Current Regulations and Practices. *J. Nurs. Regul.* **2014**, *5*, 25–30. [CrossRef]
22. Hayter, M.; Jackson, D. Pre-registration undergraduate nurses and the COVID-19 pandemic: Students or workers? *J. Clin. Nurs.* **2020**. [CrossRef] [PubMed]
23. Fontaine, G.; Cossette, S.; Maheu-Cadotte, M.-A.; Mailhot, T.; Deschênes, M.-F.; Mathieu-Dupuis, G.; Côté, J.; Gagnon, M.-P.; Dubé, V. Efficacy of adaptive e-learning for health professionals and students: A systematic review and meta-analysis. *BMJ Open* **2019**, *9*, e025252. [CrossRef] [PubMed]
24. Voutilainen, A.; Saaranen, T.; Sormunen, M. Conventional vs. e-learning in nursing education: A systematic review and meta-analysis. *Nurse Educ. Today* **2017**, *50*, 97–103. [CrossRef] [PubMed]
25. Pather, N.; Blyth, P.; Chapman, J.A.; Dayal, M.R.; Flack, N.A.M.S.; Fogg, Q.A.; Green, R.A.; Hulme, A.K.; Johnson, I.P.; Meyer, A.J.; et al. Forced Disruption of Anatomy Education in Australia and New Zealand: An Acute Response to the Covid-19 Pandemic. *Anat. Sci. Educ.* **2020**, *13*, 284–300. [CrossRef] [PubMed]
26. University of Murcia The Notica. Newsletter of ÁTICA of the University of Murcia [La Notica. *Boletín informativo de ÁTICA de la Universidad de Murcia*]. Available online: https://www.um.es/notica/boletin14/prestamo.htm (accessed on 29 May 2020).
27. University of Granada 1,000 Internet Connection Lines for Students Who Have Difficulty Connecting [1.000 Líneas de Conexión a Internet Para los Estudiantes con Dificultades Para Conectarse]. Available online: https://covid19.ugr.es/noticias/1000-lineas-conexion-internet-estudiantes-dificultades (accessed on 29 May 2020).
28. McCormack, B. What value nursing knowledge in a time of crisis? *J. Clin. Nurs.* **2020**. [CrossRef] [PubMed]
29. Hodges, C.; Moore, S.; Lockee, B.; Trust, T.; Bond, A. The Difference Between Emergency Remote Teaching and Online Learning. Available online: https://er.educause.edu/articles/2020/3/the-difference-between-emergency-remote-teaching-and-online-learning (accessed on 13 May 2020).
30. Means, B.; Bakia, M.; Murphy, R. *Learning Online: What Research Tells Us about Whether, When and How*; Routledge: New York, NY, USA, 2014.

Permissions

All chapters in this book were first published by MDPI; hereby published with permission under the Creative Commons Attribution License or equivalent. Every chapter published in this book has been scrutinized by our experts. Their significance has been extensively debated. The topics covered herein carry significant findings which will fuel the growth of the discipline. They may even be implemented as practical applications or may be referred to as a beginning point for another development.

The contributors of this book come from diverse backgrounds, making this book a truly international effort. This book will bring forth new frontiers with its revolutionizing research information and detailed analysis of the nascent developments around the world.

We would like to thank all the contributing authors for lending their expertise to make the book truly unique. They have played a crucial role in the development of this book. Without their invaluable contributions this book wouldn't have been possible. They have made vital efforts to compile up to date information on the varied aspects of this subject to make this book a valuable addition to the collection of many professionals and students.

This book was conceptualized with the vision of imparting up-to-date information and advanced data in this field. To ensure the same, a matchless editorial board was set up. Every individual on the board went through rigorous rounds of assessment to prove their worth. After which they invested a large part of their time researching and compiling the most relevant data for our readers.

The editorial board has been involved in producing this book since its inception. They have spent rigorous hours researching and exploring the diverse topics which have resulted in the successful publishing of this book. They have passed on their knowledge of decades through this book. To expedite this challenging task, the publisher supported the team at every step. A small team of assistant editors was also appointed to further simplify the editing procedure and attain best results for the readers.

Apart from the editorial board, the designing team has also invested a significant amount of their time in understanding the subject and creating the most relevant covers. They scrutinized every image to scout for the most suitable representation of the subject and create an appropriate cover for the book.

The publishing team has been an ardent support to the editorial, designing and production team. Their endless efforts to recruit the best for this project, has resulted in the accomplishment of this book. They are a veteran in the field of academics and their pool of knowledge is as vast as their experience in printing. Their expertise and guidance has proved useful at every step. Their uncompromising quality standards have made this book an exceptional effort. Their encouragement from time to time has been an inspiration for everyone.

The publisher and the editorial board hope that this book will prove to be a valuable piece of knowledge for researchers, students, practitioners and scholars across the globe.

List of Contributors

Lianping Yang, Wenmin Liao, Na Zhang and Cunrui Huang
School of Public Heath, Sun Yat-sen University, Guangzhou 510080, China

Chaojie Liu
School of Psychology and Public Health, La Trobe University, Melbourne 3086, Australia

Shuang Zhong
Center for Chinese Public Administration Research, School of Government, Sun Yat-sen University, Guangzhou 510275, China

Tatjana Fischer
Institute of Spatial Planning, Environmental Planning and Land Rearrangement, University of Natural Resources and Life Sciences Vienna, Peter-Jordan-Straße 82, 1190 Vienna, Austria

Markus Jobst
Department for Geodesy and Geoinformation, Research Group Cartography, Vienna University of Technology, Erzherzog-Johann-Platz 1/120-6, 1040 Vienna, Austria

Elena Ortega-Campos
Faculty of Psychology, University of Almería. Carretera de Sacramento s/n, 04120 Almería, Spain

Guillermo A. Cañadas-De la Fuente and Luis Albendín-García
Faculty of Health Sciences, University of Granada, Avenida de la Ilustración, 18016 Granada, Spain

Carolina Monsalve-Reyes
Departamento de Ciencias Sociales, Universidad Católica de La Santísima Concepción, Avenida Alonso de Ribera, 2850 Concepción, Chile

E. Inmaculada de la Fuente-Solana
Brain, Mind and Behaviour Research Center (CIMCYC), University of Granada, Campus Universitario de Cartuja, 18071 Granada, Spain

María González-García and Yolanda Valcárcel-Álvarez
Health Care Service of Asturias, Central University Hospital of Asturias, Avda. Roma, s/n, 33011 Oviedo, Spain
Department of Medicine, School of Medicine and Health Sciences, University of Oviedo, Avda. Julián Clavería, s/n, 33006 Oviedo, Spain
Healthcare Research Area, Health Research Institute of Asturias (ISPA), Avda. Roma, s/n, 33011 Oviedo, Spain

Alberto Lana and Ana Fernández-Feito
Department of Medicine, School of Medicine and Health Sciences, University of Oviedo, Avda. Julián Clavería, s/n, 33006 Oviedo, Spain
Healthcare Research Area, Health Research Institute of Asturias (ISPA), Avda. Roma, s/n, 33011 Oviedo, Spain

Paula Zurrón-Madera
Department of Medicine, School of Medicine and Health Sciences, University of Oviedo, Avda. Julián Clavería, s/n, 33006 Oviedo, Spain
Healthcare Research Area, Health Research Institute of Asturias (ISPA), Avda. Roma, s/n, 33011 Oviedo, Spain
Mental Health Center of La Corredoria, Health Care Service of Asturias (Spain), C. Alfredo Blanco, s/n, 33011 Oviedo, Spain

Ana Fernandez-Araque and Julia Gomez-Castro
Department of Nursing, Faculty of Health Sciences, University of Valladolid, 42004 Soria, Spain

Andrea Giaquinta-Aranda
Department of Nursing, Faculty of Health Sciences, University of Valladolid, 42004 Soria, Spain
Haemodialysis Service, Santa Bárbara Hospital, 42005 Soria; Spain

Zoraida Verde
Department of Biochemistry, Molecular Biology and Physiology, University of Valladolid, 42004 Soria, Spain

Clara Torres-Ortega
Department of Nursing, Faculty of Health Sciences, University of Valladolid, 42004 Soria, Spain
Emergency Service of the Hospital Santa Bárbara, 42005 Soria, Spain

Rosario Fernández-Peña
Department of Nursing, University of Cantabria (Spain), SALBIS Research Group, Nursing Research Group IDIVAL, 39008 Santander, Spain

José Luis Molina
Department of Social and Cultural Anthropology, GRAFO, Universitat Autònoma de Barcelona, 08193 Barcelona, Spain

Oliver Valero
Servei d'Estadística Aplicada, Universitat Autònoma de Barcelona, 08193 Barcelona, Spain

Jison Ki
College of Nursing, Seoul National University, 103, Daehak-ro, Jongno-gu, Seoul 03080, Korea

Jaegeum Ryu and Jihyun Baek
The Research Institute of Nursing Science, Seoul National University, 103, Daehak-ro, Jongno-gu, Seoul 03080, Korea

Iksoo Huh and Smi Choi-Kwon
College of Nursing, Seoul National University, 103, Daehak-ro, Jongno-gu, Seoul 03080, Korea
The Research Institute of Nursing Science, Seoul National University, 103, Daehak-ro, Jongno-gu, Seoul 03080, Korea

Yudai Kobayashi, Misari Oe, Tetsuya Ishida, Michiko Matsuoka, Hiromi Chiba and Naohisa Uchimura
Department of Neuropsychiatry, Kurume University School of Medicine, Asahi-machi 67, Kurume 830-0011, Japan

Pantaleo Greco
Department of Medical Sciences, University of Ferrara, 44121 Ferrara, Italy
Obstetrics and Gynecology Unit, Azienda Ospedaliero-Universitaria S. Anna, 44121 Ferrara, Italy

Rosaria Cappadona
Department of Medical Sciences, University of Ferrara, 44121 Ferrara, Italy
Obstetrics and Gynecology Unit, Azienda Ospedaliero-Universitaria S. Anna, 44121 Ferrara, Italy
Department of Nursing, Instituto Maimónides de Investigación Biomédica de Córdoba (IMIBIC), 14071 Córdoba, Spain

Marco Di Muzio
Department of Clinical and Molecular Medicine, Sapienza University of Rome, 00185 Rome, Italy

Alfredo De Giorgi and Benedetta Boari
Clinica Medica Unit, Azienda Ospedaliero-Universitaria S. Anna, 44121 Ferrara, Italy

Emanuele Di Simone
Department of Clinical and Molecular Medicine, Sapienza University of Rome, 00185 Rome, Italy
Clinica Medica Unit, Azienda Ospedaliero-Universitaria S. Anna, 44121 Ferrara, Italy

Roberto Manfredini and Fabio Fabbian
Department of Medical Sciences, University of Ferrara, 44121 Ferrara, Italy
Department of Nursing, Instituto Maimónides de Investigación Biomédica de Córdoba (IMIBIC), 14071 Córdoba, Spain
Clinica Medica Unit, Azienda Ospedaliero-Universitaria S. Anna, 44121 Ferrara, Italy

Pablo Jesús López-Soto and María Aurora Rodríguez-Borrego
Department of Nursing, Instituto Maimónides de Investigación Biomédica de Córdoba (IMIBIC), 14071 Córdoba, Spain
Department of Nursing Pharmacology and Physiotherapy, University of Córdoba, 14071 Córdoba, Spain

Luis Miguel Dos Santos
Woosong Language Institute, Woosong University, Daejeon 34514, Korea

Ólöf Kristjánsdóttir and Gudrún Kristjánsdóttir
Faculty of Nursing, University of Iceland, Eirberg, Eiriksgata 34, 101 Reykjavík, Iceland

Annica Sjöström-Strand
Department of Health Sciences, Faculty of Medicine, Lund University, Box 157, 22100 Lund, Sweden

María José Pujalte-Jesús
Faculty of Nursing, Universidad Católica de Murcia UCAM, 30107 Murcia, Spain

José Luis Díaz Agea
Faculty of Nursing, Catholic University of Murcia, 30107 Murcia, Spain

Virginia Navajas-Romero
Department of Statistics, Management and Applied Economy. Universidad de Córdoba, 14014 Córdoba, Spain

Antonio Ariza-Montes
Management Departament, Universidad Loyola Andalucía, 14014 Córdoba, Spain

Felipe Hernández-Perlines
Departament of Business Administration; Universidad de Castilla La Mancha, 13071 Ciudad Real, Spain

Macrina Tortajada-Soler
Facultad de Ciencias de la Salud, Campus de Vegazana, Universidad de León, s/n, C.P. 24071 León, Spain

Leticia Sánchez-Valdeón, Cristina Liébana-Presa and Enrique Bayón-Darkistade
SALBIS Research Group, Facultad de Ciencias de la Salud, Campus de Ponferrada, Universidad de León, Avda/ Astorga s/n, C.P. 24402 Ponferrada (León), Spain

Marta Blanco-Nistal
Complejo Asistencial Universitario de León, C/ Altos de nava s/n, C.P. 24001 León, Spain

José Alberto Benítez-Andrades
SALBIS Research Group, Department of Electric, Systems and Automatics Engineering, University of León, s/n, 24071 León, Spain

Filipa Maria Reinhardt Andrade
Institute of Health Sciences, Doctorate Student of the Doctorate Degree in Nursing, Universidade Católica Portuguesa, 1649-023 Lisbon, Portugal

Amélia Simões Figueiredo, Manuel Luís Capelas, Zaida Charepe and Sérgio Deodato
Institute of Health Sciences, Centre for Interdisciplinary Research in Health (CIIS), Universidade Católica Portuguesa, 1649-023 Lisbon, Portugal

Alberto González García
Department of Nursing and Physiotherapy, Universidad de León, 24401 Ponferrada, Spain

Arrate Pinto-Carral
SALBIS Research Group, Department of Nursing and Physiotherapy, Universidad de León, 24001 Ponferrada, Spain

Jesús Sanz Villorejo
Director of the University Dental Clinic, European University of Madrid, 28670 Madrid, Spain

Pilar Marqués-Sánchez
SALBIS Research Group, Department of Nursing and Physiotherapy, Universidad de León, 24401 Ponferrada, Spain

Antonio Jesús Ramos-Morcillo, César Leal-Costa and María Ruzafa-Martínez
Faculty of Nursing, University of Murcia, 30100 Murcia, Spain

José Enrique Moral-García
Physical Activity and Sports Sciences, Faculty of Education, Pontifical University of Salamanca, Street Henry Collet, 52-70, 37007 Salamanca, Spain

Index

A

Absenteeism, 42, 98, 119, 170, 176, 208

Alzheimer's Disease, 34, 185, 187-189, 194-199

B

Burnout, 35-44, 98-99, 101-102, 104-108, 110-111, 123, 138, 169, 171-172, 179-183

C

Cardiopulmonary Resuscitation, 157-158, 165-167

Career Development, 123, 125, 129-139, 179

Cataracts, 185, 190-191, 196

Chest Compression, 157, 159, 162-163, 165, 167

Chronic Disease, 72, 85

Chronic Illness, 66, 71-74, 84-86

Chronic Pain, 59, 65, 68, 71-74, 76, 80-87

Chronotype, 112-122

Circadian Rhythm, 96, 112, 119-120, 182

Clinical Placements, 45-46, 48-49, 55-56

Clinical Practice, 46-48, 54-56, 138, 234

Cognitive Appraisal, 60-61, 65

Comorbidity, 59, 89-90, 96-97, 100, 185, 188, 196-197

Content Analysis, 48, 57, 141-142, 145, 153-156

Control Group, 157-160, 164, 185, 188-193, 196-197

Control Population, 190, 195

Core Competencies, 214-216, 219-223

Cultural Perspective, 123

D

Decision-Making Process, 123, 136, 138

Dementia, 17, 32-34, 108, 185, 187, 195-196, 198-199

Depression, 35-41, 44, 65, 68-69, 89, 91-92, 94, 96-100, 102-103, 110, 113, 118, 120, 141, 149, 170-172, 178, 180, 185-187, 193, 196

E

Effective Coping, 66

Effective Ventilation, 162-163

Emergency Department, 46-49, 51-54, 56, 120, 122, 187-188

Emotional Disorder, 26, 59-60, 65, 69

Emotional Experience, 45, 48-49, 53-54, 56

F

Fatigue, 35, 44, 65-66, 70, 89, 91-92, 94, 96-100, 110, 113-114, 117-118, 120-121, 149, 159, 161, 176, 181

Fibromyalgia, 59-62, 66-67, 69-71, 86

Filial Piety, 123-126, 133-139

Finding Closure, 141, 145, 150

H

Health Organization, 33-34, 85, 103, 105, 110, 114, 120, 155, 170, 176, 180, 242

Health Problems, 4, 8, 10, 89-92, 94, 96-98, 114, 120, 141, 149-150, 153, 202, 208

Health System, 37, 66-67, 69, 89, 169, 214-215, 220

Healthcare Worker, 158-159

Healthy Transition, 147, 150-151

Heart Surgery, 141-148, 151, 154, 156

Hierarchical Clustering, 75, 89, 92, 94

Humanization, 45-46, 51-53, 55-56

Hypoacusis, 190-191

I

Intensive Care Unit, 43, 56-57, 91, 93, 100, 141, 154

J

Job Control, 168-177, 179, 181

Job Demands, 89, 168-177, 179, 181-183

L

Learning Experience, 14, 46, 85

M

Midwives, 112, 114-119, 121-122, 179

Musculoskeletal Pain, 89, 91, 94, 97, 100

N

Near Misses, 112, 114-115, 118, 121

Nervousness, 49, 54

Nurse Manager, 181, 214-223, 225-228

Nurse Preceptor, 55, 181

Nursing Care, 15-17, 19-24, 27, 45-47, 55, 109, 175, 180, 194, 202, 211, 215, 217, 232-233

Nursing Education, 14, 45, 57, 123, 125-126, 136, 138, 233, 242-243

Nursing Personnel, 40, 98, 169, 171-172

Nursing Professional, 50, 123

Nursing Students, 1, 4, 6-12, 45-49, 54-57, 123-126, 131, 135-136, 138, 182, 229-230, 239-240, 243

O

Osteoarthritis, 185, 190-191, 196, 199

Osteoporosis, 185, 190-191, 196, 199

P

Pathologies, 47, 52, 188, 190, 192

Personality Disorder, 191

Progressive Confidence, 50, 54
Protective Factor, 108

Q
Qualitative Research, 59, 63, 69, 125, 136, 139, 141-142, 200, 205-207, 209, 229, 231, 242

R
Risk Factor, 43, 108, 122, 186

S
Scoping Review, 32, 59-60, 121, 221, 226
Secondary Traumatic Stress, 101-102, 104-107
Shift Work, 39, 89-94, 96-99, 112-114, 116-122, 176
Social Support, 32-34, 41, 44, 66, 72-88, 117-118, 141, 151-152, 168-177, 179-180, 182, 202, 208
Stigma, 59-60, 65-67, 200-201, 207-208, 211
Supportive Environment, 145, 147

T
Turnover Intention, 89-94, 96-97, 102, 108, 110, 120, 181

U
Uncertainty, 26, 59-61, 65-70, 142, 146, 183, 229-230, 232-235, 240
Urinary Incontinence, 185, 190-191, 196, 199

V
Verbal Abuse, 101-102, 109
Vulnerable Population, 200, 203, 212

W
Work-Life Balance, 168, 173, 178, 180-183
Workplace Violence, 101, 104-107, 109-111

www.ingramcontent.com/pod-product-compliance
Lightning Source LLC
LaVergne TN
LVHW080947210926
848485LV00004B/791